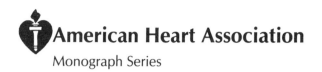

American Heart Association
Monograph Series

Cardiovascular Response to Exercise

Previously published:

Cardiovascular Applications of Magnetic Resonance.
Edited by Gerald M. Pohost, MD.

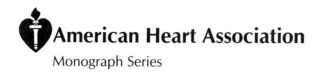

American Heart Association
Monograph Series

Cardiovascular Response to Exercise

Edited by

Gerald F. Fletcher, MD
Professor and Chairman,
Department of Rehabilitation Medicine,
Professor in Medicine (Cardiology),
Emory University School of Medicine,
The Robert W. Woodruff Health Sciences Center,
Atlanta, Georgia

FUTURA

**Futura Publishing
Company, Inc.**
Mount Kisco, NY

Library of Congress Cataloging-in-Publication Data

Cardiovascular response to exercise / [edited by] Gerald F. Fletcher.
    p.   cm.—(American Heart Association monograph series)
    Includes bibliographical references and index.
    ISBN 0-87993-559-6
    1. Heart—Physiology. 2. Exercise—Physiological effect.
    3. Heart—Pathophysiology. I. Fletcher, Gerald F., 1935– .
    II. Series.
    [DNLM: 1. Cardiovascular System—physiology. 2. Exercise—
    physiology. WG 102 C2675 1993]
    OP114.E9C37   1993
    612.1—dc20
    DNLM/DLC
    for Library of Congress   93-22393
                                            CIP

Published by
Futura Publishing Company, Inc.
2 Bedford Ridge Road
Mount Kisco, New York 10549

LC #: 93-22393
ISBN #: 0-87993-559-6

Every effort has been made to ensure that the information in this book is as up to date and accurate as possible at the time of publication. However, due to the constant developments in medicine, neither the author, nor the editor, nor the publisher can accept any legal or any other responsibility for any errors or omissions that may occur.

Printed in the United States of America.

Printed on acid-free paper.

The editor would like to express his warmest thanks and
appreciation to the following contributors
who were instrumental in the development of
this volume.

Colin M. Bloor, MD
Michael Crawford, MD
Victor Froelicher, MD
James Muller, MD
James Scheuer, MD
Peter Wood, MD

Contributors

Gary J. Balady, MD Associate Professor of Medicine, Boston University School of Medicine, Director, Cardiovascular Exercise Center and Cardiac Rehabilitation, Boston University Medical Center/The University Hospital, Boston, Massachusetts

Carolyn E. Barlow, MD Division of Epidemiology, Institute for Aerobics Research, Dallas, Texas

Gerald G. Blackwell, MD Assistant Professor of Medicine, Division of Cardiovascular Disease, The University of Alabama at Birmingham, Birmingham, Alabama

Steven N. Blair, PED Division of Epidemiology, Institute for Aerobics Research, Dallas, Texas

Colin M. Bloor, MD Professor of Pathology and Director, Molecular Pathology, Graduate Program, University of California, San Diego, School of Medicine, La Jolla, California

Robert O. Bonow, MD Professor of Medicine, Chief, Division of Cardiology, Northwestern University Medical School, Chicago, Illinois

Claude Bouchard, PhD Professor of Exercise Physiology, Physical Activity Sciences Laboratory, Laval University, Ste-Foy, Quebec

Thomas Brand, PhD Molecular Cardiology Unit, Departments of Medicine, Cell Biology, and Molecular Physiology, Baylor College of Medicine, Houston, Texas

Peter M. Buttrick, MD Division of Cardiology, Montefiore Medical Center, Albert Einstein College of Medicine, Bronx, New York

Victor A. Convertino, PhD Laboratory for Aerospace Cardiovascular Research, Brooks Air Force Base, Texas

Michael H. Crawford, MD Chief, Division of Cardiology, University of New Mexico School of Medicine, Department of Medicine/Cardiology Division, University of New Mexico Hospital, Albuquerque, New Mexico

Arthur C. De Graff, Jr., MD Director of the Pulmonary Laboratory at Hartford Hospital and Clinical Professor of Medicine at

The University of Connecticut School of Medicine, Hartford, Connecticut

Louis J. Dell'Italia, MD   Division of Cardiovascular Disease, The University of Alabama at Birmingham, Birmingham, Alabama

Jerome L. Fleg, MD   Senior Investigator, Gerontology Research Center, National Institute on Aging, Associate Professor of Medicine (Cardiology), Johns Hopkins University, Baltimore, Maryland

Gerald F. Fletcher, MD   Professor and Chairman, Department of Rehabilitation Medicine, Professor in Medicine (Cardiology), Emory University School of Medicine, The Robert W. Woodruff Health Sciences Center, Atlanta, Georgia

Robert S. Flinn   Chief, Division of Cardiology, University of New Mexico Medical School, Albuquerque, New Mexico

Robert F. Grover, MD, PhD   Professor Emeritus, and former Director of the Cardiovascular-Pulmonary Research Laboratory at The University of Colorado Health Science Center in Denver, Denver, Colorado

David M. Herrington, MD   Section of Cardiology, Bowman Gray School of Medicine, Wake Forest University, Winston-Salem, North Carolina

C. David Ianuzzo, PhD   Exercise and Health Sciences, and Biology, Faculty of Pure and Applied Science, York University, and Cardiovascular Surgery, University of Toronto, Toronto, Canada

Harold W. Kohl, III   Division of Epidemiology, Institute for Aerobics Research, Dallas, Texas

Robert L. Johnson, Jr., MD   Professor of Medicine, Pulmonary Research Division, University of Texas Southwestern Medical Center at Dallas, Dallas, Texas

M. Harold Laughlin, PhD   Department of Veterinary Biomedical Sciences, Department of Physiology, Department of Internal Medicine, and The Dalton Cardiovascular Research Center, University of Missouri, Columbia, Missouri

William Little, MD   Section of Cardiology, Bowman Gray School of Medicine, Wake Forest University, Winston-Salem, North Carolina

J. D. MacDougall, PhD   Department of Physical Education and Department of Medicine, McMaster University, Hamilton, Ontario, Canada

M. Dan McKirnan, PhD   School of Medicine, Department of Pathology, University of California, San Diego, La Jolla, California

Murray Mittleman, MD   Teaching Fellow, Harvard University School of Public Health; Research Fellow, Institute for Prevention of Cardiovascular Disease, Deaconess Hospital, Boston, Massachusetts

Judy M. Muller, PhD   Department of Veterinary Biomedical Sciences, Department of Physiology, Department of Internal Medicine, and The Dalton Cardiovascular Research Center, University of Missouri, Columbia, Missouri

James E. Muller, MD   Associate Professor of Medicine, Harvard Medical School; Chief, Cardiovascular Division, Deaconess Hospital, Boston, Massachusetts

Paul Murray, MD   Section of Cardiology, Bowman Gray School of Medicine, Wake Forest University, Winston-Salem, North Carolina

P. Robert Myers, MD, PhD   Department of Veterinary Biomedical Sciences, Department of Physiology, Department of Internal Medicine, and The Dalton Cardiovascular Research Center, University of Missouri, Columbia, Missouri

Navin C. Nanda, MD   Professor of Medicine and Director, Heart Station and Echocardiography, Graphics Labs, Department of Medicine, Division of Cardiovascular Disease, The University of Alabama at Birmingham, Birmingham, Alabama

Peter J. O'Brien, DVM, PhD, DVSc   Pathology, Ontario Veterinary College, University of Guelph, Guelph, Ontario, Canada

Christine L. Oltman, PhD   Department of Veterinary Biomedical Sciences, Department of Physiology, Department of Internal Medicine, and The Dalton Cardiovascular Research Center, University of Missouri, Columbia, Missouri

Janet L. Parker, PhD   Department of Veterinary Biomedical Sciences, Department of Physiology, Department of Internal Medicine, and The Dalton Cardiovascular Research Center, University of Missouri, Columbia, Missouri

Gerald M. Pohost, MD   Division of Cardiovascular Disease, The University of Alabama at Birmingham, Birmingham, Alabama

Steven M. Rosenthal, MD   Division of Cardiovascular Disease, The University of Alabama at Birmingham, Birmingham, Alabama

Tomas A. Salerno, MD   Cardiovascular Surgery, University of Toronto, Toronto, Canada

James Scheuer, MD   Division of Cardiology, Department of Medicine, Albert Einstein College of Medicine, and Montefiore Medical Center, Bronx, New York

Michael D. Schneider, MD   Molecular Cardiology Unit, Departments of Medicine, Cell Biology, and Molecular Physiology, Baylor College of Medicine, Houston, Texas

David S. Siscovick, MD, MPH   Associate Professor, Departments of Medicine and Epidemiology, Co-director, Cardiovascular Health Research Unit, University of Washington, Seattle, Washington

Marcia L. Stefanick, PhD   Stanford Center for Research in Disease Prevention, Stanford University, Palo Alto, California

Martin J. Sullivan, MD   Department of Medicine, Division of Cardiology and the Center for Living, Duke University Medical Center and the Durham Veterans Administration Medical Center, Durham, North Carolina

Paul D. Thompson, MD   Cardiovascular Disease Prevention Center, Pittsburgh Heart Institute, The University of Pittsburgh, Pittsburgh, Pennsylvania

Geoffrey Tofler, MBBS   Assistant Professor of Medicine, Harvard Medical School; Co-Director, Institute for Prevention of Cardiovascular Disease, Deconess Hospital, Boston, Massachusetts

John Zornosa, MD   Section of Cardiology, Bowman Gray School of Medicine, Wake Forest University, Winston-Salem, North Carolina

Preface

Society has honored athletic achievements for thousands of years. Knowledge of the general benefits of exercise and exercise conditioning to the individual also has a long history. Although Professor Ernst Jokl established the first Institute of Sports Medicine in Breslau in 1931, both physicians and nonphysicians have been relatively slow in accepting and applying the full benefits of sport activities for all individuals in society, including many medical patients. In recent years, however, many physicians have recognized that individuals who exercise throughout their lives may benefit both psychologically and physically from such activity. While the possibility of preselection bias cannot be excluded in many such studies, other studies have clearly shown short-term benefits that can be expected to persist and to influence long-term physical well-being with continued exercise activity.

Future studies will elaborate the molecular mechanisms responsible for the beneficial effects of exercise and exercise training. Of particular interest will be studies of the effects of exercise and exercise training upon hematologic factors, lipid metabolism, the endothelium, and skeletal blood vessels. This knowledge will permit a more accurate use of exercise, both for the general population and for patients with many forms of illness, including cardiovascular, orthopedic, and psychological disorders.

Robert C. Schlant, MD
Atlanta, Georgia

xi

Introduction

In recent years, there has been increasing clinical interest and more scholarly research in the important area of exercise and the cardiovascular system. This research activity, both in animals and humans, has provided substantial data toward the understanding and implementation of exercise as a diagnostic and management modality in the care of patients. This book on the *Cardiovascular Response to Exercise* includes and encompasses experiences in research from the "bench" laboratory to the clinical setting with regard to cardiovascular function and exercise. The book is divided into six parts to address these important topics.

Part 1 addresses **Cellular Level Dynamics and Ventricular Function.** Initially myocardial metabolism and exercise and ventricular function in experimental animals' response to exercise is discussed. Exercise is then discussed with regard to ventricular function in humans followed by a specific emphasis on Doppler echocardiography with regard to left ventricular flow during exercise both in systole and diastole.

Next, Part 2 incorporates **Genetic, Biochemical, and Physiological Responses of the Heart to Factors Related to Long-Term Exercise.** This basic part discusses in depth the molecular control of muscle growth, exercise-associated mechanical loading, and heart rate effects on the myocardium. These topics are followed by a clear summary of the synthesis of isolated factors into a long-term exercise pattern.

Part 3 details the **Systemic Responses to Exercise and Results of Training.** In this are included blood pressure responses to isometric, resistive, and dynamic exercise. In addition, there are discussions on the adaptation of the coronary circulation to exercise training, blood volume response to training, and high altitude effects on exercise training.

In a clinically and timely manner, Part 4 addresses **Exercise as a Trigger of Onset of Acute Cardiovascular Disease.** Herein, the triggering of onset of myocardial infarction and sudden cardiac death are addressed in detail. Sudden cardiac death during jogging and the relative risk of morning versus evening exercise are then addressed. Last, the relative risk of myocardial infarction during jogging is covered in explicit detail.

Part 5 delves more in prevention and the important topic of **Modification of Cardiovascular Risk by Exercise.** In this particular part, cardiovascular fitness versus cardiovascular disease is discussed as well as the relationship of exercise, lipoproteins, and cardiovascular disease. Endurance exercise and coronary artery "bore" are then addressed, followed by a description of the genetic determinants of cardiovascular fitness and response to exercise.

Appropriately in Part 6, **Clinical Applications** brings together the topics addressed in previous parts. In this part, exercise and the failing heart are discussed as an important clinical topic. Magnetic resonance imaging with regard to exercise evaluation and the effects of aging on the cardiovascular response to exercise are detailed. Exercise echocardiology to assess left ventricular size and performance is then discussed, followed by practical guidelines for exercise in patients with normal left ventricular function.

In a broad-spectrum manner, this book addresses various components of the cardiovascular functional process and reactivity to physical activity or exercise. It brings together data from the "bench" and basic science researcher to the level of the clinician who has been involved in clinical trials and clinical evaluations. A number of these chapters can be taken by the reader as single entities for a satisfying knowledge procurement. However, for the most part, each of the six parts of the book stands alone, and readers should consider these as distinct, specific entities for their satisfaction.

In essence, the material in this book provides a broad base of information at various levels for the application of exercise in cardiovascular health and in patients with cardiovascular disease. With the growing interest in exercise and the designation by the American Heart Association of physical inactivity being the fourth major modifiable coronary risk factor, this publication should provide significant information to the clinician and/or the basic scientist. Exercise as opposed to other management modalities has not been addressed in the past as "scientifically" as one would so desire. However, based on the contents of this book and the endeavors that many are addressing with regard to this, it is felt that the future is bright with regard to basic and clinical research in this important segment of health care.

Gerald F. Fletcher, MD

Contents

Part 1. Cellular Level Dynamics and Ventricular Function

Part 2. Genetic, Biochemical, and Physiological Responses of the Heart to Factors Related to Long-Term Exercise

Part 5. Modification of Cardiovascular Risk by Exercise

Part 6. Clinical Applications

Part 1

Cellular Level Dynamics and Ventricular Function

Chapter 1

Myocardial Metabolism During Exercise

Joseph W. Starnes, PhD

When you are resting, your heart is at work. It never rests and thus always needs an adequate supply of energy. Although representing only 0.5% of the total adult body weight, the heart accounts for 10% of the total resting oxygen consumption. Each minute the left ventricle of the average resting person, athlete and nonathlete alike, pumps the entire blood volume of approximately 5 liters. During most forms of exercise, the heart demands more and more energy as it is called on to pump more blood in proportion to the intensity of the exercise. In the case of strength-training types of exercises, the blood will have to be pumped against greatly elevated peripheral resistance. A healthy untrained individual typically can increase his resting cardiac output about fourfold to an average maximum of 20 to 22 liters of blood per minute. This pales by comparison with highly trained endurance athletes, whose hearts are capable of pumping 40 liters per minute. The factors that influence myocardial energy demand and supply during exercise in the untrained and trained individual are the subject of this chapter.

Myocardial Energy Demands

Cardiac output is the product of heart rate and stroke volume. Stroke volume is influenced by three variables: afterload, preload, and intrinsic contractility. Thus, cardiac output is a multifactorial variable with four major determinants, all of which are increased

From Fletcher GF, (ed): *Cardiovascular Response to Exercise.* Mount Kisco, NY, Futura Publishing Company, Inc., © 1994.

during exercise. However, only two of these variables, heart rate and afterload (often estimated by systolic blood pressure [SBP]), are responsible for almost all of the energy demanded by the heart during exercise. Preload has a small impact on myocardial energy utilization but a large impact on cardiac output; an increased filling pressure or increased filling time leads to increased end-diastolic left ventricular volume, which results in increased stroke volume according to the law of Starling.[1] Over a wide range of exercise intensities, myocardial energy demand has been found to be strongly related to either heart rate (HR; $r = 0.88$) or aortic peak systolic pressure ($r = 0.75$); when the two are combined into a rate–pressure product (HR × SBP) the correlation coefficient is higher than for either individually.[2] A conclusion reached by several studies is that the rate–pressure product is a good indicator of the amount of energy being used by the heart during all types of exercise,[2–4] even in the presence of β-blockers.[3] The linear relationship of rate–pressure product and VO_2 has been fitted into the following equations by Nelson et al.[4]

$$MVO_2 = 11.5 + 0.0018 \, (HR \times \text{brachial SBP}) \qquad (1)$$

$$MVO_2 = 5.3 + 0.0017 \, (HR \times \text{aortic SBP}) \qquad (2)$$

where MVO_2 is in units of ml O_2/min/100 g left ventricle and correlation coefficients are .85 and .86, respectively. Thus, myocardial metabolic activity is not always related to cardiac output per se, but to two of its determinants, that is, HR and SBP.

Unlike skeletal muscle, the heart is designed to use aerobic energy transfer pathways during all types of exercises. Thus, in general the metabolic efficiency of contraction is greater in heart than skeletal muscle, but as discussed above the heart does not always pump the same amount of blood for any given contractile effort or energy expenditure. In weight-training and other resistance/training exercises, the peripheral arterial network becomes quite compressed, causing a sudden and dramatic increase in resistance to left ventricle ejections. For example, performing a bench press with a weight representing 50% of maximum voluntary contraction has been reported to elevate systolic and diastolic blood pressure to 232 and 154 mm Hg, respectively.[5] As a result, the metabolic and contractile activity of the myocardium must increase dramatically simply to *maintain* cardiac output. During endurance types of exercise such as jogging or bicycling, which employ rhythmic activity of large muscle groups, increased cardiac metabolic activity is accompanied by elevated cardiac output. This is caused by vasodilatation in the active muscles, which decreases peripheral resistance and to the alternate contraction and relaxation of the active muscles aiding in the return of blood to the heart, thus providing significant elevation of preload or volume loading. The increase in cardiac output itself causes an elevation of SBP because the more rapid blood flow causes greater expansion in the elastic components of the major blood vessels. However, the increase in SBP typically is less than in resistance-type exercises and diastolic pressure usually is not increased. Heart rate increases rapidly in both types of exercises in an intensity-related manner associated with an increase in sympathetic drive and a withdrawal of parasympathetic activity.[5] Overall, the key point is that the amount of metabolic work necessary to pump a given amount of blood varies considerably with the type and intensity of exercise.

Myocardial Energy Supply

At all levels of metabolic work, cardiac muscle maintains an essentially constant concentration of high energy phosphates, adenosine triphosphate (ATP), and creatine phosphate.[6,7] This is not the case for skeletal muscle, which incurs a significant decrease in creatine phosphate during high energy demands.[8] The two muscle types differ in that the heart cannot afford the luxury of an inactive rest period to replete its high energy phosphate levels; it must beat continuously for the survival of its host. The stored amounts of high energy compounds in the left ventricle are quite low, approximately 5 μmol/g for ATP and 8 μmol/g for creatine phosphate.[7] This represents only enough energy to support cardiac work for about 15 seconds at rest or about 4 seconds during maximum work (the actual times will be much shorter, however, because work would cease before total depletion of the high energy phosphates). Thus, the myocardium relies on a very close temporal matching of oxidative metabolism to changes in metabolic demand. It has little tolerance for an oxygen debt and even a brief interruption or lag in oxidative metabolism adversely affects cardiac function.

The small size of the cardiac cell (relative to skeletal muscle) plays an important role in function and metabolism.[8] Its small size enhances the spread of electrical activity throughout the myocardium to provide a synchronous contraction. More relevant to the topic of this discussion is that the small size of the cardiac cell prevents an oxygen debt during rapid increases in work load. In all muscle types, mitochondrial ATP production is spatially separated from the myosin ATPase. In skeletal muscle, large cell diameter and low mitochondrial density result in a large diffusion distance between ATP-synthesizing reactions and ATP-utilizing reactions. Consequently, the ATP concentration in the cell is maintained constant during brief bursts of activity by hydrolysis of creatine phosphate. The relatively small diameter of cardiac muscle, coupled with a lower myosin ATPase activity and much larger mitochondrial density, serves to reduce drastically the diffusion distance between the mitochondria and the contractile apparatus. As a result, the metabolic demands of the heart can be met exclusively by mitochondrial oxidative phosphorylation as long as the blood flow through the coronary circulation is sufficient.

It has been estimated that there are more than 2500 capillaries/mm^2 left ventricle.[9] The amount of oxygen extracted from the blood as it passes through the myocardium is near the physiological maximum even in the resting state; thus, increasing the volume of blood flowing through the coronary circulation is absolutely required for myocardial metabolism to produce enough ATP for exercise-induced cardiac work. We,[7] as well as others,[10] have reported that over a broad range of cardiac work, oxygen extraction changes little and coronary flow varies linearly with oxygen consumption. Seeking the underlying mechanisms of vasoregulation is an active area of research in cardiology; a discussion of potential mechanisms is beyond the scope of this discussion. Most relevant to this chapter is the awareness of the crucial importance of adequate coronary vasodilatation during exercise. This point was demonstrated quite clearly in a recent study by Weiss et al.[11] employing isometric exercise in coronary patients. Cardiac energy demand was estimated by the rate–pressure product (HR × SBP) and myocardial energetic status was evaluated with phosphorus 31 nuclear magnetic resonance spectroscopy. Figure 1 displays the creatine phosphate/ATP ratios at rest, during exercise (7–8 minutes of single handgrip at 30% of maximum force), and after 2 minutes of recovery. The exercise resulted in a modest increase in HR × SBP from approximately 10,000 to 13,000 in all groups. In normal individuals this 30% increase did not alter left ventricular energetic

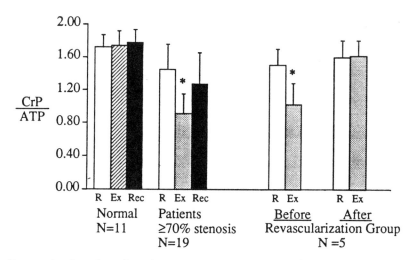

FIGURE 1. *Creatine phosphate (CrP) to ATP ratios in the anterior myocardium during rest (R), exercise (Ex), and after 2 minutes of recovery (Rec) in 11 normal persons and in 19 patients with severe stenosis of the left anterior descending or left main coronary arteries and during rest (R) and exercise (Ex) in five patients before and after successful revascularization. Exercise consisted of 7–8 minutes of single hand-grip exercise at 30% of maximum force. *Ratios during exercise significantly less than during rest. Data redrawn from values reported by Weiss et al.[11]*

status, whereas in patients with coronary stenosis the same increase in cardiac work resulted in a significant decline of high-energy phosphates. Proof that these metabolic changes were due specifically to inadequate blood flow was obtained by evaluating the exercise in a group of patients before and after revascularization procedures. As seen in Figure 1, this group displayed the typical exercise-induced decline in energetic status before revascularization but was able to increase cardiac work without compromising energetic status after revascularization.

The selection of substrates taken from the blood supplying the heart plays an important role in myocardial metabolism. For more than 20 years we have known that changes occur in the variety and quantities of exogenous substrates used by the human heart during exercise. This knowledge comes primarily from two studies using the technique of coronary sinus catheterization, in which myocardial substrate extraction is calculated by measuring the concentration difference between arterial and coronary venous blood and multiplying by the coronary flow rate.[12,13] During prolonged endurance exercise, represented by the two columns on the right in Figure 2, free fatty acid levels rise high enough relative to the other substrates to make it the major fuel source. Similarly, during acute and intense exercise, represented by the two columns on the left, lactate levels increase and lactate becomes the major fuel source. Furthermore, since blood glucose concentration is essentially fixed at 4–5 mM at all times, its relative contribution to the total fuel mixture decreases during all forms of exercise. It should be noted, however, that the *absolute* rate of glucose uptake actually may increase because of the increased overall energy demand.

Although it is now well established that shifts in substrate preference occur during exercise, there remains some uncertainty regarding the absolute quantification of the changes because of methodological limitations associated with in vivo human studies. Such studies are limited because they typically measure substrate

EXERCISE CONDITION

Arterial Substrate, mM	Keul, 1971			Lassers et al., 1971
	100 W 6 min	200 W 6 min	Moderate 2 hrs	Moderate 2 hrs
Glucose	4.9	4.5	5.0	3.4
Lactate	3.0	9.0	1.8	1.4
FFA	0.9	1.2	2.8	1.3
HR, beats/min		180	160	142

CONTRIBUTION TO VO2

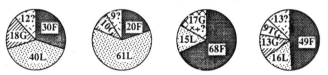

FIGURE 2. **Top:** *Concentrations of glucose, lactate, and free fatty acids (FFA) in the arterial blood during three intensities of exercise: 100 watts for 6 minutes, 200 watts for 6 minutes, and a moderate intensity that could be maintained for 2 hours. Heart rate (HR) during some exercises is also displayed.* **Bottom:** *The percentage contribution of various substrates when present in the arterial concentrations and exercise conditions given in the top panel. G, glucose; L, lactate; F, free fatty acids; TG, triglyceride; ?, unknown. Data estimated from the studies of Keul[12] and Lassers et al.[13]*

extraction and assume that it provides a good estimate of substrate *oxidation.* Extraction (or consumption) can be defined as the disappearance of substrate from arterial blood into the myocardium whereas oxidation is defined as the conversion of substrate to CO_2 and H_2O. Extraction and oxidation may not be the same if some of the substrate is diverted to other pathways. How a substrate is actually used after it is extracted can be measured by labeling the substrate with isotopes and following the conversion of the labeled substrate to labeled end products. Such experiments can be readily carried out in isolated heart preparations, but at the present time are difficult to carry out in exercising animals and humans. The extraction versus oxidation problem as well as the considerable technical difficulty of accurately measuring very small differences in blood substrate levels on the arterial and venous sides of the heart may partially explain the apparent discrepency in free fatty acid use during prolonged exercise reported by Lassers et al.[13] and Keul[12] (Figure 2).

Experiments carried out by Drake and colleagues[14,15] have demonstrated the powerful role of arterial lactate concentration on myocardial metabolism. Their studies, using intact resting dogs, indicate that lactate extraction increases linearly with increases in arterial concentration up to about 4.5 mM, at which maximum extraction is reached. Lactate levels exceeding 4.5 mM often are reached by exercising humans (note values displayed in Figure 2). Furthermore, Drake reported that the linear relationship between lactate use and lactate availability did not appear to be affected by changes in arterial glucose or fatty acid concentrations. Lactate has been reported to inhibit lipolysis directly[16,17]; thus, when both lactate and fatty acid levels are high, lactate is the preferred substrate. At arterial lactate concentrations of 4.5 mM and above, exogenous lactate was found to account for about 85% of myocardial oxygen consumption, glucose for about 5% to 6%, and other substrates for the remaining 9% to 10%.[15]

Although Drake and colleagues[15] maintained that anytime arterial lactate exceeds 4.5 mM it will account for 85% of the myocardial energy source, one must keep in mind that the data were collected on resting dogs. Caution should be advised in the extrapolation of these data to the exercising human. Recall that Keul reported that lactate accounts for 61% of the myocardial energy source during intense exercise with arterial lactate levels of 9 mM (Figure 2). Evidence from experiments by Noakes and Opie[18] using the isolated perfused working rat heart, in which substrate extraction and oxidation can be evaluated with much greater precision than in intact animals, indicated that lactate use is much less than that estimated by either Drake[15] or Keul.[12] Noakes and Opie reported that even when the only exogenous substrate is 10 mM lactate, it accounts for only 53% of the myocardial oxygen consumption at high levels of cardiac work. When glucose is added to the 10-mM lactate perfusate, the lactate use by the heart drops to only 28% of the total energy source (with glucose accounting for the remainder). This contribution of lactate to the total energy production is far less than the 85% reported by Drake. Perhaps Drake's values were higher because the hearts were performing very low levels of work and, thus, a slow rate of lactate oxidation was adequate to meet the energy needs. There is evidence that at a sufficiently high level of cardiac work, flux through lactate dehydrogenase will become limited by accumulation of NADH produced when the enzyme converts lactate to pyruvate for entry into the mitochondria.[19] At this level of work, an inability to supply additional energy will prevent any further increase in cardiac work. Consistent with this notion is the observation that maximum cardiac performance is lower in hearts perfused with lactate alone compared with hearts perfused with lactate plus glucose.[18]

Exercise Training Effects on Energy Demand and Supply

Regularly performed aerobic types of exercise produce adaptations that serve to decrease myocardial energy demand and improve its energy supply. The decrease in energy demand is realized by the well-known bradycardia observed at rest and during submaximal exercise intensities.[5] Cardiac output is maintained at the lower heart rate because the longer diastolic period allows greater ventricular filling, which produces a greater stroke volume according to the law of Starling.[1] Since energy demand is determined primarily by the rate–pressure product (HR × SBP), and is affected only minimally by stroke volume, the magnitude of the energy savings approaches the magnitude of the decline in heart rate. Well-conditioned endurance athletes typically have resting and submaximum exercise heart rates at least 30% less than untrained individuals.[5] From a clinical point of view, this may be the most important adaptation resulting from a program of regular exercise. The reason for this statement is that many acute cardiac episodes are due to energy demand exceeding energy supply; thus, a lowering of energy demand will lessen this possibility. Furthermore, most of the exercise-related bradycardia is realized within the first 4 to 8 weeks of training.[20] The answer to why the bradycardia occurs so rapidly may lie at least partially in the fact that heart rate is influenced by sympathetic and parasympathic systems and that outflow from these systems may acclimatize rapidly to changes in activity patterns and stress.

In addition to the decrease in energy demand, there may be changes in substrate metabolism that provide an improvement in energy supply. There is an increase in stored glycogen content[21] and glucose uptake is significantly enhanced[22] in rat hearts after swim training. The enhanced glucose uptake occurs independently of cardiac work load or the availability of other exogenous substrates, which suggests an adaptation at the level of the glucose transporter.[22] Switching away from fats and lactate and toward glucose as a substrate for energy metabolism improves the energy supply in two ways: First, maximum cardiac performance is depressed when hearts primarily use lactate as an energy source[18,19] and in vivo situations do indeed occur in which lactate is the primary substrate.[12,13] Second, efficiency of mechanical work becomes progressively less and coronary blood flow needs greater as substrate use shifts toward fat and away from glucose.[7] This is the general trend in substrate use during prolonged endurance exercise[12,13]; thus, an adaptation that would attenuate the substrate shift would be beneficial to the heart. The explanation for the fat-induced decline in efficiency and increase in coronary flow is that the metabolic routes taken by fats result in more oxygen required for each ATP molecule produced compared with the routes taken by glucose. Potentially, the effect could be considerable when one considers that a heart using fatty acid alone would need about 16% more oxygen to produce the same amount of ATP than when using only glucose.

References

1. Starling EH: The Linacre Lecture on the Law of the Heart. London, Longmans, Green and Co, 1918
2. Kitamura K, Jorgensen CR, Gobel FL, Taylor HL, Wang Y: Hemody-

namic correlates of myocardial oxygen consumption during upright exercise. *J Appl Physiol* 1972;32:516–522

3. Jorgensen CR, Wang K, Wang Y, Gobel FL, Nelson RR, Taylor HL: Effects of propranolol on myocardial oxygen consumption and its hemodynamic correlates during upright exercise. *Circulation* 1973;48:1173–1182

4. Nelson RR, Gobel FL, Jorgensen CR, Wang K, Taylor HL: Hemodynamic predictors of myocardial oxygen consumption during static and dynamic exercise. *Circulation* 1974;50:1179–1189

5. McArdle WD, Katch FI, Katch VL: *Exercise Physiology.* Philadelphia, Lea & Febiger, 1991, pp 292–325

6. Balaban RS: Regulation of oxidative phosphorylation in the mammalian cell. *Am J Physiol* 1990;258:C377–C389

7. Starnes JW, Wilson DF, Erecinska M: Substrate dependence of metabolic state and coronary flow in perfused rat heart. *Am J Physiol* 1985;246:H799–H806

8. Krisanda JM, Moreland TS, Kushmerick MJ: ATP supply and demand during exercise, in Horton ES, Terjung RL (eds): *Exercise, Nutrition, and Energy Metabolism.* New York, Macmillan, 1988, pp 27–44

9. Opie LH: *The Heart.* New York, Grune & Stratton, 1984, pp 154–165

10. Nuutinen EM, Nishiki K, Erecinska M, Wilson DF: Role of mitochondrial oxidative phosphorylation in regulation of coronary blood flow. *Am J Physiol* 1982;243:H159–H169

11. Weiss RG, Bottomly PA, Hardy CJ, Gerstenblith G: Regional myocardial metabolism of high-energy phosphates during isometric exercise in patients with coronary artery disease. *N Engl J Med* 1990;323:1593–1600

12. Keul J: Myocardial metabolism in athletes, in Pernow B, Saltin B (eds): *Muscle Metabolism During Exercise.* New York, Plenum, 1971, pp 447–455

13. Lassers BW, Kaijser L, Wahlqvist ML, Carlson LA: Myocardial metabolism in man at rest and during prolonged exercise, in Pernow B, Saltin B (eds): *Muscle Metabolism During Exercise.* New York, Plenum, 1971, pp 457–467

14. Drake AJ, Haines JR, Noble MIM: Preferential uptake of lactate by the normal myocardium of dogs. *Cardiovasc Res* 1980;14:65–72

15. Drake AJ: Substrate utilization in the myocardium. *Basic Res Cardiol* 1982;77:1–11

16. Boyd AE, Giamber SR, Mager M, Lebovitz HE: Lactate inhibition of lipolysis in exercising man. *Metabolism* 1974;23:531–542

17. Shepherd RE, Noble EG, Klug GA, Goldnick PD: Lipolysis and cAMP accumulation in adipocytes in response to physical training. *J Appl Physiol* 1981;50:143–148

18. Noakes TD, Opie LH: Substrates for maximum mechanical function in isolated perfused working rat heart. *J Appl Cardiol* 1989;4:391–405

19. Kabayashi K, Neely JR: Control of maximum rates of glycolysis in rat cardiac muscle. *Circ Res* 1979;44:166–175

20. Mary DASG: Exercise training and its effects on the heart. *Rev Physiol Biochem Pharmacol* 1987;109:61–144

21. Scheuer J, Penpargkul S, Bhan AK: Experimental observations on the effects of physical training upon intrinsic cardiac physiology and biochemistry. *Am J Cardiol* 1974;33:744–751
22. Kainulainen H, Virtanen P, Ruskoaho H, Takala TES: Training increases cardiac glucose uptake during rest and exercise in rats. *Am J Physiol* 1989;257:H839–H845

Chapter 2

Ventricular Function in Experimental Animals:
Response to Exercise

Colin M. Bloor, MD and
M. Dan McKirnan, PhD

We have conducted cardiovascular pathophysiological studies in chronically instrumented, conscious animal models for a number of years. In describing those studies related to the ventricular function responses to exercise in these models, we separated our discussion into several topics, namely, selection of the animal model, the normal ventricular function responses to exercise, ventricular function responses associated with exercise-induced hypertrophy, and the regional dysfunctional changes that occur in the heart's ischemic region during exercise stress.

The selection of animal models for studying ventricular function changes in response to exercise depends on appropriate physiological comparisons to humans. We selected the pig as a model for our studies for several reasons: 1) the heart size and heart weight/body weight ratio of the pig are similar to those of humans;[1] 2) the pig's physiological response to exercise is similar to that of humans;[2] 3) the pig is easily exercise trained;[3] 4) the innate coronary collateral circulation in the pig heart is sparse, similar to that of humans;[4,5] 5) the coronary artery anatomy of the pig heart is similar to that of the human heart;[4,6] and 6) pigs are a cost-effective animal model in biomedical research.

Swine possess a sparse innate coronary collateral circulation[4]

Supported by NIHLBI grants HL-32670, HL-07104, HL-20190, HL-40649, and AHA California Affiliate grant 88-S125.

From Fletcher GF, (ed): *Cardiovascular Response to Exercise.* Mount Kisco, NY, Futura Publishing Company, Inc., © 1994.

consisting of an anastomotic network of endomural vessels similar to the endomural coronary collateral vessels present in humans.[5] However, swine can develop additional coronary collateral vessels after gradual occlusion of a coronary artery.[7,8] These coronary collaterals function adequately, that is, they provide normal resting myocardial blood flow and function 3 to 4 weeks after the occlusion occurs. However, during exercise myocardial perfusion through these collaterals is not adequate to support regional myocardial function in the collateral-dependent myocardium. This exercise-induced underperfusion of the collateral-dependent region and accompanying myocardial dysfunction persists for at least 16 weeks after the onset of gradual coronary artery occlusion.[8] Humans with coronary artery disease demonstrate similar persistent regional myocardial dysfunction and ischemia in collateral-dependent myocardium during exercise stress.[9] Thus, gradual coronary artery occlusion in the pig, characterized by persistent myocardial ischemia during exercise stress, provides a good animal model for studying the effects of various interventions on regional myocardial function and blood flow in the collateral-dependent myocardium.

An additional advantage of the pig model for cardiovascular physiology studies is the similarity of the pig's coronary artery anatomy to that of humans[4,6] and the similarity of its heart size and heart weight/body weight ratio to that of humans.[1] Also, the pig model's adaptation to exercise is markedly similar to that of man.[2] After exercise training pigs we have seen an increase in $\dot{V}O_2$max of about 25% above the pretraining levels similar to changes reported in young men.[1]

In cardiovascular experiments breed selection and size of the pigs used may be important considerations. In our studies we have used both Yucatan minipigs and farm pigs (ie, Hampshire pigs) for different reasons. We have used the Yucatan minipig in most of our chronic animal experiments[10] because of their gentle disposition, slow growth, and easy adaptation to exercise. However, we usually use Hampshire pigs for acute experiments because of their availability and low cost.

This chapter focuses on the use of the pig in our laboratory as an animal model of ventricular function changes occurring in response to exercise. Results from various studies are reviewed, with particular emphasis on regional myocardial function changes in the collateral-dependent myocardium and the potential use of this model to mimic the clinical setting of myocardial "stunning" seen in humans.

Methods

Our laboratory uses anesthesia and surgical procedures similar to those described for swine by Swindle.[11] We handle animals similarly for both acute procedures and chronic instrumentation. Our exception is the maintenance of surgical sterility during surgical instrumentation in the chronic studies. Avoidance of undue excitement before surgery is an important consideration. We accomplish this by adjusting the pig to the laboratory environment before surgery and using appropriate doses of preanesthetic drugs (eg, ketamine or rompun). We induce surgical anesthesia with ketamine (25 mg/kg, i.m.) plus atropine (1/30 g) and thiamylal (20 mg/kg, i.v. in an ear vein) and maintain it with a combination of 1% halothane and oxygen. We administer lidocaine (80 mg i.v.) as a bolus before manipulation and instrumentation of the heart. A left lateral thoracotomy is performed in the fifth intercostal space. We place Silastic catheters in the aorta, left atrium, and pulmonary artery to measure hemodynamic parameters. For cardiac output measurements, we place aortic flow transducers (Biotronex 18 mm) on the root of the aorta. For regional myocardial function measurements, we implant piezoelectric discs in the heart wall to determine wall thickness and internal left ventricular diameter.[12] When dimensional measurements are made, a high-fidelity micromanometer (Konigsberg-P7) and a small calibration catheter are placed in the left ventricular chamber through a stab wound near the apex for measurements of left ventricular pressure and dP/dt (used as an index of contractility). In our myocardial ischemia models, we place either a cuff occluder or an ameroid occluder on the proximal left circumflex coronary artery.[7,12]

In chronic experiments the animals are given buprenorphine (0.01 mg/kg i.m.) for the first 24 hours postsurgery. After 1 week we reintroduced the animals to the laboratory. We maintain catheter patency by flushing weekly with a heparin solution. To maintain catheters chronically in the pig requires special consideration and care to assure tissue healing around the catheter.[13] Usually we can start acute exercise experiments or exercise training 2 weeks after surgery.

Our methods of determining functional and morphological critical cardiovascular parameters, including ventricular weight, coronary blood flow, coronary collateral flow, and regional myocardial function, have been described in detail.[1,8,14] Frequently we use exercise as both an acute physiological stress and as a chronic condition (ie, exercise training). The procedures briefly described here are available in more detail elsewhere.[14,15] Our acute exercise stress test for swine using a motorized treadmill is as follows: there are successive 2- to 3-minute stages of increasing workload; the speed (mph) and incline (% grade) are listed respectively for each consecutive stage: 2 mph/5%; 3 mph/5%; 4 mph/10%; 4 mph/15%; 4 mph/15%; and 4 mph/20%. Maximal oxygen consumption ($\dot{V}O_2$max) and maximal work are determined when increased effort no longer elicits further increases in heart rate or oxygen consumption.[16,17] An electrically charged grid at the rear of the treadmill discourages halting before exhaustion. Previous studies from our laboratory have shown that the pig can achieve and sustain maximal heart rate for several minutes while measurements are being taken.[4] Also, the parameters observed at maximal performance are constant for individual animals when studied on multiple occasions.

Our typical exercise training protocol is as follows: after surgery, the animals are rested for 2 weeks and then gradually allowed to begin or resume training. Animals are trained on a treadmill 5 days per week for 10 weeks with two training regimens defined as "continuous training" and "interval training." Continuous training is defined as follows: animals are initially trained to run for 20 min/day, increasing to 30 min/day by the end of week 2. Subsequently the duration of training is increased by 5 to 10 min/day until a maximum of 60 min/day for 5 days per week is achieved by week 6. After 6 weeks of continuous training, interval training begins on Tuesday and Thursday of each week. Exercise intensity for continuous training is set at 65% to 85% of the heart rate range ([HRmax − HR rest] × [0.7 − 0.85] + HR rest). For interval training, 5-minute exercise bouts alternate between 80% and 100% of the heart range for the 30 to 40-minute exercise bout. We follow the intensity closely and adjust for training responses by weekly electrocardiographic monitoring. Occasionally, during hot weather, if heart rates are excessive, the external workloads are reduced to achieve the appropriate heart rate. We also use fans and spray bottles of water to facilitate cooling during training in warm temperatures. Body temperature during exercise typically ranges between 39° and 40° C.[16]

Our discussion of pig training studies includes four animal groups previously reported.[15] Control animals consisted of nine Yucatan and three Hampshire pigs. Animal groups trained for 10 weeks were as follows: group 1, nine Yucatan pigs exercised at a moderate intensity (65%–75% of the heart rate range); group 2, seven Yucatan pigs exercised at higher intensities (75%–85% of the heart rate range plus interval training); group 3, four Yucatan pigs and three farm pigs trained at higher intensities (75%–85% of the heart rate range plus interval training).

We have exercised pigs during and after gradual coronary artery occlusion.[7] Mortality during all exercise studies in our laboratory is less than 1%. We evaluated the response to exercise training by measuring oxygen consumption, heart rate at a fixed workload, and measurements of citrate synthase in biopsies of the biceps femoris muscle both before and after training.

Results

Normal Physiological Responses to Exercise

Figure 1 shows the pig's responses to exercise and exercise training compared with the dog's for $\dot{V}O_2$max changes. The post-training results were measured after 10 weeks of exercise training. We measured maximal oxygen consumption in the pig by using a respiratory mask and open circuit techniques.[17] The time of each exercise stress test ranged from 12 to 18 minutes. These data show that dogs and pigs have marked differences in exercise capacities. Also, the exercise capacity of the Yucatan pig is greater than that of the Hampshire pig. The greater exercise capacity of the Yucatan pig may relate to the higher red blood cell packed volume of the Yucatan breed (39% vs. 33%). Also, the observed breed differences could reflect differences in age and maturity of individual animals rather than distinct breed differences in response to exercise training

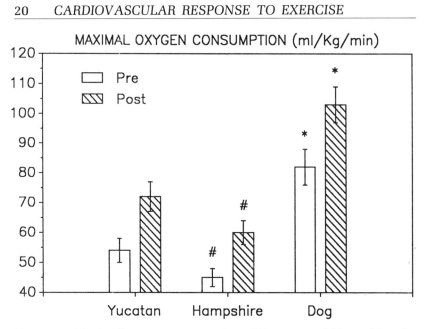

FIGURE 1. *Maximal oxygen consumption of Yucatan and Hampshire pigs and dogs before (Pre) and after (Post) 10 weeks of exercise training. Values are means ± SEM. #P<0.05 Hampshire (N = 7) vs. Yucatan (N = 7) pigs; *P<0.05 dog (N = 6) vs. both Yucatan and Hampshire pigs.*

(Figure 2).[15] These data also show that exercise training increases $\dot{V}O_2$max in both the dog and pig (Figures 1 and 2).

Ventricular Function Responses Associated with Exercise-Induced Hypertrophy

Exercise training for 10 weeks in pigs results in significant enhancement of aerobic capacity associated with compensated ventricular hypertrophy and markedly reduced systemic resistance, but no indication of increased contractile performance of the myocardium.[15] Left ventricle/body weight (LV/BW) ratios increased by 15% to 30% above sedentary control animal values depending on the intensity of the exercise training (Figure 3). The hypertrophy

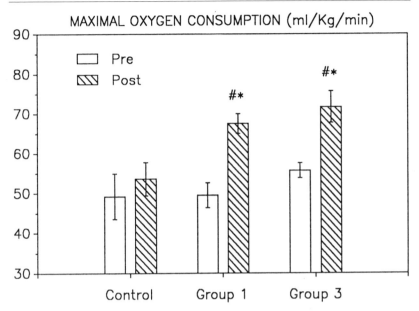

FIGURE 2. *Maximal oxygen consumption of control and exercise trained pigs (groups 1 and 3) before (Pre) and after (Post) 10 weeks of exercise training. Values are mean ± SEM. #P<0.05 trained vs. control; *P<0.05 before vs. after training.*

induced with these exercise training protocols was physiological since the increases in end-diastolic diameter were matched by increased wall thickness, thereby normalizing wall stress and O_2 demands.[15] Wall stress either decreased or remained constant in these animals, which suggested that an appropriate increase in wall thickness adequately compensated for the increase in internal diameter and that with this wall stress normalization in the exercise-trained heart, the work of the heart at matched heart rates did not increase. Other important adaptive changes occurring with exercise training were increased stroke volume, ejection fraction, and end-diastolic volume at rest and during exercise (Figures 4 and 5). The increased stroke volume with exercise training appears to be caused by an increase in the two end-diastolic dimensions rather than by a more vigorous ventricular contraction. These findings are similar to those reported in men.[18]

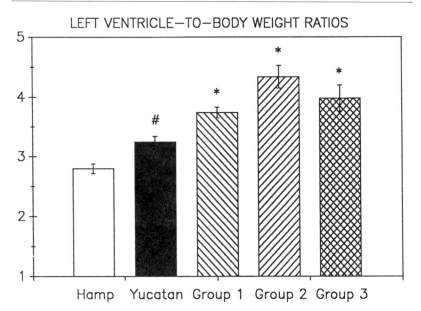

FIGURE 3. *Left ventricle/body weight ratios in control (Hampshire [Hamp] and Yucatan) and trained pigs (groups 1–3). Values are means ± SEM. #P<0.05 Yucatan vs. Hampshire; *P<0.05 trained groups vs. both Hampshire and Yucatan.*

Regional Myocardial Dysfunction During Gradual Coronary Artery Occlusion

We have determined changes occurring in regional myocardial function during gradual coronary artery occlusion.[19] We used changes in myocardial wall thickening in the collateral-dependent region as a measure of regional myocardial function. Regional myocardial wall thickening at rest significantly decreased during the time of gradual coronary artery occlusion. Some recovery of function occurred during the ensuing weeks. These results show that the pig model, with a sparse innate coronary collateral circulation, develops regional dysfunction at rest during progressive coronary artery occlusion that resembles the phenomenon of myocardial "stunning" or "hibernating myocardium" observed in humans with chronic, episodic myocardial ischemia.

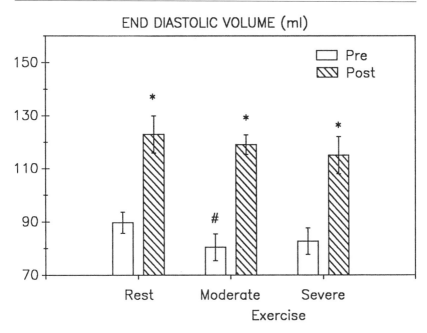

FIGURE 4. *End-diastolic volume before (Pre) and after (Post) 10 weeks of exercise training in group 1. Values are mean ± SEM for N = 5. #P<0.05 moderate vs. rest for pretraining; *P<0.05 before vs. after training for the same condition.*

Effect of Exercise Training on Regional Myocardial Function in the Collateral-Dependent Myocardium

During gradual coronary artery occlusion pigs were divided into sedentary and exercise-trained groups. When we measured changes in regional myocardial function and coronary collateral development, significant differences were noted in the exercise-trained animals compared with the sedentary controls.[19] Regional myocardial function and coronary collateral reserve in the collateral-dependent myocardium during exercise stress improved in the exercise-trained group. These results showed a beneficial effect of long-term exercise on regional myocardial function and collateral perfusion primarily at intense exercise levels, thus demonstrating that long-term exercise improves the ability of the collateral circulation and the collateral-

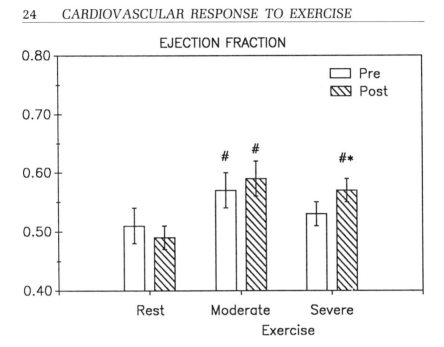

FIGURE 5. *Ejection fraction before (Pre) and after (Post) 10 weeks of exercise training in group 1. Values are mean ± SEM for n = 5. #p<0.05 vs. rest; *p<0.025 vs. pretraining.*

dependent myocardium to withstand the increased myocardial tissue pressures associated with tachycardia (Figure 6).

Discussion

The pig has several advantages as a model for cardiovascular studies. These include 1) an adaptation to exercise, which is markedly similar to that of man;[2] 2) a coronary anatomy similar to that of man;[4,6] and 3) a sparse innate coronary collateral circulation.[4,20,21]

Hemodynamic and metabolic adaptations to acute and chronic exercise in pigs are quite similar to those observed in humans.[1,15–17] Acute hemodynamic responses are described as proportional increments in left ventricular dP/dt_{max}, heart rate, and cardiac output with modest increases in stroke volume. Similar responses are present in

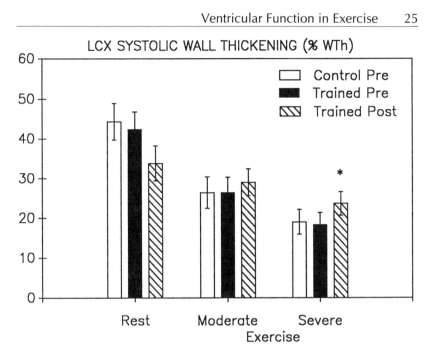

FIGURE 6. *Systolic wall thickening (WTh) in the left circumflex (LCX) region of myocardium in control and trained pigs before (Pre) and after (Post) 5 weeks of exercise training. Values are mean ± SEM for n = 9 control and n = 10 trained pigs. *p<0.05 significant difference from pretraining for the same condition.[19]*

dogs,[22,23] whereas greater increases in stroke volume occur in humans who exercise in the upright posture.[18] Considerable interest exists in the mechanisms responsible for increasing stroke volume and cardiac output when the time for diastolic filling of the ventricle greatly diminishes at higher exercise heart rates. The increased stroke volumes observed in dogs[24] and our pigs relate to increased contractility and reduced left ventricular end-systolic volume because left ventricular end-diastolic dimensions (Figure 4) were unchanged.[15] However, increased end-diastolic dimensions appear after both moderate[25] and severe exertion[24] in dogs. Recently, moderate exercise in dogs revealed a downward shift of the early diastolic portion of the left ventricular pressure–volume loop.[25] This fall in early diastolic left ventricular pressure pro duced more rapid mitral valve flow in early diastole and maintained left ventricular filling despite the shortening of diastole during exercise.[25]

Exercise-training pigs produces hemodynamic and metabolic adaptations similar to those found in humans (Figure 2).[1,15] Our moderately trained pigs (group 1) did not exhibit the improvement in intrinsic myocardial function observed after training in dogs (Figure 7).[15,26] Dogs trained at high intensities exhibited an increased myocardial contractility during exercise and a 30% increase in left ventricular mass.[26] Group 1 pigs had only a 15% increase in left ventricular mass. These data support the hypothesis that intrinsic improvements in cardiac function require high intensity training. Such adaptations also have been reported in a select group of patients with coronary artery disease.

Although the existence of collateral circulation in the heart has been known for centuries, few studies have been conducted on factors promoting collateral growth. A significant problem has been the lack of an appropriate model. The dog has many collaterals that develop

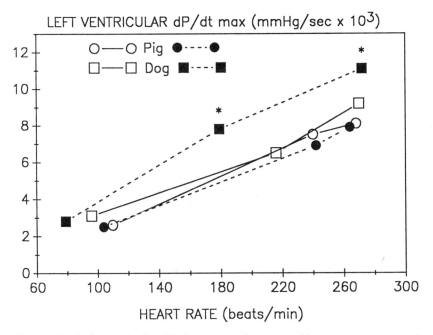

FIGURE 7. *Left ventricular dP/dt max as a function of heart rate at rest and during exercise in untrained (open symbols) and trained (solid symbols) pigs. Values are mean for n = 7 pigs and n = 4 trained and 13 untrained dogs. *p<0.05 significantly different from pretraining for the same exercise condition.[15,26]*

rapidly during periods of ischemia,[27] but there is strong clinical evidence that such collaterals do no exist in any great abundance in humans.[6] Thus, a model that nearly mimics the collateral scarceness of the human heart has been needed. Rapid occlusion of a coronary artery in a heart with sparse collaterals usually leads to complete infarction of the vascular bed at risk. This model does not provide an opportunity to study the growth of the collateral circulation. The collaterals present in such hearts are thin-walled vessels with little growth potential.[27] What we need is a collateral-dependent vascular bed at risk in which most of the tissue could be salvaged and in which collateral development could be monitored. Our experiments in pigs with slow gradual occlusion of the left circumflex coronary artery by an ameroid occluder confirmed the potentiality of this model.[7] We found the collateral reserve of this ischemic bed to be 40% of the normal bed. Over a period of 16 weeks we found that collateral circulation changed little.[8] After the initial rapid growth of collaterals, subsequent growth slows, perhaps because of a lack of ischemic stimulus. Thus, this model is appropriate for studying changes in collateral circulation.

We have characterized the pig as an appropriate model for cardiovascular studies of coronary physiology, coronary collateral circulation, and exercise physiology. We compared both Yucatan pigs and Hampshire pigs in experiments concerning myocardial ischemia, gradual coronary artery occlusion, and regional myocardial function during infarction and exercise. The Yucatan pig was vigorous and docile. The exercise capacity of the Yucatan pig was greater than that of the similar weight Hampshire pig, presumably because of its higher hematocrit and larger heart size. Both breeds increased their $\dot{V}O_2$max by 25% after 10 weeks of exercise training. The maximal coronary vascular capacity of these pigs was similar to that of humans, but less than that of the dogs.[4] Acute occlusion of a pig's coronary artery infarcted most of the tissue in the vascular bed at risk. Gradual occlusion of the left circumflex coronary artery produces a collateral-dependent vascular bed with only 5% infarct. At rest, collateral flow is sufficient to meet demands, but during exercise stress severe ischemia and regional dysfunction are unmasked. These persist for up to 16 weeks after occlusion. These observations of limited infarction, along with limited collateral vessel development, show that this is a good model for investigating the growth and development of coronary collateral circulation in humans.

Echocardiographic studies in patients during acute coronary artery occlusion show myocardial dysfunction in the region of myocardium distal to the occlusion.[28] This regional myocardial dysfunction was not present in experiments in dogs during a period of progressive coronary artery occlusion with an ameroid occluder.[29] The generally abundant epicardial innate collateral circulation of the dog[27] most likely preserved ventricular function at rest in the region of myocardium jeopardized by the coronary artery occlusion. Given the similarities of the innate collateral circulation of pigs and humans, the pig may serve as an appropriate model for the study of therapeutic interventions designed for use in patients with ventricular dysfunction related to myocardial ischemia.

Our investigations of the coronary physiology of the pig have led to the following conclusions: 1) collateral circulation of the pig is sparse; 2) acute occlusion of the coronary artery results in infarction of most of the bed at risk and is associated with a high mortality; 3) maximal coronary blood flow of the pig is less than the dog but similar to that of humans; 4) collateral blood flow in the left circumflex coronary artery may be sufficient to prevent a major infarction if the occlusion is slow; 5) the limited development of the collateral circulation in the pig provides a suitable environment in which to study factors that control collateral growth; 6) the distribution of coronary blood flow in the pig during stenosis is similar to that found in other mammals; and 7) regional myocardial dysfunction persists after gradual coronary artery occlusion when the animal is exercise stressed.

References

1. White FC, Roth DM, Bloor CM: The pig as a model for myocardial ischemia and exercise. *Lab Anim Sci* 1986;36:351–356
2. Hastings AB, White FC, Sanders TM, Bloor CM: Comparative physiological responses to exercise stress. *J Appl Physiol* 1982;52: 1077–1083
3. Bloor CM, White FC, Roth DM: The pig as a model of myocardial ischemia and gradual coronary artery occlusion, in Swindle MM (ed): *Swine as Models in Biomedical Research.* Ames, Iowa State University Press, 1992, pp 163–175
4. White FC, Sanders TM, Bloor CM: Coronary reserve at maximal heart rate in the exercising swine. *J Cardiac Rehab* 1981;1:31–40
5. Cohen MV: *Coronary Collaterals. Clinical and Experimental Observations.* New York, Futura Publishing Co, Inc, 1992, pp 251–258

6. Baroldi G, Mantero O, Scomazzoni G: The collaterals of the coronary arteries in normal and pathologic hearts. *Circ Res* 1992;4:223–229

7. O'Konski MS, White FW, Longhurst JC, Roth DM, Bloor CM: Ameroid constriction of the proximal left circumflex coronary artery in swine. *Am J Cardiovasc Pathol* 1987; 1:69–77

8. Roth DM, Mauroka Y, Rogers J, White FC, Longhurst JC, Bloor CM: Development of the coronary collateral circulation in left circumflex ameroid occluded swine myocardium. *Am J Physiol* 1987;253: H1279–H1288

9. Kolibash AJ, Bush CA, Wepsic RA, Schroeder DP, Tetalmen MR, Lewis RP: Coronary collateral vessels: Spectrum of physiological capabilities with respect to providing rest and stress myocardial perfusion, maintenance of left ventricular function and protection against infarction. *Am J Cardiol* 1982;50:230–238

10. Pantepinto LM, Phillips RW, Wheeler LP, Will DH: The Yucatan miniature pig as a laboratory animal. *Lab Anim Sci* 1978;28:308–313

11. Swindle MM: *Basic Surgical Exercises Using Swine.* New York, Praeger, 1992

12. Savage RM, Guth B, White FC, Hagan AD, Bloor CM: Correlation of regional myocardial blood flow and function with myocardial infarct size during acute myocardial ischemia in the conscious pig. *Circulation* 1981;64:699–707

13. Gray CE, White FC, Crisman RP, Wisniewski J, McKirnan MD, Bloor CM: Chronic swine instrumentation techniques utilizing the Gor-tex peritoneal catheter, in Tumbleson ME (ed): *Swine in Biomedical Research.* New York, Plenum Publishing Corp, 1987, pp 279–290

14. Bloor CM, White FC, Sanders TM: Effects of exercise on collateral development in myocardial ischemia in pigs. *J Appl Physiol* 1984;56:656–665

15. White FC, McKirnan MD, Breisch EA, Guth BD, Liu YM, Bloor CM: Adaptation of the left ventricle of exercise-induced hypertrophy. *J Appl Physiol* 1987;62:1097–1110

16. McKirnan MD, Gray CG, White FC: Plateau in muscle blood flow during prolonged exercise in miniature swine. *J Appl Physiol* 1989;66: 2101–2108

17. McKirnan MD, White FC, Guth B, Longhurst JC, Bloor CM: Validation of a respiratory mask for measuring gas exchange in exercising swine. *J Appl Physiol* 1987;61:1226–1229

18. Rowell LB: *Human Circulation: Regulation During Physical Stress.* New York: Oxford University Press, 1986

19. Roth DM, White FC, Nichols ML, Dobbs SL, Longhurst JC, Bloor CM: Effect of long-term exercise on regional myocardial function and coronary collateral development after gradual coronary artery occlusion in pigs. *Circulation* 1990;82:1778–1789

20. Millard RW: Induction of functional coronary collaterals in the swine heart. *Basic Res Cardiol* 1981;76:468–473

21. Patterson RE, Kirk ES: Analysis of coronary collateral structure, function and ischemic border zones in pigs. *Am J Physiol* 1983;244:23–31

22. Stone HL: Cardiac function and exercise training in conscious dogs. *J Appl Physiol* 1977;42:824–832
23. Horwitz LD, Lindenfeld J: Effects of enhanced ventricular filling on cardiac pump performance in exercising dogs. *J Appl Physiol* 1985;59:1886–1890
24. Vatner SF, Franklin D, Higgins CB, Patrick T, Braunwald B: Left ventricular response to severe exertion in untethered dogs. *J Clin Invest* 1972;51:3052–3060
25. Cheng CP, Igarashi Y, Little WC: Mechanism of augmented rate of left ventricular filling during exercise. *Circ Res* 1992;70:9–19
26. Barnard RJ, Duncan HW, Baldwin KM, Grimditch G, Buckberg GD: Effects of intensive exercise training on myocardial performance and coronary blood flow. *J Appl Physiol* 1980;49:444–449
27. Schaper W: *The Pathophysiology of Myocardial Perfusion.* Amsterdam: Elsevier/North-Holland, 1979
28. Gibson RS, Bishop HL, Stamm RB, Crampton RS, Beller GA, Martin RP: Value of early two-dimensional echocardiography in patients with acute myocardial infarction. *Am J Cardiol* 1982;49:1110–1119
29. Tomoike H, Franklin D, Kemper WS, McKown D, Ross J: Functional evaluation of coronary collateral development in conscious dogs. *Am J Physiol* 1981;241:H519–H524

Chapter 3

Left Ventricular Response to Exercise

Robert O. Bonow, MD

The normal human cardiovascular system rapidly adjusts to the demands of exercise by calling on a number of interrelated responses that, in concert, serve to augment cardiac output to adequate levels to meet the requirements of the exercising skeletal muscles. With increasing oxygen consumption, there is a linear increase in cardiac output that is accomplished by an increase in heart rate and the rapid response of the left ventricle to augment stroke volume. The augmentation in stroke volume is accomplished both by use of the Frank-Starling mechanism and by use of left ventricular contractile reserve (Table 1). This chapter focuses on these cardiovascular responses, with emphasis on the adaptation of the normal left ventricle during exercise in order to achieve the necessary increases in stroke volume.

Cardiovascular Response to Exercise

The cardiovascular response to dynamic, graded upright exercise for normal men studied by radionuclide angiography is shown in Figure 1. Heart rate, blood pressure, ejection fraction, and cardiac output all increase steadily with increasing workloads.[1] Although left ventricular function and cardiac output increase in a stepwise fashion at early, submaximal, and peak stages of exercise, the mechanisms responsible for the progressive increase in cardiac output differ at various levels of exercise intensity. During early stages of exercise, the initial increase in cardiac output is accomplished by increases in heart rate and stroke volume,[1-4] and the

From Fletcher GF, (ed): *Cardiovascular Response to Exercise.* Mount Kisco, NY, Futura Publishing Company, Inc., © 1994.

TABLE 1. Components of the Left Ventricular Response to Exercise

Heart rate response
Frank-Starling mechanism
   Increased venous return
   Increased rate and extent of ventricular relaxation and filling
Left ventricular contractile reserve

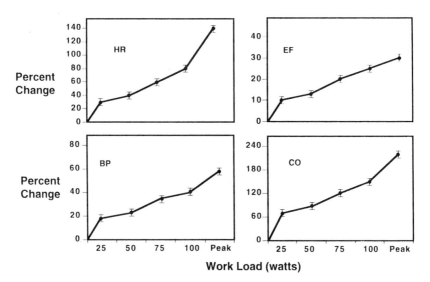

FIGURE 1. *Cardiovascular response to exercise in 30 normal men, aged 26 to 50 years. Changes in heart rate (HR), systolic blood pressure (BP), ejection fraction (EF), and cardiac output (CO) with increasing workloads during upright bicycle ergometry are expressed as percentages of the resting values. Each variable increases significantly (p<0.05) at each stage compared with the values in each preceding stage. Reproduced from Reference 1 with permission.*

augmentation in stroke volume is accomplished predominantly by a brisk increase in left ventricular end-diastolic volume (Figure 2). Thus, Frank-Starling mechanisms are responsible for the rapid and significant increase in stroke volume that occurs at low levels of exercise intensity. Stroke volume increases by 30%–50% during upright exercise,[1–3,5–9] with the greatest increase occurring during the initial minutes of exercise. After the substantial increases in end-diastolic volume and stroke volume that occur at the onset of

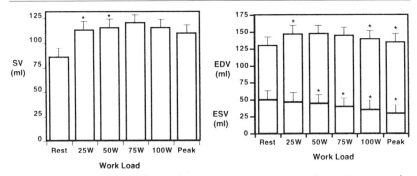

FIGURE 2. *Left ventricular volume response to exercise. Mean stroke volume (SV), end-diastolic volume (EDV), and end-systolic volume (ESV) are shown at each stage of exercise in the same 30 men illustrated in Figure 1. Asterisks indicate significant differences (p<0.05) compared with each immediately preceding stage. Reproduced from Reference 1 with permission.*

exercise, end-diastolic volume plateaus at higher intermediate levels of exercise.[1–3] Thus, the small increases in stroke volume that continue to occur during submaximal exercise develop not from further chamber dilatation, but from enhanced left ventricular contractile function with a resultant decrease in left ventricular end-systolic volume (Figure 2). At even higher, maximal levels of exercise intensity, end-diastolic volume declines significantly compared with the volume at submaximal exercise. However, despite the decrease in end-diastolic volume, stroke volume is maintained at the value achieved during submaximal exercise because greater left ventricular contractility causes significant reductions in end-systolic volume (Figure 2). Hence, stroke volume is augmented during early exercise primarily through the use of preload reserve and Frank-Starling relationships, whereas stroke volume is maintained at these levels during maximal exercise predominantly through the use of left ventricular contractile reserve.

The changes in left ventricular end-diastolic volume relative to end-systolic volume throughout the spectrum of exercise result in a progressive increase in ejection fraction at each level of exercise (Figure 1). However, as stroke volume increases only slightly at progressively higher submaximal exercise levels and then reaches a plateau at maximal intensities of exercise, the steady increase in cardiac output that occurs at the higher exercise workloads depends on the progressive increases in heart rate, until maximal heart rates are achieved. This heart rate dependence has important implications in elderly patients, in whom the reduced maximal heart rate with exercise contributes critically to the age-related decline in maximum cardiac output and oxygen consumption.

These physiological relationships between use of the Frank-Starling mechanism and the use of left ventricular contractile reserve are evident in all forms of dynamic exercise, although the relative importance of left ventricular preload and the use of Frank-Starling forces in augmenting and maintaining stroke volume depends on a number of factors. One such factor is exercise position. Maximal cardiac output is similar in both the upright and supine positions.[8] As heart rates are significantly lower during supine compared with upright exercise, the maintenance of cardiac output depends on greater stroke volumes in the supine position. This is achieved primarily by recruitment of preload reserve and use of the Frank-Starling mechanism. In the supine position under resting conditions, end-diastolic volume is greater than in the upright position.[3,8] Despite the greater supine end-diastolic volume at rest, substantial preload reserve is recruited during supine exercise, with appropriate use of the Frank-Starling mechanism at the early stages of exercise to increase stroke volume.[8] In contrast, end-systolic volume, which decreases significantly compared with resting values during upright exercise, is unchanged during maximal exercise in the supine position. As a result, the magnitude of increase in ejection fraction from rest to exercise is greater in the upright position.[8]

Prolonged Submaximal Exercise Versus Brief Maximal Exercise

The importance of Frank-Starling forces also depends on whether the exercise activity is one of gradual prolonged intensity or brief maximal activity. The left ventricular response in young men to prolonged, submaximal upright exercise compared with brief, maximal upright exercise is depicted in Figure 3, as reported by Upton et al.[9] using radionuclide ventriculography. A prolonged submaximal exercise period was terminated by 10 minutes of maximal exercise. This was followed by a second exercise period that consisted of a single 10-minute period of maximal exercise. The maximal heart

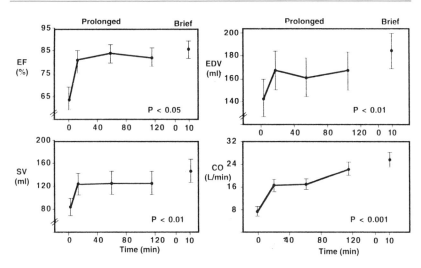

FIGURE 3. *Effects of prolonged submaximal versus brief maximal exercise on left ventricular function. Data are shown for 9 normal men, aged 20 to 32 years, who underwent two exercise studies. The first was 120 minutes of prolonged exercise, during which submaximal (60% of maximal work) was maintained for 110 minutes, with the final 10 minutes representing maximal exercise. The second study was a single 10-minute period of maximal exercise. The maximum heart rate achieved on both exercise protocols was identical (mean 180 beats per minute). However, ejection fraction (EF), end-diastolic volume (EDV), stroke volume (SV), and cardiac output (CO) were all significantly higher during the brief maximal exercise study than during the prolonged exercise study. Reproduced from Reference 9 with permission.*

rate achieved at the end of both protocols was identical (mean, 180 beats per minute). However, left ventricular end-diastolic volume was 14% higher at the end of the brief, intense exercise protocol compared with that at the end of the prolonged protocol. This, in turn, led to a 15% greater stroke volume and cardiac output during the brief, intense effort compared with the prolonged effort. The higher end-diastolic volume during brief maximal exercise despite the same maximal heart rate as that achieved during the prolonged exercise protocol suggests that preload reserve may be exhausted during long submaximal exercise, and no further increase in end-diastolic volume may be possible even when higher work levels are then added. These data add further support to the concept that the Frank-Starling mechanism is recruited early during exercise. Moreover, it appears that these mechanisms are more efficient in augmenting stroke volume when they are recruited early during maximal rather than submaximal effort. Thus, bursts of intense exercise are likely to recruit preload reserve and use the Frank-Starling mechanism more efficiently than are periods of submaximal activity or activities of graded exercise intensity.

The ventricular volume and functional responses to normal daily activities, rather than activities studied under laboratory conditions, have not been investigated in depth. However, the technology to study such activities is now available in the form of portable nonimaging scintillation probes (Figure 4) that are capable of monitoring ventricular volume and function continuously during normal ambulatory activities.[10]

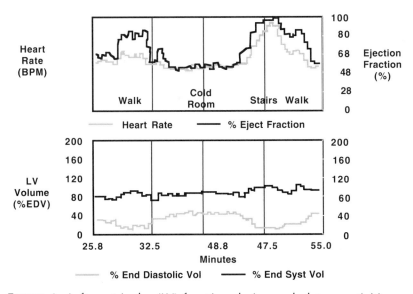

FIGURE 4. *Left ventricular (LV) function during ambulatory activities as measured by a portable nonimaging scintillation probe. Heart rate, ejection fraction, end-systolic volume, and end-diastolic volume are monitored continuously and demonstrate changes in ventricular volumes and function during normal activities such as walking and climbing stairs. Reproduced from Reference 10 with permission.*

Mechanisms for Augmentation of Diastolic Volume During Exercise

There are two mechanisms responsible for the increase in left ventricular end-diastolic volume during exercise (Table 1). The exercising skeletal muscles serve as a pump to enhance the rate of venous return to the central circulation. This is probably the initial process employed in increasing left ventricular diastolic volumes. This mechanism in and of itself, however, would be expected not only to increase left ventricular end-diastolic volume, but also to increase end-diastolic pressures substantially within the ventricular cavity. The observation in the normal heart is that the increases in end-diastolic volume during upright exercise are associated with either no change or only a slight increase in pulmonary wedge pressure.[3] Thus, additional mechanisms must also be operational during exercise to enhance left ventricular relaxation, so that the left ventricle can accommodate a significant increase in diastolic volume with little or no change in diastolic pressure. The increase in the rate and extent of left ventricular relaxation during exercise has the added salutary effect of augmenting the rate and magnitude of left ventricular filling, thereby contributing directly to the increase in end-diastolic volume.[11]

When left ventricular relaxation in the normal heart reduces ventricular pressure below left atrial pressure to achieve mitral valve opening and the onset of ventricular filling, ventricular pressure continues to fall despite the dramatic increase in ventricular volume. This paradox of a chamber that increases in size without a concomitant increase in pressure is evidence that ventricular filling in early diastole is enhanced by the continuing decline of ventricular pressure, which creates a suction effect. Thus, ventricular relaxation creates a suction pressure in early diastole to augment the left atrial–left ventricular pressure gradient across the mitral valve, which is the principal determinant of ventricular filling.[12]

This suction effect may be enhanced by the actions of sympathetic and β-adrenergic stimulation, which enhance myocardial relaxation (Figure 5), thereby increasing the rate and extent of left ventricular pressure decay to develop very low or even negative early diastolic pressures.[13] The ability of the left ventricle to develop suction and to augment the degree of suction through sympathetic drive is an important vehicle for the normal left ventricle during

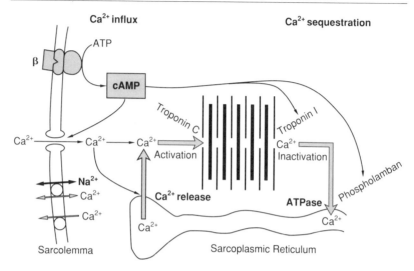

FIGURE 5. *Effect on calcium ion cycling on activation and inactivation of myocardial contractile proteins. Calcium ion flux across the sarcolemma as well as calcium released from sarcoplasmic reticulum stores allow association and cross-linking of the myofibrillar proteins actin and myosin, with resultant cellular contraction. This rapid increase in intracellular calcium concentration is then countered by rapid sequestration of calcium ion into the sarcoplasmic reticulum by calcium ATPase. The decrease in intracellular calcium concentration allows "inactivation" of the actin myosin cross-bridges with resultant cellular relaxation. Stimulation of sarcolemmal β-adrenergic receptors increases the intracellular concentration of cyclic AMP (cAMP), which not only enhances activation but also facilitates inactivation, by phosphorylating troponin I (which reduces contractile protein affinity for calcium) and of phospholamban (which augments calcium ATPase activity). Reproduced from Reference 11 with permission.*

exercise, permitting the ventricle to augment filling volume, recruit Frank-Starling mechanisms, and eject greater stroke volume. Importantly, this vehicle also allows the ventricle to fill to significantly larger volumes despite the marked reduction in diastolic filling time that occurs at high heart rates. Thus, the facilitation of the suction mechanism by sympathetic drive allows the normal left ventricle to operate efficiently at high cycling rates, thereby increasing transmitral flow while maintaining normal left atrial pressure.[11]

The importance of relaxation and diastolic suction in the

generation of preload reserve and the recruitment of Frank-Starling mechanisms is illustrated in patients with left ventricular hypertrophy. Many such patients, with impaired ventricular relaxation, are unable to increase end-diastolic volume in the face of tachycardia, are unable to use the Frank-Starling relationship effectively, and are unable to increase stroke volume adequately during exercise.[14,15]

The recruitment of left ventricular contractile reserve at submaximal and maximal levels of exercise further facilitates ventricular relaxation and diastolic suction. The degree of systolic contraction influences the process of relaxation through the restoring forces that develop as the left ventricle is compressed to a small end-systolic volume.[16] The subsequent elastic recoil after contraction is a loading factor that further enhances the rate and extent of left ventricular pressure decline during early diastole and contributes to the creation of the diastolic suction pressure. Thus, use of contractile reserve not only provides an obviously important inotropic boost, but also has a lusitropic action as well to facilitate ventricular filling at near-maximal heart rates. Even as ventricular end-diastolic volume declines at maximal heart rates (Figure 2), these factors prevent the ventricular volume from decreasing too precipitously to baseline values or below, which would have a major detrimental effect on stroke volume maintenance. Thus, these factors counter the tendency of a pure chronotropic stimulus (without concomitant sympathetic stimulation) to decrease end-diastolic volume.

Effect of Gender

Numerous studies have demonstrated that there are significant differences in the left ventricular functional response to exercise between men and women.[2,17–21] At matched workloads and at peak exercise, men achieve higher ejection fractions than do women (Figure 6), even when aerobic capacity (measured by weight-adjusted maximal oxygen consumption) is the same between the two groups.[2] In keeping with the similar aerobic capacities, the increases in stroke volume and cardiac output during exercise also are similar between men and women (Figure 7). However, the mechanisms for the increase in stroke volume differ. Women manifest a greater increase in end-diastolic volume than do men

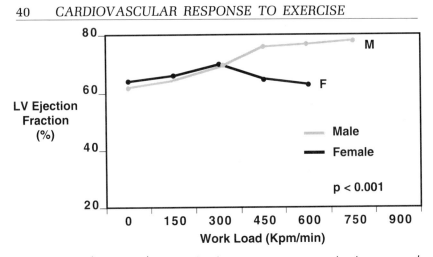

FIGURE 6. *Left ventricular (LV) ejection response to exercise in men and women. Mean ejection fractions are shown for 15 normal men and 16 age-matched normal women. Despite similar aerobic capacity (measured by weight-adjusted peak oxygen consumption), men achieved higher ejection fractions at matched submaximal workloads and at peak exercise. Reproduced from Reference 2 with permission.*

(Figure 7), explaining the differences in the ejection fraction responses.[2,20] These data suggest that women, who also have smaller end-diastolic volume indexes at rest than men,[20] rely to a greater extent on the use of the Frank-Starling mechanism to augment stroke volume than men do. These differences are not explained by differences in exercise capacity or aerobic capacity.[2,20]

Effect of Aging

The cardiovascular response to exercise is altered with aging, with blunted chronotropic and inotropic responsiveness. This results in the decline in maximal oxygen consumption and cardiac output, which has been demonstrated in numerous studies.[18,22–26] The reduced cardiac output response to exercise in the elderly reflects primarily a progressive decline in maximal heart rate with advancing age[23,24] (Figure 8). The same has been observed regarding chronotropic responsiveness to β-adrenergic stimulation; the heart

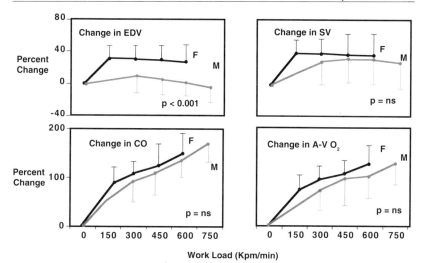

FIGURE 7. *Cardiovascular responses to progressive exercise in the same normal men and women shown in Figure 6. Men and women achieved similar increases in stroke volume (SV), cardiac output (CO), and arteriovenous O_2 difference (A-V O_2), but women did so with a significantly greater increase in end-diastolic volume (EDV) than the men. Reproduced from Reference 2 with permission.*

rate response to isoproterenol infusion steadily decreases with the process of aging.[27,28] This does not reflect altered baroreceptor function, as the same age-related chronotropic effect of isoproterenol persists even with anesthesia or with atropine administration.[27] Since age-related differences in heart rate and cardiac output responses are obliterated after β-blockade,[29] reduced β-adrenergic responsiveness is the primary mediator of the blunted heart rate and cardiac output response to exercise in the elderly.

Elderly persons manifest roughly the same stroke volume response to exercise as do young adults,[18] so the age-related reduction in cardiac output with exercise results almost purely from altered chronotropic reserve. However, inotropic reserve also is diminished with aging. In contrast to young adults, there is little or no reduction in end-systolic volume with higher levels of exercise intensity in the elderly, and augmented stroke volume is accomplished by left ventricular cavity dilatation, augmented end-diastolic

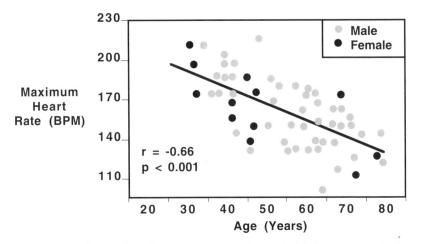

FIGURE 8. *Relationship between age and maximal heart rate during upright exercise in healthy persons free of cardiac disease. Reproduced from Reference 18 with permission.*

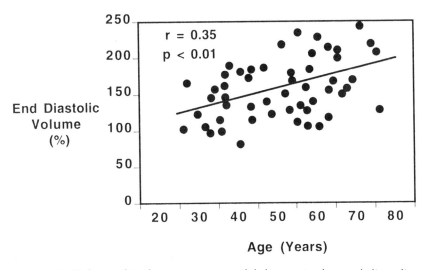

FIGURE 9. *Relationship between age and left ventricular end-diastolic volume during maximal upright exercise in the same healthy persons shown in Figure 8. Reproduced from Reference 18 with permission.*

volume (Figure 9), and use of the Frank-Starling mechanism.[18,25,26] As a result of the greater increase in end-diastolic volume with similar stroke volumes in the elderly compared with the young adult, there is less of an increase (or an actual decrease) in ejection fraction during exercise in elderly persons (Figure 10). Several studies have, in fact, demonstrated a progressive, linear decline in the ejection fraction response to exercise from young adulthood through old age.[18,21,26,30] The gender-related differences in left ventricular functional responses are maintained throughout this age range[18,21] (Figure 10).

Two factors contribute to the age-related reduction in ejection performance and the relative increase in end-systolic volume with exercise. Aortic impedance is heightened during exercise in the elderly,[31] resulting from the structural changes and reduced β-adrenergic responsiveness of the aorta with aging. Augmented impedance to ejection reduces shortening, resulting in a relative increase in end-systolic volume. The second factor is related to

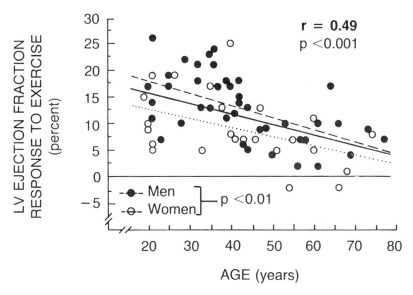

FIGURE 10. *Magnitude of the change in left ventricular ejection from rest to exercise in normal healthy men and women ages 18 through 77 years. Reproduced from Reference 21 with permission.*

reduced contractile reserve of the left ventricle with aging.[27] This reflects in large part the attenuated end-organ response to β-adrenergic stimulation, such that β-adrenergic modulation of contractility is reduced progressively with increasing age.[27,28,32,33] The importance of this effect is underscored by studies demonstrating that the age-related difference in contractile performance during exercise is abolished by β-blockade.[29] Reduced β-adrenergic responsiveness also may affect the efficiency with which preload reserve can be recruited during exercise in the elderly, particularly if the lusitropic effect of β-adrenergic stimulation (Figure 5) is similarly affected by aging. However, the available data suggest that there is a dissociation between inotropic responsiveness and lusitropic responsiveness in the aged heart, with maintenance of the responsiveness of left ventricular relaxation to β-adrenergic stimuli.[33] Thus, in contrast to the marked decrease in inotropic response to catecholamines, the lusitropic response is selectively well maintained. This would account for the efficient use of preload reserve and Frank-Starling mechanisms in the elderly to augment left ventricular stroke volume during exercise.

Conclusion

The normal heart adjusts to exercise by recruiting chronotropic reserve, preload reserve, and contractile reserve to augment cardiac output. The balance of these three components of the exercise response varies considerably, depending on a number of factors, most notably gender, age, the type and intensity of exercise, and the suddenness with which the cardiovascular response to exercise is demanded. In a number of these circumstances, the recruitment of preload reserve with use of Frank-Starling forces to augment stroke volume plays a dominant role. This is the case in the early stages of the exercise response, during sudden intense exercise, and during supine exercise, and this is especially the case in women and in the elderly. This mechanism, governed by increased venous return and enhanced left ventricular relaxation, provides a rapid and efficient means to achieve the required increase in ventricular function to meet the demands of exercise.

References

1. Plotnick GD, Becker LC, Fisher ML, Gerstenblith G, Renlund DG, Fleg JL, Weisfeldt ML, Lakatta EG: Use of the Frank-Starling mechanism during submaximal versus maximal upright exercise. *Am J Physiol* 1986;251:H1101–H1105

2. Higginbotham MB, Morris KG, Coleman RE, Cobb FR: Sex-related differences in the normal cardiac response to upright exercise. *Circulation* 1984;70:357–366

3. Higginbotham MB, Morris KG, Williams RS, McHale PA, Coleman RE, Cobb FR: Regulation of stroke volume during submaximal and maximal upright exercise in normal man. *Circ Res* 1986;58:281–291

4. Weiss JL, Weisfeldt ML, Mason SJ, Garrison JB, Livingood SV, Fortuin NJ: Evidence of Frank-Starling effect in man during severe semisupine exercise. *Circulation* 1979;59:655–661

5. Astrand PO, Cuddy TE, Saltin B: Cardiac output during submaximal and maximal work. *J Appl Physiol* 1964;19:268–274

6. Grimby G, Nillson NJ, Saltin B: Cardiac output during submaximal and maximal exercise in active middle-aged athletes. *J Appl Physiol* 1966;21:1150–1156

7. Ekblom B, Astrand PO, Saltin B, Steinberg J, Wallstrom B: Effect of training on circulatory response to exercise. *J Appl Physiol* 1968;24:518–528

8. Poliner LR, Dehmer GJ, Lewis SE, Parkey RW, Blomqvist DG, Willerson JT. Left ventricular performance in normal subjects: a comparison of the response to exercise in the upright and supine position. *Circulation* 1980;62:528–534

9. Upton ME, Rerych SK, Roeback JR, Newman GE, Douglas JM, Wallace AG, Jones RH: Effect of brief and prolonged exercise on left ventricular function. *Am J Cardiol* 1980;45:1154–1160

10. Tamaki N, Gill JB, Moore RH, Yasuda T, Boucher CA, Strauss HW: Cardiac response to daily activities and exercise in normal subjects assessed by an ambulatory ventricular function monitor. *Am J Cardiol* 1987;59:1164–1169

11. Bonow RO, Udelson JE: Left ventricular diastolic dysfunction as a cause of congestive heart failure: mechanisms and management. *Ann Intern Med* 1992;117:502–510

12. Yellin EL, Sonnenblick EH, Frater RWM. Dynamic determinants of left ventricular filling: an overview, in Baan J, Artezius AC, Yellin EL (eds): *Cardiac Dynamics*. Boston: Martinus Nijhoff Publishing, 1980, pp 145–158

13. Udelson JE, Bacharach SL, Cannon RO, Bonow RO: Minimum left ventricular pressure during beta-adrenergic stimulation in human subjects: evidence for elastic recoil and diastolic "suction" in the normal heart. *Circulation* 1990;82:1174–1182

14. Cuocolo A, Sax FL, Brush JE, Maron BJ, Bacharach SL, Bonow RO: Left

ventricular hypertrophy and impaired left ventricular filling in essential hypertension: diastolic mechanisms for systolic dysfunction during exercise. *Circulation* 1990;81:978–986

15. Kitzman DW, Higginbotham MB, Cobb FR, Sheikh KH, Sullivan MJ: Exercise intolerance in patients with heart failure and preserved left ventricular systolic function: failure of the Frank-Starling mechanism. *J Am Coll Cardiol* 1991;17:1065–1072

16. Tyberg JV, Keon WJ, Sonnenblick EH, Urschell CW: Mechanics of ventricular diastole. *Cardiovasc Res* 1970;4:423–428

17. Gibbons RJ, Lee KL, Cobb F, Jones RH: Ejection fraction response to exercise in patients with chest pain and normal coronary arteriograms. *Circulation* 1981;64:952–957

18. Rodeheffer RJ, Gerstenblith G, Becker LC, Fleg JL, Weisfeldt ML, Lakatta EG: Exercise cardiac output is maintained with advancing age in healthy human subjects: cardiac dilatation and increased stroke volume compensate for a diminished heart rate. *Circulation* 1984;69:203–214

19. Adams KF, Vincent LM, McAllister SM, El-Ashmawy H, Sheps DS: The influence of age and gender on left ventricular response to supine exercise in asymptomatic normal subjects. *Am Heart J* 1987;113:732–742

20. Hanley PC, Zinsmeister AR, Clements IP, Bove AA, Brown ML, Gibbons RJ: Gender-related differences in cardiac responses to supine exercise assessed by radionuclide angiography. *J Am Coll Cardiol* 1989;13:624–629

21. Bonow RO: Gated equilibrium blood pool imaging: current role for diagnosis and prognosis in coronary artery disease, in Zaret BL, Beller GA (eds): *Nuclear Cardiology.* St. Louis: CV Mosby Co, 1992, pp 123–136

22. Dehn M, Bruce RA: Longitudinal variations in maximal oxygen uptake with age and activity. *Am J Physiol* 1972;83:805

23. Gerstenblith G, Lakatta EG, Weisfeldt ML. Age changes in myocardial function and exercise response. *Prog Cardiovasc Dis* 1976;19:1–21

24. Strandell T: Cardiac output in old age, in Caird FI, Dall JL, Kennedy RD (eds): *Cardiology in Old Age.* New York: Plenum Publishing Corp, 1976, pp 81–100

25. Higginbotham MB, Morris KG, Williams, Coleman RE, Cobb FR: Physiologic basis for the age-related decline in aerobic work capacity. *Am J Cardiol* 1986;57:1374–1379

26. Mann DL, Denenberg BS, Gash AK, Makler PT, Bove AA: Effects of age on ventricular performance during graded supine exercise. *Am Heart J* 1986;111:108–115

27. Lakatta EG: Alterations in the cardiovascular system that occur in advanced age. *Fed Proc* 1979;38:163–167

28. Lakatta EG: Age-related alterations in the cardiovascular response to adrenergic mediated stress. *Fed Proc* 1980;39:3173–3177

29. Conway J, Wheeler R, Sannerstedt R: Sympathetic nervous activity during exercise in relation to age. *Cardiovasc Res* 1971;5:577–581

30. Port S, Cobb FR, Coleman RE, Jones RH: Effect of age on the response

of the left ventricular ejection fraction to exercise. *N Engl J Med* 1980; 303:1133–1137

31. Yin FC, Weisfeldt ML, Milnor WR: Role of aortic input impedance in the decreased cardiovascular response to exercise with aging in dogs. *J Clin Invest* 1981;68:28–38

32. Guarnieri T, Filburn CR, Zitnik G, Gerstenblith G, Weisfeldt ML, Lakatta EG: Contractile and biochemical correlates of beta-adrenergic stimulation of the aged heart. *Am J Physiol* 1980;239:H501

33. Lakatta EG, Gerstenblith G, Angell CS, Weisfeldt ML: Diminished inotropic response of aged myocardium to catecholamines. *Circ Res* 1979;44:517–523

Chapter 4

Doppler Echocardiographic Assessment of Left Ventricular Systolic and Diastolic Flow During Exercise

Michael H. Crawford, MD
and Robert S. Flinn

Left ventricular flow is customarily measured as the stroke volume per heart beat. Stoke volume per beat multiplied by the heart rate equals the cardiac output. Exercise-induced increases in cardiac output directly correlate with increases in oxygen uptake.[1] The ability to increase oxygen consumption is a major determinant of exercise performance. Systolic left ventricular flow is the stroke volume delivered to the aorta. Diastolic left ventricular flow is the stroke volume delivered to the left ventricle from the left atrium. These two stroke volumes reflect the systolic and diastolic performance of the left ventricle, respectively. Both can be readily measured by Doppler echocardiography and are the subject of this chapter.

Doppler Echocardiography

Doppler echocardiography is a technique whereby ultrasound is beamed at moving blood elements at a known frequency. Echoes returning from the moving blood elements are at a different frequency because of the effect of the movement of the blood elements (the Doppler effect). This frequency change is proportional to the velocity of blood flow at the site being sampled. There are two types of devices

From Fletcher GF, (ed): *Cardiovascular Response to Exercise.* Mount Kisco, NY, Futura Publishing Company, Inc., © 1994.

for delivering ultrasound: continuous wave and pulsed wave. Continuous wave sends ultrasound almost continuously and is dominated by the fastest velocity it encounters. Because of its high sampling rate, it can resolve the rapid velocities encountered in the aorta caused by exercise. The disadvantage of this technique is that the location of the fastest velocity along the sound beam is not known.

The other technique, pulsed Doppler, samples at a specific location (the sample volume). This range-gating ability sacrifices sample frequency and, thus, limits the velocities that can be resolved. Pulsed Doppler cannot resolve the rapid aortic velocities encountered during exercise, but it is adequate for measuring mitral valve velocity, even during exercise. The sample volume can be placed in the mitral inflow stream to avoid contamination from the faster velocities in the left ventricular outflow tract. Thus, for exercise studies, continuous wave Doppler is used to assess systolic flow at the aortic valve, and pulsed wave Doppler is used to assess diastolic flow at the mitral valve.

Velocity data are not sufficient for measuring volume flow. The area through which the blood is moving also needs to be measured.[2] According to the simplified Bernoulli principle, volume flow equals the velocity multiplied by the area. When applied to heart flow, there is acceleration and deceleration of blood during the systolic and diastolic periods. Pulsatile cardiac flow must be averaged to obtain the mean stroke volume. Average velocity is estimated by measuring the velocity-time integral. The velocity-time integral is readily measured from the velocity signal recorded over time. The area must be measured from the two-dimensional echocardiographic image of the heart, which is used to guide the Doppler probe. For pulsed wave Doppler, the site at which blood velocity is sampled must be measured. For continuous wave Doppler, the presumed smallest area through which the sound beam is sampling blood flow is measured, since it is assumed that the most rapid velocities are encountered at the smallest area in the flow stream.

The major technical pitfall in measuring the velocity of blood flow by the Doppler technique is that the Doppler beam must be angled within 20° of the flow stream in order to ignore this angle in calculating the velocity. If the beam deviates by more than 20°, then the angle must be considered. Also, the greater the angle of the Doppler beam in relationship to the flow stream, the smaller the velocity signal encountered and the more difficulty there is in accurately measuring flow. The other limitation of this technique is the ability to measure the flow area accurately from the two-dimensional echocardiographic image. This is most accurate for the aortic valve, is done with some difficulty with the pulmonic valve, and is most difficult to measure at the mitral and tricuspid valves. Thus, if one is merely interested in cardiac output, then the most accurate measurement is obtained at the aortic valve site. However, other considerations such as valve regurgitation and shunts may dictate measuring cardiac output at a different cardiac site.

Systolic Left Ventricular Flow

Left ventricular systolic flow is measured at the aortic valve. Customarily, the continuous wave Doppler probe is placed in the suprasternal notch and the sound beamed toward the aortic valve until the highest velocities are observed. In individuals with a more horizontal heart position, the direction of the ascending aortic systolic jet may be more toward the right clavicle. Thus, the transducer should be moved to the right supraclavicular area or the right parasternal area in such individuals. It is important to record the fastest velocities obtainable because presumably these reflect the attainment of an ultrasound beam angle to the flow stream of less than 20°, thus permitting the actual angle to be ignored. Doppler velocity recordings are easily done at rest and during exercise, with little discomfort to the patient (Figure 1, top).

The appropriate flow area for the maximum velocity recorded is assumed to be the aortic valve, which usually is smaller than the left ventricular outflow tract or the ascending aorta. Aortic valve area can be measured from two-dimensional echocardiography by measuring its diameter during systole, or from an M-mode tracing of the aortic valve by measuring leaflet separation. The area is then calculated from standard formulas for the area of a circle. One source of error in this measurement is that the diameter of the aortic valve changes during systole. However, most of the change is early and late in systole, when the valve is opening and closing. During the majority of systole, the valve is wide open and its area changes little. For practical purposes, the rapid changes in area during opening and closing are ignored and the maximum area measured during early systole is used. The maximum systolic aortic valve area also may change during exercise as stroke volume increases. However,

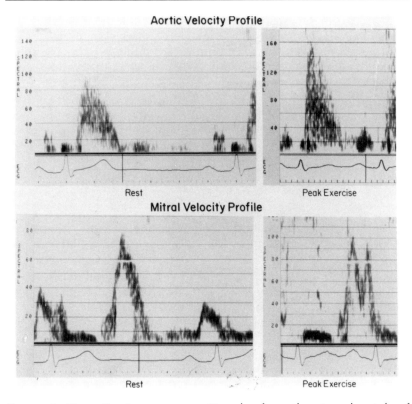

FIGURE 1. Top: *Continuous wave Doppler from the sternal notch of ascending aortic velocity at rest and at peak exercise. Note the doubling of peak aortic velocity. Velocity scale cm/sec, ECG at bottom.* **Bottom:** *Pulsed Doppler recording of mitral inflow velocity at the leaflet tips. Note the merger of the E and A velocities at peak exercise and the small increase in peak E velocity (25%).*

measurements of aortic valve area made during exercise have shown that this change in area during maximum exercise is negligible.[3] Thus, another simplification is to measure only the area at rest and assume that there is no significant change during exercise. This simplifies the exercise measurements required. In fact, if one is interested mainly in changes in stroke volume during exercise, one can assume that the aortic valve area is a constant and simply examine the velocity-time integral as a reflection of stroke volume.

Experimental studies at rest and during exercise have shown the accuracy of this approach for measuring stroke volume as compared with other accepted methods.[2-5] Stroke volume also can be measured by two-dimensional echocardiographic volume measurements at end systole and diastole (their difference is the stroke volume). Although volume measurements by two-dimensional echocardiography are quite accurate at rest, they are less so with exercise.[6] Also, the variability in left ventricular volume measurements is greater than that of Doppler velocity measurements. Thus, Doppler aortic velocity measurements are superior to echocardiographic left ventricular volume measurements for estimating stroke volume.

Studies in normal individuals have confirmed that stroke volume increases with exercise, especially during the early stages. Also, stroke volume is greater in the supine position than in the upright position. However, during upright exercise, the stroke volume increases more than during supine exercise, when it may increase very little.[7] Thus, the results of Doppler echocardiographic measurements of left ventricular systolic flow during exercise are comparable to those that have been obtained with other techniques. This simple technique is readily applied to patients and has the possibility of providing a great deal of physiological information concerning left ventricular systolic performance during exercise.

Left Ventricular Diastolic Flow

Left ventricular diastolic flow is measured at the mitral valve by pulsed Doppler echocardiography. The estimation of stroke volume at the mitral valve area during diastole is much more complex than measuring stroke volume during systole at the aortic area. First, the velocity profile in diastole is biphasic, with an early passive filling component and a late active filling component caused by atrial contraction. In general, the mitral valve orifice area parallels the flow velocity during diastole, with the exception of mid-diastole during slow heart rates when there is no velocity recordable by Doppler, but the mitral valve is wide open. Thus, techniques for estimating velocity area during diastole must be adjusted for this discrepancy.[8]

Second, the mitral valve orifice area changes during diastole with changes in flow. Also, the area changes more with exercise when stroke volume increases. In fact, mean mitral valve area increases during upright isotonic exercise by approximately 34%.[7]

Thus, mitral valve area cannot be considered a constant during exercise, nor can it be considered constantly related to flow during a single diastolic period since the mitral valve may be open when there is very little flow occurring.

Third, during the rapid heart rates encountered with exercise, the mitral valve early and late filling peaks merge, thus making the separation of these two components of the diastolic flow velocity signal difficult at heart rates greater than 110 beats per minute (Figure 1, bottom). Therefore, this technique may not be as accurate during periods of high heart rates during maximum exercise.

Another problem is that the incidence of mitral regurgitation increases progressively with age, such that many individuals in mid-life have some mild mitral regurgitation. Many elderly individuals have moderately severe mitral regurgitation, such that measurements of diastolic stroke volume in this area may be inaccurate because of the regurgitant flow in systole.[9] This is less of a problem at the aortic valve because aging does not result in any significant aortic regurgitation until over age 65 years. Also, in many patients it is not known whether mitral regurgitation occurs or worsens during exercise, especially in those with ischemic heart disease.

For the reasons mentioned above, the velocity-time integral from the Doppler recording is not a reliable index of stroke volume at the mitral valve area. In fact, studies during exercise in normal individuals have shown a decrease in the velocity-time integral during exercise, as the heart rate increases and shortens diastole.[7] Thus, the major reason for increased stroke volume at the mitral area during exercise is an increase in mitral valve area rather than a change in average velocity over diastole. The difficulty with determinations of diastolic mitral valve orifice area complicates the use of mitral Doppler recordings to measure flow during exercise. However, stroke volume can be estimated relatively accurately at the mitral valve if these factors are considered.[10] However, values at the mitral valve probably are less accurate than those recorded at the aortic valve.

Conclusions

Doppler echocardiography provides a simple method to assess left ventricular systolic flow at rest and during exercise. This technique also can provide volume flow information during diastole, but less accurately because of the complexities of diastolic left ventricular inflow. To the extent that volume flow measurements are valuable, Doppler echocardiography provides a simple method to provide this information at rest and during exercise. Finally, it must be kept in mind that since the stroke volume of the right and left ventricles are the same on the average during the respiratory cycle, if there are difficulties in measuring stroke volume at the aortic and mitral valve areas the pulmonary and tricuspid valve areas can be used. These are especially valuable when there are problems with valvular regurgitation or shunts that render stroke volume measurements on the left side of the heart inaccurate. However, area measurements of the pulmonary artery and tricuspid orifice area are more difficult than the corresponding measures in the left side of the heart. Thus, it is generally believed that stroke volume measurements from the right side of the heart are less accurate than those derived from the left side of the heart.

References

1. Donald KW, Bishop JM, Cumming G, Wade OL: The effect of exercise on the cardiac output and circulatory dynamics of normal subjects. *Clin Sci* 1955;14:37–73
2. Huntsman LL, Steward DK, Barnes SR, Franklin SB, Colocousis JS, Hessel EA: Noninvasive doppler determination of cardiac output in man. *Circulation* 1983;67:593–602
3. Ihlen H, Amlie JP, Dale J, Forfang K, Nitter-Hauge S, Oherstad JE, Simonson S, Myhre E: Determination of cardiac output by doppler echocardiography. *Br Heart J* 1984;51:54–60
4. Ihlen H, Myhre E, Amlie JP, Forfang K, Larson S: Changes in left ventricular stroke volume measured by doppler echocardiography. *Br Heart J* 1985;54:378–383
5. Daley PJ, Sagar KB, Wann LS: Doppler echocardiographic measurement of flow velocity in the ascending aorta during supine and upright exercise. *Br Heart J* 1985;54:562–567
6. Crawford MH, Petru MA, Rabinowitz C: Effect of isotonic exercise training on left ventricular volume during upright exercise. *Circulation* 1985;72:1237–1243
7. Rassi, A Jr., Crawford MH, Richards KL, Miller JF: Differing mechanisms of exercise flow augmentation at the mitral and aortic valves. *Circulation* 1988;77:543–551
8. Miller WE, Richards KL, Crawford MH: Accuracy of mitral doppler echocardiographic cardiac output determinations in adults. *Am Heart J* 1990;119:905–910

9. Zhang Y, Nitter-Hauge S, Ihlen H, Myhre E: Doppler echocardiographic measurement of cardiac output using the mitral orifice method. *Br Heart J* 1985;53:130–136

10. Lewis JF, Kuo LC, Nelson JG, Limacher MC, Quinones MA: Pulsed doppler echocardiographic determination of stroke volume and cardiac output: clinical validation of two new methods using the apical window. *Circulation* 1984;70:425–431

Part 2

Genetic, Biochemical, and Physiological Responses of the Heart to Factors Related to Long-Term Exercise

Chapter 5

Peptide Growth Factors as Determinants of Myocardial Development and Hypertrophy

Thomas Brand, PhD and Michael D. Schneider, MD

Insight into the fundamental mechanisms that control the growth and development of cardiac muscle cells is a prerequisite to manipulating the cardiac phenotype in order to achieve a therapeutic benefit. This clinical imperative is obvious in the context of cardiac myocytes' virtual complete loss of potential for proliferative growth[1] and corresponding meager capacity to regenerate after infarction. However, the potential for growth by cell enlargement remains intact in adult ventricular myocardium, and hypertrophy provoked by mechanical load is a hallmark of hypertension, valvular heart disease, and congenital anomalies. A primary role for mechanical forces is clinically self-evident from entities like aortic and pulmonic stenosis, although in some coarctation and renovascular models of hypertension it may be harder to discriminate between the role of load per se and associated trophic substances, notably angiotensin. Increasingly, it is recognized that myocardial hypertrophy entails not only the quantitative growth response, but also more particular, specific perturbations in the expression of many constituents of the cardiac cell.[2–4] The prototypes for this plasticity of gene expression are transitions among isoforms for two indispensable components of the sarcomere, myosin and actin, with selective up-regulation, at least in small mammals, of developmentally regulated varieties that ordinarily are abundant in embryonic but not adult heart—β-myosin heavy chain (βMHC),[5] skeletal muscle α-

From Fletcher GF, (ed): *Cardiovascular Response to Exercise.* Mount Kisco, NY, Futura Publishing Company, Inc., © 1994.

actin,[6] and vascular smooth muscle α-actin.[7] The notion that hypertrophy recapitulates ontogeny, that is, a program of gene regulation that resembles the fetal myocardium in key respects also gains support from reciprocal changes observed in two genes whose expression is more clearly abnormal during end-stage heart failure in humans—induction of atrial natriuretic factor (ANF)[8,9] and partial suppression of the cardiac sarcoplasmic reticulum calcium adenosine triphosphatase (Ca^{2+}ATPase).[10,11]

Four questions are prompted by this complexly orchestrated response to load (Figure 1):

What is the sensor for mechanical stress? Postulated initiating signals include load-sensing cytoskeletal elements or, alternatively, mechanosensitive ion channels[12] and forms of adenylate cyclase[13] that are activated by membrane tension. Passive stretch suffices to induce not only growth but also expression of hypertrophy-related genes like βMHC, ANF, and skeletal α-actin.[14–16] Both ion channels[12,17] and calcium transients[18] activated by stretch have been detected in cardiac cells, yet it remains ambiguous whether such ion movements are either necessary or sufficient to trigger the cascade of responses associated with pressure overload.

What transduction mechanisms couple hemodynamic forces to altered cardiac gene transcription? Candidate second messengers include cyclic adenosine monophosphate (cAMP)[19] and intracellular calcium,[20] which increase in isolated hearts with elevated perfusion pressure. Activation of protein kinase C (PKC) accompanies pressure-overload hypertrophy in vivo,[21] can be provoked by passive stretch of cardiac muscle[22] or isolated cardiac myocytes[14] and, importantly, suffices to trigger multiple aspects of the hypertrophic phenotype.[23–25]

How extensive or generalized is the set of cardiac genes that are modulated during cardiac hypertrophy or failure? Newly recognized members of this ensemble include the renin-angiotensin system intrinsic to myocardium (angiotensinogen,[26] angiotensin-converting enzyme[27]) and additional components of the machinery for calcium homeostasis (phospholamban,[10] calsequestrin,[28] and the SR calcium release channel[29–31]). Immediately early induction of nuclear proto-oncogenes—c-*myc*, c-*fos*, c-*jun*, and *jun B*[7,32–35]—along with other transcription factors like Egr-1[36] furnishes a potential hierarchical mechanism for mechanical signals to govern this vast and complex series of cardiac-restricted genes. Crude extracts of hypertrophied myocardium promote protein synthesis in recipient hearts,[37] and plasticity of gene expression after pressure

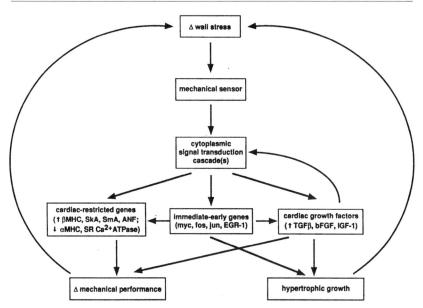

FIGURE 1. *A model of regulatory circuits postulated to mediate cardiac hypertrophy triggered by load. Mechanical stress activates cytoplasmic "second messengers" and immediate-early nuclear proteins ("third messengers") remarkably similar to those evoked by polypeptide growth factors. Altered expression of actin, myosin, ANF, and other cardiac genes after load is thought, at least in part, to depend on these immediate-early transcription factors. One component of cardiac hypertrophy in vivo is up-regulation of growth factors including TGFβ and basic FGF, which themselves induce the fetal or hypertrophic phenotype in vitro. Hypertrophic growth, by increasing wall thickness, restores wall stress toward normal. Plasticity of cardiac-restricted proteins and more direct effects of growth factors on contractility per se may impair or improve cardiac function and thus, as a net effect, either increase or reduce wall stress in the ventricle.*

overload now is known to encompass specific peptide growth factors, including basic fibroblast growth factor (FGF)[38] and type β1 transforming growth factor (TGFβ1).[39]

As *a matter of teleology, does this spectrum of gene repression and induction comprise an invariably homeostatic response, as might be extrapolated from the favorable economy of contractile work resulting from the shift from α to βMHC?*[40] Comparable functional benefit has not been proven in the case of α-actin isoform transitions; even though it is tenable that certain functional differences might elude purely biochemical methods (myosin ATPase activity, in vitro motility assays), skepticism also is urged by the seemingly normal hearts of BALB/c mice, which harbor a spontaneous mutation of the cardiac α-actin gene and thus overexpress skeletal α-actin in the heart,[41] as seen with pressure overload. Still other responses have been viewed as likely contributors to eventual ventricular *dys*function, notably the partial loss of calcium sequestering capacity.[10,11,42,43]

These divergent or frankly antagonist effects on ventricular performance have suggested a revisionist hypothesis that genes coordinately regulated by load (and even by passive stretch in culture) might share hierarchical regulatory pathways in common. Interest in the isolation, localization, and action of myocardial growth factors has been spurred by pathophysiological observations such as these, by developmental studies pointing to a remarkably intricate temporal and spatial program of growth factor expression in the primitive heart, and, increasingly, by functional evidence that peptide growth factors might govern cardiac organogenesis and differentiated gene transcription. Peptide growth factors identified in cardiac muscle include multiple members of the FGF and TGFβ gene families, insulin-like growth factors, and proteins that are less completely characterized, like myotrophin[44] and non–myocyte-derived growth factor.[45] In this chapter we examine the strengths and limitations of current knowledge concerning growth factor expression in myocardium, developmental regulation of cardiac growth factors, involvement of peptide growth factors in pressure-overload hypertrophy and other disorders of the adult heart, growth factor receptors in myocardium, mechanisms of growth factor signal transduction and their relation to mechanical load, and role of growth factors as determinants of cardiac differentiation.

Growth Factors and Their Receptors Expressed in Myocardium

Fibroblast Growth Factors

Heparin-binding growth factors have been isolated from the cardiac muscle of many species, including man, as well as from isolated cardiac myocytes of neonatal and adult rats.[46–52] One component of this mitogenic activity was proven to be basic FGF, which was localized by immunocytochemistry to multiple cell types in the myocardium, including cardiac myocytes themselves.[47,49] In each species, the abundance of basic FGF was three-to four-fold higher in the atria than in the ventricles, raising speculation that this might relate to inherent differences in the growth capacity of atrial and ventricular cells.[47] Acidic FGF also contributes to the heparin-binding fraction and is as abundant in adult myocardium (500 μg/kg) as in brain.[46,48] Acidic FGF accumulates in cardiac myocytes' extracellular matrix,[50] but also has been found by immunohisto-chemistry in cultured neonatal myocytes[48] and isolated adult ventricular muscle cells.[52] Among other characterized members of the FGF multigene family—FGF-3 (int-2), FGF-4 (hst/KS3), FGF-5, FGF-6, and FGF-7 (KGF)[53]—only FGF-6 is known to be expressed in the heart.[54] Acidic and basic FGF appear to share a similar intracellular distribution in rat cardiac myocytes and were localized to the cell membrane, myofibrillar Z-lines, and nuclei[52]; basic FGF also has been observed in association with cardiac gap junctions.[55] Although nuclear localization has been shown to occur with certain other growth factors and cytokines as well, additional proof is required to establish the physiological significance of these putative intracellular or "intracrine" pathways[56] (see ref. 57). It is nonetheless interesting that during mesoderm formation early in embryogenesis, nuclear localization of FGFs is associated with the cells that are competent to be induced to enter the skeletal muscle pathway.[58]

At least four genes encode high-affinity FGF receptors: FGFR1 (flg), -2(bek/K-sam), -3(cek2), and -4.[59] FGF receptors typically comprise a transmembrane protein with either two or three immunoglobulin-like extracellular domains, a membrane-spanning region, and a cytoplasmic tyrosine kinase, interrupted by a characteristic hydrophilic insert. Additional diversity of FGF receptors is generated by alternative ribonucleic acid (RNA) splicing, producing receptor forms that differ in the number of extracellular immunoglobulin-like domains, differ within the third immunoglobulin-like domain, or lack the transmembrane domain and are thought to be secreted. FGF receptor transcripts differ both in their patterns of expression throughout development and in their tissue distribution in adults, pointing toward functional differences. Indeed, various alternatively spliced forms of FGFR1 have equivalent affinity for acidic and basic FGF (FGFR1-IIIc), higher affinity for bFGF (FGFR1-IIIb), or higher affinity for acidic FGF (FGFR1-IIIa).[60–62] Using sensitive RNAse protection assays, two splice forms of FGFR1, having two and three immunoglobulin-like domains, have been detected in adult mouse heart.[63] FGFR1 binding sites and mRNA are almost undetectable in isolated adult rat cardiac myocytes, yet the gene and protein are up-regulated when ventricular cells are cultured in fetal bovine serum, in concert with increases of basic and acidic FGF.[52] This demonstrates that the down-regulation of FGFR expression in "terminally differentiated" adult ventricular cells is not irreversible.

Insulin-like Growth Factors

Insulin-like growth factor–I (IGF-I), IGF-II, and insulin comprise a family of peptides with both metabolic and mitogenic activity. Unlike insulin itself, however, IGF-I and -II have been isolated from a broad array of organs including cardiac, skeletal, and smooth muscle, suggesting that they might function in local paracrine or autocrine pathways.[64,65] Neonatal rat myocardium contains transcripts for both IGF-I and -II, which have been localized to cardiac myocytes by in situ hybridization.[66] In adult rat heart IGF-I mRNA is low, whereas IGF-II transcript abundance is relatively high.[64]

In contrast to the structure of FGF receptors, the insulin and IGF-I receptor each are heterotetramers, made of two extracellular α-subunits for ligand binding, each linked by a disulfide bridge to a membrane-spanning β-subunit, whose cytoplasmic domain possesses the tyrosine kinase activity.[67] The extracellular domains are marked by cysteine-rich sequences, rather than the immunoglobulin-like repeats characteristic of FGF (and PDGF) receptors. The IGF-I receptor binds IGF-I itself with highest affinity, but can also mediate the biological effects of both IGF-II and insulin, whereas the IGF-II receptor is identical to the cation-independent mannose-6-phosphate receptor and plays no known role in growth factor signal transduction.[68] IGF-I and -II receptors have been demonstrated in neonatal[66] and adult[69] rat heart by receptor cross-linking. Positive inotropic effects of IGF-I and -II have been shown in cultured fetal rat myocytes,[70] and, in adult rat cardiac myocytes,

IGF-I and -II cause phosphoinositol hydrolysis,[69] establishing that the receptors indeed are functional.

Epidermal Growth Factor

Similar physiological actions have been shown for epidermal growth factor (EGF), which stimulates contractility in both cultured myocytes and isolated perfused hearts.[71,72] EGF receptors, like FGF receptors, comprise a single polypeptide chain but differ in structural characteristics: the extracellular domain contains two cysteine-rich repeats rather than immunoglobulin-like sequences, and the tyrosine kinase domain lacks interruption by the hydrophilic inserts seen with receptors for FGF and for PDGF.[67] EGF receptors have been demonstrated to be present in cardiac myocytes by cross-linking.[73] Notwithstanding their canonical role in signal transduction via tyrosine kinase, EGF receptors in the heart are coupled via $G_{s\alpha}$ to adenylate cyclase: consequently, EGF leads to increased cAMP accumulation in cardiac muscle cells.[74] Like the vasoconstrictor and vasodilator activities reported for PDGF[75] and FGF,[76] or the ability of nominal vasoconstictors like endothelin[77] and angiotensin II,[78,79] that evoke aspects of myocardial hypertrophy, the chronotropic and inotropic effects of EGF and IGFs are memorable illustrations that peptide "growth" factors are truly multifunctional.

The Type β Transforming Growth Factor Superfamily

TGFβ1 is the prototype for a complex group of regulators of cell growth, morphogenesis, and differentiation. TGFβ1 was discovered as a sarcoma-derived protein causing anchorage-independent growth in fibroblasts, which soon was found to function in many systems, instead, as a growth inhibitor.[80,81] Like acidic and basic FGF, TGFβ is remarkably abundant in myocardium, relative to other organs.[82] Several closely related TGFβ isoforms exist with 60–80% identity among the mature, processed peptides, in addition to more distantly related family members:[80,83] activins and inhibins, bone morphogenic proteins (BMP), Müllerian inhibiting substance, the

Drosophila decaplentagenic gene product, Vg1, a maternal RNA localized to the vegetal pole of *Xenopus* oocytes, Vgr-1, and GDF-1 (growth/differentiation factor-1).

The normal adult rat ventricle contains a 2.4-kb TGFβ1 transcript, and TGFβ1 protein is found in the cardiac myocytes themselves and in the specialized conduction tissue.[84–86] TGFβ2 mRNA is expressed in virtually all tissues in the neonatal and adult mouse including the heart, at rather low abundance compared with placenta, submaxillary gland, and lung.[87] TGFβ5 mRNA, not expressed by avains or mammals, is highly abundant in the adult *Xenopus* heart.[88] Two of the more distantly related TGFβ-like transcripts also are expressed in adult rat myocardium: the inhibin α-subunit, in both atria and ventricles, and activin A (inhibin βA), in the atria alone.[89]

TGFβ1 has been localized to the mitochondria of rat and mouse cardiac muscle, by immunoelectron microscopy and cell fractionation,[90] consistent with the role in cardiac metabolism postulated from evidence that TGFβ1 can protect myocardium after ischemic injury.[91]

Covalent labeling of TGFβ receptors in a variety of cells has implicated as many as nine distinct proteins that bind TGFβ, with three principal products visualized by this technique in most cell types.[92] Analysis of the forms absent or present in variant cell lines that are insensitive to TGFβ led to the conclusion that only TGFβ receptor types I and II (TβR-I, II) mediate TGFβ signal transduction,[93] a prediction confirmed with the cloning of TβR-II and -III. The gene for TβR-III encodes the protein core of a proteoglycan, betaglycan, with no known signaling function.[94,95] Interestingly, TGFβ is recognized by this protein core, whereas basic FGF also can bind to betaglycan, via its heparan sulfate side chains[96] (FGF binding has an absolute requirement for heparan sulfate proteoglycans[97]). In contrast, TβR-II is a novel transmembrane serine/theonine kinase,[98] as are receptors for the TGFβ-like peptide, activin,[99,100] distinct from all the more familiar growth factor receptors, with protein tyrosine kinase activity. The molecular structure of TβR-I is unknown but is expected to resemble that of TβR-II. By receptor cross-linking, all three receptors—TβR-I, TβR-II, and TβR-III—have been shown to coexist in neonatal cardiac myocytes and bind all three mammalian TGFβ isoforms equivalently.[101]

Growth Factors in Cardiac Organogenesis

Growth Factors Govern Mesoderm Formation

Peptide growth factors have been implicated as important factors as determinants of cell fate and organization of the body plan.[102] Members of the FGF, TGFβ/activin, and Wnt gene families each can induce the formation of dorsal mesoderm (skeletal muscle) in the presumptive ectoderm or animal cap of primitive *Xenopus* embryos and, of equal importance, have also been detected in the embryo at the time of gastrulation. In contrast, BMP-4 induces mesoderm with ventral or posterior characteristics and overrides the effect of activin A.[103] However, neither the provocative results in explant models nor expression in a suggestive spatial and temporal pattern[104] necessarily points to the function of a peptide during development in vivo. One approach for which important initial success has been achieved in the context of skeletal muscle determination, and that points to a means to identify molecular events crucial for the onset of the cardiac lineage, is the use of dominant-suppressor mutations to extinguish the function of potential inducers and regulators in the intact embryo. Mesoderm formation is prevented in *Xenopus* embryos by forced expression of a truncated, kinase-deficient mutant of the FGF[105] or activin[106] receptor, confirming that the action of one or more endogenous members of the FGF and activin families indeed is indispensable for induction of skeletal muscle to occur.

FGFs and FGF Receptors During Cardiac Development

The remarkable abundance of several growth factors in the primitive heart—notably, basic FGF (bFGF) and TGFβ1—makes it plausible that they might play an important role in cardiac organogenesis. During avian development, bFGF is found as punctate cytoplasmic aggregates at the time the heart tube fuses (stage 9–10).[107] At stage 12 (48 hours), intense staining for basic FGF is seen only in myocytes of the developing heart. Basic FGF down-regulates in at least a portion of the myocardium between days 5 and 15 of development: immunoreactive basic FGF is diminished in subendocardial, trabeculated myocardium yet persists in the atria and subepicardial muscle.[108] In rat cardiac myocytes, acidic and basic FGF were both persistently expressed, at 11 to 20 days of development and for at least 1 month after birth.[51] Down-regulation of acidic and basic FGF by immunocytochemistry was marked in vascular smooth muscle including coronary arteries, in contrast to myocardium itself.

Expression of FGFR-1 RNA is relatively generalized throughout cardiac development in the mouse[109] and the rat,[110] detected at moderate levels in the endocardial cushions and at lower levels in the myocardium itself. FGFR-2, in contrast, is expressed exclusively in the embryonic cushions and overlying endothelium at days 9 to 12 of gestation. At embryonic day 16.5, FGFR-2 is detected within the heart only in the developing cardiac skeleton and in the atrioventricular and semilunar valves.[109.] This precise program of differential expression suggests that FGFR-1 and -2 mediate different functions of FGFs during cardiac ontogeny. In agreement with the down-regulation of FGFR RNA and protein during skeletal muscle differentiation,[111] FGF receptor sites likewise decrease during cardiac development.[112] Given the importance of alternative mRNA splicing to the functional differences among FGF receptors, a shortcoming of present knowledge is ignorance of the precise forms of FGF receptor within cardiac muscle and other components of the developing heart. Second, it is conjectural whether loss of FGF receptor is a cause or a consequence of cardiac differentiation and the attendant loss of growth capacity.

A Complex Temporal and Spatial Program of TGFβ Expression

Cardiac mesoderm comprises the first cells of the mouse embryo to contain TGFβ1 mRNA during development, at 7 days postconception, a stage when no other embryonic cell type expresses detectable TGFβ1.[113] At day 8, with the formation of recognizable endocardial and epimyocardial cell layers, TGFβ1 mRNA is highly expressed in endocardial cells but not myocardium. By day 9, endocardial expression itself becomes restricted, confined to endothelial cells of the outflow tract and atrioventricular canal,[113] sites involved in epithelial-mesenchymal transformation. TGFβ1 mRNA continues at high levels in cardiac valves even when valvular morphogenesis is complete (day 15.5 to birth), but is not detected by in situ hybridization at later stages (postnatal day 8 and the adult heart).[113] Contrasting with this restricted distribution of TGFβ1 RNA in embryonic heart, TGFβ1 protein is found throughout atrial and ventricular myocardium using an antibody, LC(1–30), that detects its intracellular form.[85,114] Indeed, after 9 days of development, intracellular TGFβ1 is essentially limited to myocardium and a few cranial mesenchymal cells.[115] Secreted, extracellular forms of TGFβ1 peptide, however, are found in the endocardium and cardiac jelly at days 9 to 10.5 postconception and become concentrated in the developing valves.[115] Both biological and technical explanations have been cited to help account for the apparent discrepancy of mRNA and peptide localization: translational control, relative thresholds for detection, masking of TGFβ epitopes by TGFβ-binding proteins, and disparities in the selectivity of reagents for TGFβ isoforms. Akhurst and coworkers, in attempting to interpret this complex pattern of expression, have postulated that TGFβ1 is synthesized in differentiating epithelia and acts as a paracrine morphogen for adjacent mesenchymal cells.[113]

TGFβ2 mRNA also is very restricted in the heart, abundant in prevalvular myocardium and mesenchyme of atrioventricular (AV) cushion and in myocardium of the outflow tract at days 9.5 to 10.5 postconception, but not in atrial or ventricular myocardium.[116] Expression of TGFβ2 RNA is sustained in the cardiac valves.[116] Immunoreactive TGFβ2 is widely distributed in the mouse embryo, including all regions of the heart at 8.5 to 9.5 days postconception, but is no longer detected after day 10.5 postconception.[115] TGFβ3 mRNA is even more restricted than TGFβ1 or TGFβ2, found at days 11.5 to 16.5 postconception only in mesenchyme of the cardiac valves.[116] Intracellular TGFβ3 protein was detected in the myocardium at day 9 postconception, whereas extracellular TGFβ3 was localized to pericardium.[115]

The predominant TGFβ transcripts in avian myocardium are TGFβ2 and TGFβ3, rather than the high levels of TGFβ1 observed in mammalian tissues including heart.[117] Contrasting with its expression in the mouse, where it is restricted to the AV canal, TGFβ2 is evenly distributed throughout avian myocardium.[117,118] However, TGFβ3 RNA is especially concentrated in the avian AV canal,[118] concurring with evidence, discussed subsequently, for the uniquely important role of TGFβ3 in valve formation.

IGFs and Their Receptors in the Developing Heart

During early mouse enbryogenesis, IFG-II gene expression first is detected in lateral mesoderm, where cardiac progenitor cells arise,[119] and is found at relatively high abundance throughout the rat heart at embryonic day 14. IGF-II[119] and the IGF-II/mannose-6-phosphate receptor[120] are highly expressed in the mammalian heart during development but not in the adult. Indeed, among embryonic rat tissues, IGF-II receptor RNA is most abundant in cardiac muscle.[120]

The pattern of IGF-I gene expression during cardiac organogenesis is more complex. In the rat heart at 14 days postconception, IGF-I mRNA is confined to an annular rim of undifferentiated atrial myocytes and is absent from more mature atrial myocytes and from ventricular myocardium, within the limits of in situ hybridization.[121] In view of the association of IGF-I RNA with sympathetic ganglia and regions of nerve outgrowth, the alternative possibility has been raised that IGF-I–expressing cells in the atria are specialized cells related to sympathetic innervation. IGF-I also is particularly abundant in mesenchymal cells or fibroblasts contributing to the truncus arteriosus, endocardial cushion, and incipient cardiac valves.[121] The low abundance of IGF-I receptor mRNA in heart at this stage contrasts with its widespread expression in the developing nervous system and skeletal muscle.[121]

Induction and Repression of Cardiac Myogenesis by Defined Growth Factors

Cardiac progenitor cells arise not in dorsal mesoderm like the skeletal muscle myotomes but rather, in common with smooth muscle and hematopoietic cells, in mesoderm of the lateral plate.[122] Extirpation of pharyngeal endoderm adjacent to cardiac progenitor cells prevents cardiac muscle formation in *Xenopus* embryos,[123,124] suggesting an important role for a signal from pharyngeal endoderm for the onset of cardiac muscle development. Likewise, dorsal mesoderm–inducing factor (activin A) inhibits heart formation when injected into the lateral plate of *Xenopus* embryos at the blastula stage.[125] At least two defined growth factors promote cardiac differentiation, that is, the appearance of beating muscle, in hanging drop cultures of presumptive cardiac mesoderm from neurulae of the axolotl—TGFβ1 and PDGF.[126] Contrasting with its ability to evoke skeletal myogenesis, basic FGF suppresses heart formation induced by TGFβ1, at least in this preparation.[126] These results highlight the important principle that peptide growth factors are both antagonists and agonists for differentiation, even in a single cell type, and their action cannot merely be inferred from the time and location of their expression.

The present evidence that positive- and negative-acting diffusible factors might impact on cardiac myogenesis in mammals as well comes from a murine embryonal carcinoma cell line, P19, which can be induced to form spontaneously beating cardiac muscle-like cells in the presence of medium conditioned by endoderm;[127] conversely, cardiac muscle formation, in this system as in *Xenopus*, is blocked by activin A.[128] Embryoid bodies derived from murine embryonal stem cells (ES cells) also form cardiac muscle cells,[129] expressing cardiac-specific genes including α- and β-MHC,[130,131] and tropomyosin,[132] providing a model with reasonable fidelity to in vivo development, with which to unravel the factors involved in heart formation in mammals. Embryonal stem cells are amenable to differentiation along a cardiac pathway in vitro, but also can be exploited for "knock-out" mutations or gene replacement by homologous recombination. Beyond the immediate importance of ES cells for in vitro differentiation, a more far-ranging use of these pluripotent cells is the construction of novel strains of mice in which cardiac growth and development are abnormal. Genetic manipulation of intact mammals offers the greatest opportunity to surmount the limitations of cell culture—real and potential anomalies concerning innervation, hormones, local interactions, and load—and to obviate the known (and unknown) disparities inherent in simpler vertebrate models.[133]

TGFβ is Required for Cardiac Valve Formation

Valve formation is initiated in the embryonic heart by an epithelial→mesenchymal transformation of endothelial cells of the endocardial cushion and requires factors produced locally and deposited in extracellular matrix.[134] In view of their precise localization to endocardium, prevalvular myocardium, and mesenchyme of the atrioventricular canal and ventricular outflow tract, members of the TGFβ superfamily have been especially intriguing as candidates for this inductive interaction. Importantly, antibodies directed against TGFβ can block the epithelial → mesenchymal transformation in avian explants, with the caveat that the antisera did not distinguish among the multiple forms of TGFβ that would be present.[134] To obviate this concern, the same investigators subsequently used oligodeoxynucleotides complementary to nonconserved regions of TGFβ1 through TGFβ4. Antisense oligonucleotides to TGFβ3 inhibited epithelial→mesenchymal transformation whereas oligonucleotides against TGFβ1, -2, or -4 were ineffective.[135] A developmentally regulated antisense mRNA, complementary to the TGFβ3 message, also has been detected in embryonic chick heart: the antisense transcript for TGFβ3 accumulates at the time myocardium of the AV canal loses the capacity to induce epithelial → mesenchymal transformation, inviting speculation that this molecule might be an endogenous regulator of TGFβ3 biosynthesis.[118] Aspects of the intracellular signaling cascade for this morphogenic event have begun to become clear. Activation of PKC induces epithelial → mesenchymal transformation; inhibitors of PKC, tyrosine kinase inhibitors, and pertussis toxin inhibit cellular transformation; myocardial-conditioned medium causes free intracellular Ca^{2+} to rise. Together, these findings suggest that this inductive interaction required for valve formation is mediated by a pertussis toxin–sensitive G protein, Ca^{2+} transients, and several protein kinase activities.[136]

Myocardial Growth Factors During Ischemia and Hypertrophy

Given the basal expression of peptide growth factors even in normal adult myocardium, their accumulation in the extracellular matrix, and evidence for increased trophic activity in crude extracts of hypertrophied heart,[37] the proposal that autocrine and paracrine mechanisms might amplify and modulate the signal initiated by load is plausible. However, the validity of an autocrine or paracrine model of pressure-overload cardiac hypertrophy ultimately requires proof that specific growth factors increase in abundance or availability after a hemodynamic load (or, as a formal possibility, that cells' responsiveness increases), in tandem with confirmation that the growth factors found can produce, in recipient cardiac cells, responses characteristic of hypertrophy in vivo.

Direct experimental evidence for increased expression of growth factors in the hypertrophied or ischemic heart is now available. Aortic coarctation produces a two- to threefold rise in TGFβ mRNA in myocardium.[39,137] Left ventricular expression of IGF-I likewise increases, during cardiac hypertrophy in a myriad of hemodynamic, genetic, and pharmacological models: suprarenal aortic banding,[138] uninephrectomy plus deoxycorticosterone and salt,[138] the spontaneously hypertensive rat,[138] renal artery stenosis,[139] and growth hormone administration.[140] Immunoreactive basic FGF in ventricular myocytes increases up to 80% in spontaneously hypertensive rats and by 70% in aortic coarctation.[38] Such findings concur with previous demonstrations, in skeletal muscle, that growth factors (IGFs and FGF) are induced by work[141] or by electrical stimulation to increase muscle activity.[142] Hypoxia, by itself, is one trigger for up-regulation of FGF gene and protein expression in cultured cardiac muscle cells.[143] Hypothyroidism[144] and isoproterenol-induced cardiac necrosis* are associated not only with increased content of basic FGF, but also with a shift to production of higher molecular weight forms of FGF, whose functional significance is examined below.

In addition to the characterized growth factors already discussed, an apparently novel peptide, designated "myotrophin," has been purified from hypertrophied hearts of spontaneously hypertensive rats and from cardiomyopathic human hearts, using a bioassay for protein synthesis by neonatal or adult cultured cardiac cells.[44] Under the conditions used, homogenates of normal rat and human heart fail to stimulate protein synthesis, leading to the interpretation that myotrophin might be up-regulated or otherwise activated in the course of hypertrophy and failure.[44]

Growth factor induction also is common to acute and chronic ischemia. In myocardium surviving ligation of a coronary artery, TGFβ is up-regulated more than sixfold[84,145] and is especially marked at the margin of the infarct.[84] In addition to up-regulation of

---

[a]E. Kardami, personal communication.

the normal 2.4-kb mRNA, infarcted areas express a 1.9-kb transcript that lacks a translational inhibitory element present in the longer RNA.[145] Implantation of ameroid constrictors around a coronary artery induces the expression of acidic FGF and TGFβ in the area of increased collateral vessel formation.[86,146] IGF-II expression likewise is induced in pig heart by this model of progressive stenosis or by microemboli.[147]

These investigations confirm the hypothesis that peptide growth factors are induced in myocardial tissue under physiological stress, like aortic coarction, ischemia, and infarction. The fact that PKC markedly up-regulates bFGF[148] and TGFβ1,[149] at least in fibroblastic cells, together with evidence discussed elsewhere for activation of PKC in cardiac myocytes by passive stretch, suggests the likelihood that a comparable mechanism might couple mechanical load to eventual production of autocrine and paracrine factors. The role of PKC in this connection raises a more general question: what intracellular circuitry links growth factor receptors to a program of growth and altered gene expression, and how do these signaling events relate to those that mediate growth produced by mechanical forces?

Induction of "Fetal" Cardiac Genes by FGFs or TGFβ1 Confirms a Prediction of Autocrine and Paracrine Models of Pressure-overload Hypertrophy

DNA Snythesis

Initial evidence for the possibility that cardiac muscle cells might be targets for the action of growth factors was the loss of differentiated properties of neonatal and adult myocytes in media containing fetal calf serum (reviewed in ref. 150), the cells' progression through increasingly differentiated states under mitogen-free conditions,[150] and the production of hypertrophy[151] or hyperplasia[150] by serum factors unrelated to thyroid hormone or adrenergic agonists. Acidic FGF is sufficient to trigger efficient proliferative growth by neonatal cardiac myocytes even in serum-free conditions, whereas FGF induces relatively little proliferative growth of cardiac muscle cells.[57,152]

Basic FGF can, however, cooperate with other serum factors to augment thymidine incorporation by neonatal ventricular cells.[47] A growth inhibitor for many cell types, TGFβ suppresses both basal and FGF-stimulated DNA synthesis in cultured cardiac muscle cells.[47]

Adult ventricular myocytes, notably, also are susceptible to exogenous growth factors, at least after prolonged culture in the presence of serum: IGF-I, FGF, and EGF each stimulate thymidine incorporation by adult cells.[153] However, as stated above, adult cardiac muscle cells can differentiate in vitro,[154] resulting in up-regulation of FGF receptor RNA and protein.[52] Whether adult ventricular myocytes inherently can respond to a growth factor or, instead, reacquire a response only after long-term culture warrants more systematic study.

Differentiated Gene Expression

FGFs and TGFβ1 have been the focus of investigations to determine the impact of growth factors on myocardial gene transcription.[57,152,155] The earlier phase of these experiments preceded much of the work cited above, detailing the expression of specific growth factors in normal myocardium, development, and disease. The impetus, instead, was persuasive evidence for the ability of these growth factors to prevent expression of essentially all muscle-specific proteins in committed myoblasts, even under conditions that do not provoke mitotic growth, and to reverse or extinguish muscle-specific gene expression in myocytes under conditions where terminal, irreversible differentiation had not occurred.[156] A strikingly distinct outcome resulted from growth factor stimulation of neonatal cardiac muscle cells, which coexpress the embryonic and adult isoforms of both α-actin and MHC. TGFβ1 and bFGF evoked a continuum of responses specifically resembling the program produced by mechanical load: induction of all four "fetal" cardiac genes tested (smooth muscle α-actin, skeletal α-actin, βMHC, and ANF), concomitant with down-regulation of αMHC and the SR Ca^{2+}ATPase.[152,155] Cardiac troponin I was likewise inhibited by TGFβ1.[157] Acidic FGF and bFGF shared comparable effects on five genes (induction of smooth muscle α-actin, βMHC, and ANF; inhibition of αMHC and the SR Ca^{2+}ATPase), yet acidic FGF suppresses both striated α-actin genes and skeletal and cardiac α-actin.[152,155] Notably, these experiments established for the first time that a single ligand could regulate as many as seven cardiac-restricted genes, highlighting interest not only in the likely importance of myocardial growth factors but also in the hierarchical mechanism enabling a single signal to modulate coordinately so many aspects of the cardiac phenotype.

To establish the molecular basis for growth factor control of the skeletal and cardiac α-actin genes, the transcription of exogenous skeletal and cardiac α-actin promoters first was analyzed, upon transfer into recipient cardiac cells (transfection). Greatly expediting the subsequent effort to map the responsible elements in detail, relatively small proximal portions of the skeletal and cardiac α-actin promoters—roughly 200 and 300 nucleotides, respectively—were sufficient to reconstruct the positive and negative effects described above, for control of the endogenous genes by TGFβ1, bFGF, and acidic FGF. Thus, TGFβ1 and basic FGF selectively upregulate the skeletal α-actin promoter, with no effect on the cardiac promoter; acidic FGF inhibits both, in agreement with the effects of all three factors on the corresponding RNAs.

This region of the skeletal α-actin promoter is noteworthy for three repeats of a $CC[A/T]_6GG$ sequence, called CArG box (for CC-A/T-rich-CG), which is shared with the cardiac α-actin promoter and has been shown to be necessary[158-161] and possibly sufficient[162,163] for basal, tissue-specific transcription of these genes in skeletal muscle (compare ref.[164]). Paradoxically, this element resembles a site in the c-fos proto-oncogene promoter (serum response element, SRE) that mediates induction by serum, defined mitogens, and other agonists,[165] and one major protein that binds this site (serum response factor)[166] and binds the related sites in the actin promoters as well.[162,167-170] Mutational analysis of the skeletal α-actin promoter by internal deletions and substitution mutagenesis pointed to the importance of the most proximal SRE, SRE1, for basal, tissue-restricted expression in cardiac cells.[57] Conversely, a synthetic promoter comprising only 28 nucleotides centered on SRE1, placed upstream from a minimal promoter, was sufficient to drive high-level tissue-specific expression in cardiac muscle cells and not in cardiac fibroblasts. Thus, an SRE can by itself result in tissue-restricted transcription in cardiac muscle. Interestingly, whereas the c-fos SRE was up-regulated in cardiac muscle cells both by basic and acidic FGF, the skeletal α-actin SRE1 distinguishes between these signals. This element was sufficient for induction by bFGF, yet showed little or no response to acidic FGF. Thus, this single SRE, or immediately contiguous sequences within the 28-bp fragment, can discriminate between intracellular messages produced in cardiac cells by basic versus acidic FGF. In addition, this site clearly fails to account for the suppressive effect of acidic FGF on transcription of the longer promoter or steady-state expression of the endogenous skeletal α-actin gene.

A second SRE-binding protein, the multifunctional transcription factor YY1, is a competitive antagonist of SRF in skeletal muscle,[171,172] binding asymmetrically to the 3' arm of the CArG box palindrome. Both SRF and YY1 are readily detected in cardiac myocyte extracts (W. R. MacLellan and M. D. Schneider, *unpublished results*). The c-*fos* SRE mediates *fos* induction in cardiac muscle cells subjected to passive mechanical stretch.[14,16] Consequently, with the caveat that its function is evident thus far only from cell culture models, SRF appears likely to mediate both the global growth response in myocardial hypertrophy and control of at least skeletal α-actin among the genes induced by mechanical load. At present it is unknown whether the skeletal α-actin SRE likewise is a target for mechanical induction, how accessory SRE-binding proteins including YY1 function in cardiac cells, whether activation of the *fos* and actin SREs in cardiac cells requires inducible changes in the abundance of SRF or post-translational modifications of the protein, or how growth factor–dependent signals and mechanically activated signals converge on this transcription factor.

Growth Factor Signal Transduction, Mechanical Signal Transduction, and Cardiac Gene Transcription

Ligand-induced Dimerization Causes Association of Activated Receptor with Downstream Signaling Molecules: Assembly of the Signal Transfer Particle

For growth factor receptors with tyrosine kinase activity, ligand-induced activation is mediated by receptor dimerization and autophosphorylation, via intermolecular cross-phosphorylation, on tyrosine residues of the tyrosine kinase domain itself and other cytoplasmic sites.[67] Kinase-deficient forms of PDGF,[173] EGF,[174] and FGF[105,175] receptor inhibit the function of the respective wild-type receptor, presumably because of this requirement for cross-phosphorylation. Autophosphorylation enables the activated receptor to associate physically with cellular substrates and effectors including phospholipase C-γ1 and -γ2, the *ras* GTPase-activating protein (GAP), the tyrosine kinases *src, fyn,* and *yes,* the serine/threonine kinase *raf,* and phosphatidyl-inositol-3-kinase.[176] Association of these proteins with activated receptor typically is mediated by SH-2 and SH-3 (*src* homology) domains resembling a conserved noncatalytic domain of pp60[c-src].[177] Each SH domain recognizes specific phosphorylated tyrosine residues, via short motifs adjacent to each phosphotyrosine,[178] allowing the assembly of effectors on the receptor (and the resultant signal) to possess specificity. For example, PDGF and FGF receptors each associate with GAP, whereas phosphatidyl-inositol-3-kinase does not bind to FGFR1.[179]

That p21[ras] plays a central role in growth factor signal transduction first was substantiated by inhibiting proliferative responses by microinjecting anti-*ras* antibodies,[180] and more recently through the dominant negative forms of *ras* that inhibit signal transduction through tyrosine kinase receptors in cultured cells.[181–183] Beyond merely implicating *ras* in mitogenic signals that result in cell proliferation, dominant inhibitory *ras* alleles also have shown an obligatory role for *ras* in certain interactions that govern morphogenesis: vulval induction in *C. elegans*[184] and, in *Xenopus,* mesoderm induction by either bFGF or activin.[185] Consequently, *ras* is now presumed to mediate the signals not only of receptors with tyrosine kinase activity but also the more limited set of transmembrane serine/threonine kinases. Precisely how *ras* becomes activated after growth factor binding is unclear, although promising mediators include the mammalian homologues of a *Drosophila* protein, *son of sevenless,* which catalyzes exchange of GDP for GTP on *ras* protein and is postulated to couple tyrosine kinases to *ras.*[186] GAP may function downstream of *ras,*[187–189] apart from its ability to inhibit *ras* function. GAP associates with p62 and p190, postulated to be an hnRNA-binding protein and transcriptional repressor, respectively, implicating a direct pathway between the surface membrane and transcriptional control.[190,191] *Ras* also regulates a cascade of protein kinases, via the serine/threonine microtublule-associated protein (MAP) kinases also known as ERK-1 and -2.[192] Phosphorylated MAP kinase is translocated to the nucleus,[193] where its substrates include c-*jun*, c-*fos*, and histone H3.[194] Translocation also may be important for signaling by PKC,[195] whose activated form is sufficient to induce at least βMHC, ANF, and cardiac myosin light chain–2 among the genes associated with myocardial hypertrophy.[24,25]

As the receptors for TGFβ and activin are serine/threonine kinases, signal transduction for peptides of the TGFβ family is expected to differ at least in its initial stages from the scheme for FGF receptor and other receptor tyrosine kinases. Nonetheless, there is evidence that these signaling pathways might converge quite early in the cascade, since *ras* mediates effects of both FGFs and the TGFβ superfamily.[185,196,197] Features of the FGF and TGFβ signaling cascades are summarized in Figure 2. Precisely where and how events initiated by mechanical load might intervene with this circuitry for signal transduction remains a paramount issue in cardiovascular molecular biology.

Immediate-early Genes Can Regulate Muscle-specific Transcription

The cascade of events involving membrane-associated and cytoplasmic signaling molecules activated by growth factors in turn causes the virtually immediate induction of a battery of transcription factors, which are thought to couple growth factor ligand binding to long-term changes in structure and function.[4,176] These nuclear proteins with immediate-early kinetics of induction include the products of numerous proto-oncogenes (c-*myc*, c-*fos*, *fosB*, c-*jun*, *junB*) and can be triggered in cultured cardiac myocytes by an array of trophic signals including serum factors,[150,198] adrenergic agonists,[199,200] endothelin,[77] FGFs,[201] or passive mechanical stretch.[14,15] In vivo, this set of genes is activated with analogously rapid kinetics by aortic banding,[7,32–34,36] adrenergic agonists,[202] or ischemia.[203] c-*Fos* and c-*jun* are the prototypes of two structurally related "AP-1" transcription factor families that share a leucine zipper domain as an interface for dimerization. Differentiated gene transcription in skeletal muscle is inhibited or prevented by forced expression of c-*myc*,[204–206] c-*fos*,[207,208] or c-*jun*.[208] As one mechanism for repressing myogenesis, *fos* and *jun* block the expression of myogenin and MyoD,[207–209] muscle-specific basic helix-loop-helix

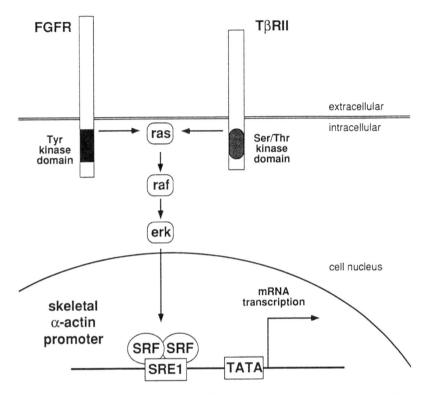

FIGURE 2. *Partial model of a cascade for FGF and TGFβ signal transduction. The cytoplasmic signaling domains of FGF and type II TGFβ receptors (FGFR, TβRII) possess intrinsic tyrosine kinase and serine/ threonine kinase activity, respectively. Dominant-suppressor mutations and measurements of ligand-induced GTP binding implicate ras proteins in signaling by both generic classes of receptor. The protein kinases raf and erk (MAP kinase) act sequentially, downstream of ras, at least for FGF receptor and other receptor tyrosine kinases; the cytoplasmic mediators of TGFβ signal transduction are conjectural at present. In cardiac muscle cells, basic FGF and TGFβ signaling cascades both converge on the same sequence-specific DNA-binding protein, serum response factor (SRF), and the same DNA sequence, the proximal serum response element (SRE1), for transcriptional activation of the skeletal α-actin promoter. Repression of the promoter by acidic FGF requires elements in addition or as an alternative to SRE1 alone.*

(HLH) proteins that can activate muscle-specific transcription when introduced into nonmuscle cells.[210,211] As a second mechanism for negative regulation of myogenesis, *jun* directly prevents *trans*-activation by MyoD and myogenin.[208,209]

Thus, in principle, *fos* and *jun* proteins induced by growth factors or mechanical load might regulate cardiac gene expression either by (1) direct binding to target sequences or (2) functional interaction with other cardiac transcription factors. An illustration of the first case is ANF, whose promoter contains a *fos/jun* recognition site[212] and is regulated in *trans* by exogenous *fos* and *jun* expression vectors.[213] A likely example of the second is the skeletal α-actin promoter, which lacks a consensus AP-1 binding site yet nevertheless can be activated by cotransfected *fos* and *jun*.[214] Alternative means to demonstrate the functional significance of cardiac nuclear proteins as "third messengers" for hypertrophy are antisense oligonucleotides to block a specific protein's expression, dominant inhibitors to block protein function (eg, truncated forms of *fos* or *jun* that dimerize but cannot bind to DNA), and ectopic or forced expression in transgenic mice. Endogenous c-*myc* in myocardium ordinarily is rapidly downregulated late in gestation, along with the loss of proliferative capacity,[198] whereas overexpression of c-*myc* causes ventricular hyperplasia.[133] Conversely, endothelin-dependent protein synthesis is suppressed in cardiac myocytes exposed to antisense oligonucleotides for *Egr*-1,[215] a zinc finger transcription factor induced as another immediate-early response to hypertrophic signals.[36,77,200] Thus, substantial evidence exists to support the conclusion that the transcription factors evoked as immediate-early responses to load or to cardiac agonists indeed are causally related to the more delayed changes in growth and cardiac-specific transcription.

Synopsis and Future Directions

Peptide growth factors, especially members of the FGF and TGFβ superfamilies, have been isolated from adult myocardium, are subject to intricate temporal and spatial programs of expression during early development, and are susceptible to hemodynamic and pharamacological cues that trigger adaptive cardiac growth and influence a host of cardiac genes and gene products. Beyond their mere presence and regulated expression, the probability that myocardial growth factors possess functional importance is upheld by both positive and negative effects on cardiac organogenesis, and by a continuum of stimulatory and inhibitory effects on cardiac-restricted genes. This spectrum of modulatory activities—selective induction of fetal cardiac genes—resembles, strikingly, the program of gene regulation found in cardiac hypertrophy produced by mechanical load. Concomitantly, growth factors including bFGF, PDGF-BB, and, in particular, TGFβ maintain the contractile function of cardiac myocytes in cell culture[101] and thus might affect mechanical performance in vivo as well, by mechanisms distinct from their control of cardiac gene transcription.

Among the prominent issues that will likely attract scrutiny as research into cardiac growth factors evolves is the cross-talk among trophic signaling pathways. A few examples are already evident: 1) induction of bFGF in myocardium during hypothyroidism and a shift toward use of an alternative upstream site for initiation of translation, producing forms that are preferentially localized to the nucleus[144] (conceivably, bFGF may account at least for part of the upregulation of βMHC with hypothyroidism.); 2) induction if IGF-I, conversely, by thyroid hormone excess[216]; 3) induction of endothelin, at least in endothelial cells, by TGFβ[217]; 4) upregulation of TGFβ1 mRNA in adult rat heart by norepinephrine[218]; 5) induction of both TGFβ3[219] and nonmyocyte-derived growth factor[220] in cardiac fibroblasts by β-adrenergic signals. A β-adrenergic, paracrine circuit for production of myocardial growth factors by cardiac fibroblasts may help explain the finding that, in cardiac myocytes at high density, activation of the skeletal α-actin promoter by norepinephrine occurs through β-adrenergic receptors (vs. β-adrenergic receptors in sparse cultures, even though the myocytes' β-adrenergic pathway is functional).[221] Apart from cross-induction of one another, these distinct classes of trophic factors might be expected to exert cooperative[222] or antagonistic effects.

A second, related question concerns potential unforeseen and consequently untested actions of familiar peptides in the heart. As one illustration, ANF might have a direct role as a growth inhibitor apart from its function in volume regulation. In vascular smooth muscle cells, proliferative growth induced by serum and hypertrophic growth induced by angiotensin II were each inhibited by ANF, with similar effects on endothelium.[223] This antiproliferative effect of ANF is mimicked by 8-bromo-cyclic GMP, suggesting the involvement of cGMP cascade for growth inhibition. Whether cardiac myocytes also are targets for ANF as a growth inhibitor has not been studied directly, although ANF is reported to reduce cell volume in rabbit atrial or ventricular myocytes.[224]

Third, more fundamentally, exactly which classes of trophic stimuli converge on which *cis*-acting motifs, and what elements or transcription factors might be proved to serve in a common pathway? The SRE mediates induction of c-*fos* both by FGFs[57] and passive stretch.[14,16] Similarly, as detailed earlier, the proximal SRE of the skeletal α-actin gene mediates induction by bFGF[57] and TGFβ1 (W. R. MacLellan and M. D. Schneider, *unpublished results*), whereas other sequences have been reported to mediate this promoter's induction by norepinephrine[225] and thyroid hormone.[226] Even where a single element and, indeed, a single transcription factor such as SRF can be implicated as a conduit for multiple signaling events, the responsible sites within the molecule and their associated post-translational modifications will remain to be defined.[194]

Fourth, and finally, the currently available data and their implication that growth factor signaling cascades have importance in the heart are predicated on a relatively small number of model systems and investigations. Despite substantial data for control of the cardiac phenotype by FGFs and TGFβ1 in neonatal cells, discrepancies exist between neonatal and adult cardiac myocytes[227,228] and current results predict the impact of growth factors on adult cells only by hazardous extrapolation. Even though adult ventricular muscle obviously can modulate differentiated gene expression (in whole-animal studies), there is no indication whether mechanical load also can provoke any or all of the "fetal" program in isolated adult ventricular myocytes. Whether passive stretch can upregulate genes encoding growth factors, their receptors, or both in adult cardiac myocytes likewise is unknown. Although significant progress has been made toward deciphering what portions of cardiac promoters are responsible for tissue-specific expression and for induction by trophic ligands, understanding the pathway for coupling mechanical load to long-term changes in the cardiac phenotype ultimately requires determining the *cis*-acting elements responsive to load, in the context of adult ventricular cells.[36,229] Recently, adult ventricular myocytes in culture have proved to be amenable to gene transfer by recombinant, replication-defective adenovirus (L. A. Kirshenbaum, W. R. MacLellan, B. A. French, and

M. D. Schneider, *unpublished results*): thus, a means exists for efficiently and uniformly modifying adult ventricular muscle cells with foreign DNA. A further step in the evolution of knowledge regarding signal transduction in myocardium will be provided by in vivo genetic methods—transgenic mouse technology,[133] homologous recombination in embryonal stem cells, and, conceivably, insertional mutagenesis—to engineer gain-of-function and loss-of-function mutations in the components of these putative cascades.[230]

Acknowledgments

The authors are grateful to Drs. Seigo Izumo, Elissavet Kardami, and Anita Roberts for their suggestions and for discussions of unpublished work, and to Drs. Brent French, David Friedman, and Lorrie Kirshenbaum for comments.

References

1. Anversa P, Palackal T, Sonnenblick EH, Olivetti G, Meggs LG, Capasso JM: Myocyte cell loss and myocyte cellular hyperplasia in the hypertrophied aging rat heart. *Circ Res* 1990;67:871–885
2. Nadal-Ginard B, Mahdavi V: Molecular basis of cardiac performance: plasticity of the myocardium generated through protein isoform switches. *J Clin Invest* 1989;84:1693–1700
3. Swynghedauw B (ed): *Cardiac Hypertrophy and Failure.* London: John Libbey & Co Ltd, 1990
4. Parker TG, Schneider MD: Growth factors, proto-oncogenes, and plasticity of the cardiac phenotype. *Annu Rev Physiol* 1991;53:179–200.
5. Izumo S, Lompre AM, Matsuoka R, Koren G, Schwartz K, Nadal-Ginard B, Mahdavi V: Myosin heavy chain messenger RNA and protein isoform during cardiac hypertrophy: interaction between hemodynamic and thyroid hormone-induced signals. *J Clin Invest* 1987;79:970–977
6. Schwartz K, de la Bastie D, Bouveret P, Oliviero P, Alonso S, Buckingham M: α-Skeletal muscle actin mRNAs accumulate in hypertrophied adult rat hearts. *Circ Res* 1986;59:551–555
7. Black FB, Packer SE, Parker TG, Michael LH, Roberts R, Schwartz RJ, Schneider MD: The vascular smooth muscle alpha-actin gene is reactivated during cardiac hypertrophy produced by load. *J Clin Invest* 1991;88:1581–1588
8. Lee RT, Bloch KD, Pfeffer JM, Pfeffer MA, Neer EJ, Seidman CE: Atrial

natriuretic factor gene expression in ventricles of rats with spontaneous biventricular hypertrophy. *J Clin Invest* 1988;81:431–434

9. Saito Y, Nakao K, Arai H, Nishimura K, Okumura K, Obata K, Takemura G, Fujiwara H, Sugawara H, Yamada T, Itoh H, Mukoyama M, Hosoda K, Kawai C, Ban T, Yasue H, Imura H: Augmented expression of atrial natriuretic polypeptide gene in ventricle of human failing heart. *J Clin Invest* 1989;83:298–305

10. Nagai R, Zarain-Herzberg A, Brandl CJ, Fujii J, Tada M, MacLennan DH, Alpert NR, Periasmy M: Regulation of myocardial Ca^{2+}-ATPase and phospholamban mRNA expression in response to pressure overload and thyroid hormone. *Proc Natl Acad Sci USA* 1989;86:2966–2970

11. Mercadier J-J, Lompre A-M, Duc P, Boheler KR, Fraysse J-B, Wisnewsky C, Allen PD, Komajda M, Schwartz K: Altered sarcoplasmic reticulum Ca^{2+}-ATPase gene expression in the human ventricle during end-state heart failure. *J Clin Invest* 1990;85:305–309

12. Bustamante JO, Ruknudin A, Sachs F: Stretch-activated channels in heart cells: relevance to cardiac hypertrophy. *J Cardiovasc Pharmacol* 1991;17:S110–S113

13. Watson PA, Giger KE, Frankenfield CM: Activation of adenylate cyclase during swelling of S49 cells in hypotonic medium is not involved in subsequent volume regulation. *Mol Cell Biochem* 1991;104:51–56

14. Komuro I, Katoh Y, Kaida T, Shibazaki Y, Kurabayashi M, Hoh E, Takaku F, Yazahi Y: Mechanical loading stimulates cell hypertrophy and specific gene expression in cultured rat cardiac myocytes. Possible role of protein kinase C activation. *J Biol Chem* 1991;266:1265–1268

15. Komuro I, Kaida T, Shibazaki Y, Kurabayashi M, Katon Y, Hoh E, Takaku F, Yazaki Y: Stretching cardiac myocytes stimulates protoonco-gene expression. *J Biol Chem* 1990;265:3595–3598

16. Sadoshima J, Jahn L, Takahashi T, et al: Molecular characterization of the stretch-induced adaptation of cultured cardiac cells. An in vitro model of load-induced cardiac hypertrophy. *J Biol Chem* 1992;267:10551–10560

17. Sadoshima J, Takahashi T, Jahn L, Sadoshima J, Jahn I, Takahashi T, Kulik TJ, Izumo S: Roles of mechanosensitive ion channels, cytoskeleton, and contractile activity in stretch-induced immediate-early gene expression and hypertrophy of cardiac myocytes. *Proc Natl Acad Sci USA* 1992;89:9905–9909

18. Sigurdson W, Ruknudin A, Sachs F: Calcium imaging of mechanically induced fluxes in tissue-cultured chick heart: role of stretch-activated ion-channels. *Am J Physiol* 1992;262:H1110–H1115

19. Watson PA, Haneda T, Morgan HE: Effect of higher aortic pressure on ribosome formation and cAMP content in rat heart. *Am J Physiol* 1989;256:C1257–C1261

20. Kitakaze M, Marban E: Cellular mechanism of the modulation of contractile function by coronary perfusion pressure in ferret hearts. *J Physiol (Lond)* 1989;414:455–472

21. Kwiatkowska PB, Domanska JK: Increased 19 kDa protein phosphorylation and protein kinase-C activity in pressure-overload cardiac hypertrophy. *Basic Res Cardiol* 1991;86:402–409

22. von Harsdorf R, Lang RE, Fullerton M, Woodcock EA: Myocardial stretch stimulates phosphatidylinositol turnover. *Circ Res* 1989;65:494–501
23. Dunnmon PM, Iwaki K, Henderson SA, Sen A, Chien KR: Phorbol esters induce immediate-early genes and activate cardiac gene transcription in neonatal rat myocardial cells. *J Mol Cell Cardiol* 1990;22:901–910
24. Kariya K, Karns LR, Simpson PC: Expression of a constitutively activated mutant of the beta-isozyme of protein kinase-C in cardiac myocytes stimulates the promoter of the beta-myosin heavy chain isogene. *J Biol Chem* 1991;266:10023–10026
25. Shubeita HE, Martinson EA, Vanbilsen M, Chien KR, Brown JH: Transcriptional activation of the cardiac myosin light chain-2 and atrial natriuretic factor genes by protein kinase-C in neonatal rat ventricular myocytes. *Proc Natl Acad Sci USA* 1992;89:1305–1309
26. Baker KM, Chernin MI, Wixson SK, Aceto JH: Renin-angiotensin system involvement in pressure-overload cardiac hypertrophy in rats. *Am J Physiol* 1990;259:H324–332
27. Schunkert H, Dzau VJ, Tang SS, Hirsch AT, Apstein CS, Lorell BH: Increased rat cardiac angiotensin converting enzyme activity and mRNA expression in prssure overload left ventricular hypertrophy. Effects on coronary resistance, contractility, and relaxation. *J Clin Invest* 1990;86:1913–1920
28. Takahashi T, Schunkert H, Isoyama S, Wei JV, Nadal-Ginard B, Grossman W, Izumo S: Age-related differences in the expression of proto-oncogene and contractile protein genes in response to pressure overload in the rat myocardium. *J Clin Invest* 1992;89:939–946
29. Arai M, Otsu K, MacLennan DH, Alpert NR, Periasmy M: Effect of thyroid hormone on the expression of mRNA encoding sarcoplasmic reticulum proteins. *Circ Res* 1991;69:266–276
30. Naudin V, Oliviero P, Rannou F, Saintepeuve C, Charlemagne D: The density of ryanodine receptors decreases with pressure overload-induced rat cardiac hypertrophy. *FEBS Lett* 1991;285:135–138
31. Brillantes AM, Allen P, Takahashi T, Izumo S, Marks AR: Differences in cardiac calcium release channel (ryanodine receptor) expression in myocardium from patients with end-stage heart failure caused by ischemic versus dilated cardiomyopathy. *Circ Res* 1992;71:18–26
32. Mulvagh SL, Michael LH, Perryman MB, Roberts R, Schneider MD: A hemodynamic load in vivo induces cardiac expression of the cellular oncogene, c-*myc*. *Biochem Biophys Res Commun* 1987;147:627–636
33. Izumo S, Nadal-Ginard B, Mahdavi V: Proto-oncogene induction and reprogramming of cardiac gene expression produced by pressure overload. *Proc Natl Acad Sci USA* 1988;85:339–343
34. Komuro M, Kurabayashi M, Takaku F, Yazaki V: Expression of cellular oncogenes in the myocardium during the developmental stage and pressure-overload hypertrophy of the rat heart. *Circ Res* 1988;62:1075–1079
35. Schunkert H, Jahn L, Izumo S, Apstein CS, Lorell BH: Localization and regulation of c-*fos* and c-*jun* proto-oncogene induction by systolic wall stress in normal and hypertrophied rat hearts. *Proc Natl Acad Sci USA* 1991;88:11480–11484

36. Rockman HA, Ross RS, Harris AN, Knowlton KU, Steinhelper ME, Field LJ, Ross J, Chien KR: Segregation of atrial-specific and inducible expression of an atrial natriuretic factor transgene in an invivo murine model of cardiac hypertrophy. *Proc Natl Acad Sci USA* 1991;88:8277–8281

37. Hammond GL, Wieben E, Markert CL: Molecular signals for initiating protein synthesis in organ hypertrophy. *Proc Natl Acad Sci USA* 1979;76:2455–2459

38. Chiba M, Sakai S, Nakata M, Tashima H: The role of basic fibroblast growth factor in myocardial hypertrophy (abstract). *Circulation* 1990;82:III–761

39. Villarreal FJ, Dillmann WH: Cardiac hypertrophy-induced changes in messenger RNA levels for TGF-betal, fibronectin, and collagen. *Am J Physiol* 1992;262:H1861–H1866

40. Alpert NR, Mulieri LA: Increased myothermal economy of isometric force generation in compensated cardiac hypertrophy induced by pulmonary artery constriction in rabbits. *Circ Res* 1982;50:491–500

41. Garner I, Sassoon D, Vandekerchkove J, Alonso S, Buckingham M: A developmental study of the abnormal expression of α-cardiac and α-skeletal actins in the striated muscle of a mutant mouse. *Dev Biol* 1989;134:236–245

42. Gwathmey JK, Slawsky MT, Hajjar RJ, Briggs GM, Morgan JM: Role of intracellular calcium handling in force-interval relationships of human ventricular myocardium. *J Clin Invest* 1990;85:1599–1613

43. Bailey BA, Houser SR: Calcium transients in feline left ventricular myocytes with hypertrophy induced by slow progressive pressure overload. *J Mol Cell Cardiol* 1992;24:365–373

44. Sen S, Kundu G, Mekhail N, Castel J, Misono K, Healy B: Myotrophin: purification of a novel peptide from spontaneously hypertensive rat heart that influences myocardial growth. *J Biol Chem* 1990;265:16635–16643

45. Long CS, Henrich CJ, Simpson PC: A growth factor for cardiac myocytes is produced by cardiac nonmyocytes. *Cell Reg* 1991;2:1081–1095

46. Quinckler W, Maasberg M, Bernotat-Danielowski S, Luthe N, Sharma HS, Shaper W: Isolation of heparin-binding growth factors from bovine, porcine and canine hearts. *Eur J Biochem* 1989;181:67–73

47. Kardami E, Fandrich RR: Basic fibroblast growth factor in atria and ventricles of the vertebrate heart. *J Cell Biol* 1989;109:1865–1875

48. Sasaki H, Hoshi H, Hong Y-M, Karube K, Konno S, Onodera M, Saito T, Aoyagi S: Purification of acidic fibroblast growth factor from bovine heart and its localization in the cardiac myocytes. *J Biol Chem* 1989;264:17606–17612

49. Casscells W, Speir E, Sasse J, Klagsburn M, Allen P, Lee M, Calvo M, Chiba M, Haggroth L, Folkman J, Epstein SE: Isolation, characterization, and localization of heparin-binding growth factors in the heart. *J Clin Invest* 1990;85:434–445

50. Weiner HL, Swain JL: Acidic fibroblast growth factor mRNA is expressed by cardiac myocytes in culture and the protein is localized to the extracellular matrix. *Proc Natl Acad Sci USA* 1989;86:2683–2687

51. Speir E, Yi-Fu Z, Lee M, Shrivastar S, Casscells W: Fibroblast growth factors are present in adult cardiac myocytes in vivo. *Biochem Biophys Res Commun* 1988;157:1336–1340

52. Speir E, Tanner V, Gonzalez AM, Farris J, Baird A, Casscells W: Acidic and basic fibroblast growth factors in adult rat heart myocytes: localization, regulation in culture, and effects on DNA synthesis. *Circ Res* 1992;71:251–259

53. Baird A, Klagsbrun M (ed): *The Fibroblast Growth Factor Family.* New York: New York Academy of Sciences, 1991

54. deLapeyriere O, Rosnet O, Benharroch D, Raybaud F, Marchetto S, Panche J, Galland F, Mattei MG: Structure, chromosome mapping and expression of the murine Fgf-6-gene. *Oncogene* 1990;5:823–831

55. Kardami E, Stoski RM, Doble BW, Yamamoto T, Hertzberg EL, Nagy JI: Biochemical and ultrastructural evidence for the association of basic fibroblast growth factor with cardiac gap junctions. *J Biol Chem* 1991;266:19551–19557

56. Imamura T, Engleka K, Zhan X, Tokita Y, Forough R, Roeder D, Jackson A, Maier JAM, Maciag T: Recovery of mitogenic activity of a growth factor mutant with a nuclear translocation sequence. *Science* 1990;249:1567–1570

57. Parker TG, Chow KL, Schwartz RJ, Schneider MD: Positive and negative control of the skeletal alpha-actin promoter in cardiac muscle: a proximal serum response element is sufficient for induction by basic fibroblast growth factor (FGF) but not for inhibition by acidic FGF. *J Biol Chem* 1992;267:3343–3350

58. Godsave SF, Shiurba RA: Xenopus blastulae show regional differences in competence for mesoderm induction: correlation with endogenous basic fibroblast growth factor levels. *Dev Biol* 1992;151:506–515

59. Partanen J, Vainikka S, Korhonen J, Armstrong E, Alitalo K: Diverse receptors for fibroblast growth factors. *Prog Growth Factor Res* 1992;4:69–83

60. Yayon A, Zimmer Y, Shen GH, Awiwi A, Yarden Y, Givol D: A confined variable region confers ligand specificity on fibroblast growth factor receptors: Implications for the origin of the immunoglobulin fold. *EMBO J* 1992;11:1885–1890

61. Werner S, Duan D, Devries C, Peters KG, Johnson DE, Williams LT: Differential splicing in the extracellular region of fibroblast growth factor receptor-1 generates receptor variants with different ligand-binding specificities. *Mol Cell Biol* 1992;12:82–88

62. Duan D-SR, Werner S, Williams LT: A naturally occuring secreted form of fibroblast growth factor (FGF) receptor 1 binds basic FGF in preference over acidic FGF. *J Biol Chem* 1992;267:16076–16080

63. Bernard O, Li M, Reid HH: Expression of two different forms of fibroblast growth factor receptor 1 in different mouse tissues and cell lines. *Proc Natl Acad Sci USA* 1991;88:7625–7629

64. Murphy LJ, Bell GI, Friesen HG: Tissue distribution of insulin-like growth factor I and II messenger ribonucleic acid in the adult rat. *Endocrinology* 1987;120:1279–1282

65. Han VKM, D'Ercole AJ, Lund PK: Cellular localization of somatomedin

(insulin-like growth factor) messenger RNA in the human fetus. *Science* 1987;236:193–197

66. Engelmann GL, Boehm KD, Haskell JF, Khairallan PA, Ilan J: Insulin-like growth factors and neonatal cardiomyocyte development: ventricular gene expression and membrane receptor variations in normotensive and hypertensive rats. *Mol Cell Endocrinol* 1989;63:1–4

67. Ullrich A, Schlessinger J: Signal transduction by receptors with tyrosine kinase activity. *Cell* 1990;61:203–212

68. Morgan DO, Edman JC, Standring DN, et al: Insulin-like growth factor-II receptor as a multifunctional binding protein. *Nature* 1987;329:301–307

69. Guse AH, Kiess W, Funk B, Kessler U, Berg I, Gercken G: Identification and characterization of insulin like growth factor receptors on adult rat cardiac myocytes: linkage to inositol 1,4,5-triphosphate formation. *Endocrinology* 1992;130:145–151

70. Vetter U, Kupferschmid C, Lang D, Pentz S: Insulin-like growth factors and insulin increase the contractility of neonatal rat cardiocytes in vitro. *Basic Res Cardiol* 1988;83:647–654

71. Rabkin SW, Sunga P, Myrdal S: The effect of epidermal growth factor on chronotopic response in cardiac cells in culture. *Biochem Biophys Res Commun* 1987;146:889–897

72. Nair BG, Rashed HM, Patel TB: Epidermal growth factor stimulates adenylate cyclase through a GTP-binding regulatory protein. *Biochem J* 1989;264:563–571

73. Yu Y, Nair BG, Patel TB: Epidermal growth factor stimulates cAMP accumulation in cultured rat cardiac myocytes. *J Cell Physiol* 1992;150:559–567

74. Nair BG, Parikh B, Milligan G, Patel TB: G$_s$-alpha mediates epidermal growth factor-elicited stimulation of rat cardiac adenylate cyclase. *J Biol Chem* 1990;265:21317–21322

75. Sachinidis A, Locher R, Hoppe J, Vetter W: The platelet-derived growth factor isomers, PDGF-AA, PDGF-AB and PDGF-BB, induce contraction of vascular smooth muscle cells by different intracellular mechanisms. *FEBS Lett* 1990;275:95–98

76. Cuevas P, Carceller F, Ortega S, Zazo M, Nieto I, Gimenez-Gallego G: Hypotensive activity of fibroblast growth factor. *Science* 1991;254:1208–1210

77. Shubeita HE, McDonough PM, Harris AN, Knowlton KU, Glembotski CC, Brown JH, Chien KR: Endothelin induction of inositol phospholipid hydrolysis, sarcomere assembly, and cardiac gene expression in ventricular myocytes. A paracrine mechanism for myocardial cell hypertrophy. *J Biol Chem* 1990;265:20555–20562

78. Baker KM, Aceto JF: Angiotensin II stimulation of protein synthesis and cell growth in chick heart cells. *Am J Physiol* 1990;2589:276–280

79. Dostal DE, Baker KM: Angiotensin II stimulation of left ventricular hypertrophy in adult rat heart. Mediation by the AT1 receptor. *Am J Hypertens* 1992;5:276–280

80. Roberts AR, Sporn MB: The transforming growth factor-betas, in Sporn MB, Roberts AR (ed): *Peptide Growth Factors and their Receptors.*

Handbook of Experimental Pharmacology. Heidelberg: Springer-Verlag, 1990, vol 95, part 1, pp 419–472

81. Moses HL, Yang EY, Pietenpol JA: TGF-beta stimulation and inhibition of cell proliferation: new mechanistic insights. *Cell* 1990;63:245–247

82. Roberts AB, Frolik CA, Anzano MA, Sporn MB: Transforming growth factors from neoplastic and non-neoplastic tissues. *Fed Proc* 1983;42:2621–2626

83. Massague J: The transforming growth factor-beta family. *Annu Rev Cell Biol* 1990;6:597–641

84. Thompson NL, Bazoberry F, Speir EH, Casscells W, Ferrans VJ, Flanders KC, Kondaiah P, Geiser AG, Sporn MB: Transforming growth factor beta-1 in acute myocardial infarction in rats. *Growth Factor* 1988;1:91–99

85. Thompson NL, Flanders KC, Smith JM, Ellingsworth LR, Roberts AB, Sporn MB: Expression of transforming growth factor-beta 1 in specific cells and tissues of adult and neonatal mice. *J Cell Biol* 1989;108:661–669

86. Wunsch M, Sharma HS, Markert T, Bernotat-Danielowski S, Schott RJ, Kremer P, Bleese N, Shaper W: In situ localization of transforming growth factor beta 1 in porcine heart: enhanced expression after chronic coronary artery constriction. *J Mol Cell Cardiol* 1991;23:1051–1062

87. Miller DA, Lee A, Pelton RW, Chen EV, Moses HL, Derynck R: Murine transforming growth factor-β2 cDNA sequence and expression in adult tissues and embryos. *Mol Endocrinol* 1989;3:1108–1114

88. Kondaiah P, Sands MJ, Smith JM, Fields A, Roberts AB, Sporn MB, Melton DA: Identification of a novel transforming growth factor-β (TGF-β5) mRNA in *Xenopus laevis. J Biol Chem* 1990;265:1089–1093

89. Meunier H, Wu B: Inhibin α- and βA-subunits are selectively expressed in the rat heart (abstract). *J Cell Biochem* 1991;15C:172

90. Heine UI, Burmester JK, Flanders KC, Danielpour D, Munoz EF, Roberts AB, Sporn MB: Localization of transforming growth factor-beta-1 in mitochondria of murine heart and liver. *Cell Reg* 1991;2:467–477

91. Lefer AM, Tsao P, Aoki N, Palladino MA Jr: Mediation of cardioprotection by transforming growth factor-beta. *Science* 1990;249:61–64

92. Massagué J: Receptors for the TGF-β family. *Cell* 1992;69:1067–1070

93. Laiho M, Weis FMB, Boyd FT, Ignotz R, Massague J: Responsiveness to transforming growth factor-β (TGF-β) restored by genetic complementation between cells defective in TGF-β receptors I and II. *J Biol Chem* 1991;266:9108–9112

94. Wang XF, Lin HY, Ng-Eaton E, Weinberg RA, Lodish HF: Expression cloning and characterization of the TGF-beta type-III receptor. *Cell* 1991;67:797–805

95. Lopez-Casillas F, Cheifetz S, Doody J, Andres JL, Lane WS, Massague J: Structure and expression of the membrane proteoglycan betaglycan, a component of the TGF-beta receptor system. *Cell* 1991;67:785–795

96. Andres JL, DeFalcis D, Noda M, Massague J: Binding of two growth

factor families to separate domains of the proteoglycan betaglycan. *J Biol Chem* 1992;267:5927–30

97. Ornitz DM, Yayon A, Flanagan JG, Burmester JK, Sporn MB: Heparin is required for cell-free binding of basic fibroblast growth factor to a soluble receptor and for mitogenesis in whole cells. *Mol Cell Biol* 1992;12:240–247

98. Lin HY, Wang XF, Ng-Eaton E, Weinberg RA, Lodish HF: Expression cloning of the TGF-beta type II receptor, a functional transmembrance serine/threonine kinase. *Cell* 1992;68:775–85

99. Mathews LS, Vale WW: Expression cloning of an activin receptor, a predicted transmembrane serine kinase. *Cell* 1991;65:973–82

100. Attisano L, Wrana JL, Cheifetz S, Massague J: Novel activin receptors: distinct genes and alternative mRNA splicing generate a repertoire of serine/theonine kinase receptors. *Cell* 1992;68:97–108

101. Roberts AB, Roche NS, Winokur TS, Burmester J, Sporn MB: Role of TGF-β in maintenance of function of cultured neonatal cardiac myocytes: autocrine action and reversal of damaging effects of inter-leukin-1. *J Clin Invest* 1992;90:2056–2062

102. Jessell TM, Melton DA: Diffusible factors in vertebrate embryonic induction. *Cell* 1992;68:257–270

103. Jones CM, Lyons KM, Lapan PM, Wright C, Hogan B: DVR-4 (bone morphogenetic protein-4) as a posterior-ventralizing factor in *Xenopus* mesoderm induction. *Development* 1992;115:639–647

104. Weeks DL, Melton DA: A maternal mRNA localized to the vegetal hemisphere in *Xenopus* eggs codes for a growth factor related to TGFβ. *Cell* 1987;51:861–867

105. Amaya E, Musci TJ, Kirschner MW: Expression of a dominant negative mutant of the FGF receptor disrupts mesoderm formation in *Xenopus* embryos. *Cell* 1991;66:257–290

106. Hemmati-brivanlou A, Melton DA: A truncated activin receptor inhibits mesoderm induction and formation of axial structures in *Xenopus* embryos. *Nature* 1992;359:609–614

107. Parlow MH, Bolender DL, Kokan-Moore NP, Lough J: Localization of bFGF-like proteins as punctate inclusions in the pre-septation myocardium of the chicken embryo. *Dev Biol* 1991;146:139–147

108. Joseph-Silverstein J, Consigli SA, Lyser KM, VerPaul C: Basic fibroblast growth factor in the chick embryo: immunolocalization to striated muscle cells and their precursors. *J Cell Biol* 1989;108:2459–2466

109. Peters KG, Werner S, Chen G, Williams LT: Two FGF receptor genes are differentially expressed in epithelial and mesenchymal tissues during limb formation and organogenesis in the mouse. *Development* 1992;114:233–243

110. Wanaka A, Milbrandt J, Johnson EM: Expression of FGF receptor gene in rat development. *Development* 1991;111:455–468

111. Moore JW, Dionne C, Jaye M, Swain JL: The messenger RNAs encoding acidic FGF, basic FGF and FGF receptor are coordinately

downregulated during myogenic differentiation. *Development* 1991; 111:741–748

112. Olwin BB, Hauschka SD: Fibroblast growth factor receptor levels decrease during chick embryogenesis. *J Cell Biol* 1990;110:503–509

113. Akhurst RJ, Lehnert SA, Faissner A, Duffie E: TGF beta in murine morphogenetic processes: the early embryo and cardiogenesis. *Development* 1990;108:645–656

114. Flanders KC, Thompson NL, Cissel DS, VanObberghen-Schilling E, Baker CC, Kass ME, Ellingsworth LR, Roberts AB, Sporn MB: Transforming growth factor-beta1: histochemical localization with antibodies to different epitopes. *J Cell Biol* 1989;108:653–660

115. Mahmood R, Flanders KC, Morrisskay GM: Interactions between retinoids and TGF betas in mouse morphogenesis. *Development* 1992;115:67–74

116. Millan FA, Denhez F, Kondaiah P, Akhurst RJ: Embryonic gene expression patterns of TFGβ1, β2 and β3 suggest different developmental functions *in vivo*. *Development* 1991;111:131–144

117. Jakowlew SB, Dillard PJ, Winokur TS, Flanders KC, Sporn MB, Roberts AB: Expression of transforming growth factor-betas 1–4 in chicken embryo chondrocytes and myocytes. *Dev Biol* 1991;143:135–148

118. Potts JD, Vincent EB, Runyan RB, Weeks DL: Sense and antisense TGFbeta3 messenger RNA levels correlate with cardiac valve induction. *Dev Dynam* 1992;193:340–345

119. Lee JE, Pintar J, Efstratiadis A: Pattern of the insulin-like growth factor II gene expression during early mouse embryogenesis. *Development* 1990;110:151–159

120. Senior PV, Byrne S, Brammar WJ, Beck F: Expression of the IGF-II/mannose-6-phosphate receptor mRNA and protein in the developing rat. *Development* 1990;109:67–73

121. Bondy CA, Werner H, Roberts CTJ, LeRoith D: Cellular pattern of insulin-like growth factor-I (IGF-I) and type IIGF receptor gene expression in early organogenesis: comparison with IGF-II gene expression. *Mol Endocrinol* 1990;4:1386–1398

122. Gilbert SF: *Developmental Biology*, ed 3. Sunderland, MA: Sinauer Associates, Inc, 1991

123. Cooke J: Xenopus mesoderm induction: evidence for early size control and partial autonomy for pattern development by onset of gastrulation. *Development* 1989;106:519–529

124. Jacobson AG, Sater AK: Features of embryonic induction. *Development* 1988;104:341–359

125. Cooke J, Smith JC: Gastrulation and larval pattern in Xenopus after blastocoelic injection of a Xenopus-derived inducing factor: experiments testing models for the normal organization of mesoderm. *Dev Biol* 1989;131:383–400

126. Muslin AJ, Williams LT: Well-defined growth factors promote cardiac development in axolotl mesodermal explaints. *Development* 1991;112:1095–1101

127. Mummery CL, van Achterberg TAE, van den Eijnden-van Raaij AJM,

van Haaster L, Willemse A, de Laat SW, Piersma AH: Visceral-endoderm-like cell lines induce differentiation of murine P19 embryonal carcinoma cells. *Differentiation* 1991;46:51–60

128. van den Eijnden-van Raaij AJM, van Achterberg TAE, van der Kruijssen CMM, Piersma AH, Huylebroeck D, de Laat SW, Mummery CL: Differentiation of aggregated murine P19 embryonal carcinoma cells is induced by a novel visceral endoderm-specific FGF-like factor and inhibited by activin A. *Mech Dev* 1991;33:157–166

129. Doetschman TC, Eistetter H, Katz M, Schmidt W, Lemler R: The in vitro development of blastocyst-derived embryonic stem cell lines: formation of visceral yolk sac, blood islands, and myocardium. *J Embryol Exp Morphol* 1985;87:27–45

130. Robbins J, Gulick J, Sanchez A, Howles P, Doetschman TC: Mouse embryonic stem cells express cardiac myosin heavy chain genes during development in vitro. *J Biol Chem* 1990;265:11905–11909

131. Sanchez A, Jones WK, Gulick J, Doetschman T, Robbins J: Myosin heavy chain gene expression in mouse embryoid bodies: an in vitro developmental study. *J Biol Chem* 1991;266:22419–22426

132. Wieczorek D, Howles P, Doetschman T: Regulation of α-tropomyosin expression in embryonic stem cells, in Pette D (ed): *The Dynamic State of Muscle Fibers*. Berlin: Walter de Gruyter, 1990, pp 91–101

133. Jackson T, Allard MF, Sreenan CM, Doss LK, Bishop SP, Swain JL: The c-myc proto-oncogene regulates cardiac development in transgenic mice. *Mol Cell Biol* 1990;10:3709–3716

134. Potts JD, Runyan RB: Epithelial-mesenchymal cell transformation in the heart can be mediated, in part, by transforming growth factor β. *Dev Biol* 1989;134:392–401

135. Potts JD, Dagle JM, Walder JA, Weeks DL, Runyan RB: Epithelial-mesenchymal transformation of embryonic cardiac endothelial cells is inhibited by a modified antisense oligodeoxynucleotide to transforming growth factor β3. *Proc Natl Acad Sci USA* 1991;88:1516–1520

136. Runyan RB, Potts JD, Sharma RV, Loeber CP, Chiang JJ, Bhalla RC: Signal transduction of a tissue interaction during embryonic heart development. *Cell Reg* 1990;1:301–313

137. Komuro I, Katoh Y, Hoh E, Takaku F, Yazaki Y: Mechanism of cardiac hypertrophy and injury: possible role of protein kinase C activation. *Jpn Circ J* 1991;55:1149–1157

138. Donohue TJ, Lango M, Benstein JA, Dworkin LD, Catanese VM: Hemodynamic modulation of ventricular insulin-like growth factor-I gene expression (abstract). *Clin Res* 1991;39:152A

139. Wahlander H, Isgaard J, Jennische E, Friberg P: Left ventricular insulin-like growth factor I increases in early renal hypertension. *Hypertension* 1992;19:25–32

140. Turner JT, Rotwein P, Novakofski J, Bechtel PJ: Induction of mRNA for IGF-I and IGF-II during growth hormone-stimulated muscle hypertrophy. *Am J Physiol* 1988;255:E513–E517

141. DeVol DL, Rotwein P, Sadow JL, Novakofski J, Bechtel PJ: Activation of insulin-like growth factor gene expression during work-induced skeletal muscle growth. *Am J Physiol* 1990;259:E89–E95

142. Morrow NG, Kraus WE, Moore JE, Williams RS, Swain JL: Increased expression of fibroblast growth factors in a rabbit skeletal muscle model of exercise conditioning. *J Clin Invest* 1990;85:1816–1820

143. Chiba M, Sumida E, Oka N, Nakata M: The effect of hypoxia in basic FGF synthesis of cultured myocardial cells (abstract). *Circulation* 1991;84:II–395

144. Liu L, Kardami E: Hypothryoidism favours expression of high molecular weight basic FGF in the heart (abstract). *J Cell Biochem* 1991;15C:171

145. Qian SW, Kondaiah P, Casscells W, Roberts AB, Sporn MB: A second messenger RNA species of transforming growth factor β1 in infarcted rat heart. *Cell Reg* 1991;2:241–249

146. Schaper W, Sharma HS, Zimmermann R, Mohri M, Schaper J: Ischemia-induced angiogenesis (abstract). *J Mol Cell Cardiol* 1992;24:I–S.40

147. Zimmermann R, Kluge A, Mohri M, Sack S, Verdouw P: Expression of interleukins and growth factors in ischemic pig heart (abstract). *J Mol Cell Cardiol* 1992;24:I–S.233

148. Lowe WL, Yorek MA, Karpen CW, Teasdale RM, Hovis JG, Albrecht B, Prokopiou C: Activation of protein kinase-C differentially regulates insulin-like growth factor-1 and basic fibroblast growth factor messenger RNA levels. *Mol Endocrinol* 1992;6:741–752

149. Kim SJ, Denhez F, Kim KY, Holt JT, Sporn MB, Roberts AB: Activation of the second promoter of the transforming growth factor-gene by transforming growth factor-beta 1 and phorbol ester occurs the same target sequences. *J Biol Chem* 1989;264:19373–19378

150. Ueno H, Perryman MB, Roberts R, Schneider MD: Differentiation of cardiac myocytes following mitogen withdrawal exhibits three sequential stages of the ventricular growth response. *J Cell Biol* 1988;107:1911–1918

151. Simpson P, McGrath A, Savion S: Myocyte hypertrophy in neonatal rat heart cultures and its regulation by serum and by catecholamines. *Circ Res* 1982;511:787–801

152. Parker TG, Packer SE, Schneider MD: Peptide growth factors can provoke "fetal" contractile protein gene expression in rat cardiac myocytes. *J Clin Invest* 1990;85:507–514

153. Claycomb WC, Moses RL: Growth factors and TPA stimulate DNA synthesis and alter the morphology of cultured terminally differentiated adult rat cardiac muscle cells. *Dev Biol* 1988;127:257–265

154. Eppenberger-Eberhard TM, Flamme I, Kurer V, Eppenberger HM: Re-expression of alpha-smooth muscle actin isoform in cultured adult rat cardiomyocytes. *Dev Biol* 1990;139:269–278

155. Parker TG, Chow-K-L, Schwartz RJ, Schneider MD: Differential regulation of skeletal α-actin transcription in cardiac muscle by two fibroblast growth factors. *Proc Natl Acad Sci USA* 1990;87:7066–7070

156. Florini JR, Ewton DZ, Magri KA: Hormones, growth factors, and myogenic differentiation. *Annu Rev Physiol* 1991;53:201–216

157. Dieckman LJ, Murphy AM, Engelmann GL: Transforming growth factor beta inhibits expression of cardiac TNI in cultured cardiomycytes (abstract). *J Cell Biochem* 1991;15C:168

158. Walsh K: Cross-binding of factors to functionally different promoter elements in c-fos and skeletal actin. *J Biol Chem* 1989;9:2191–2201
159. Mohun TJ, Taylor MV, Garrett N, Gurdon JB: The CArG promoter sequence is necessary for muscle-specific transcription of the cardiac actin gene in Xenopus embryos. *EMBO J* 1989;8:1153–1161
160. Chow KL, Schwartz RJ: A combination of closely associated positive and negative cis-acting promoter elements regulates transcription of the skeletal alpha-actin gene. *Mol Cell Biol* 1990;10:528–538
161. Gustafson TA, Miwa T, Boxer LM, Kedes L: Interaction of nuclear proteins with muscle-specific regulatory sequences of the human cardiac alpha-actin promoter. *Mol Cell Biol* 1988;8:4110–4119
162. Taylor M, Treisman R, Garrett N, Mohun T: Muscle-specific (CArG) and serum-responsive (SRE) promoter elements are functionally interchangeable in *Xenopus* embryos and mouse fibroblasts. *Development* 1989;106:67–78
163. Tuil D, Clergue N, Montarras D, Pinset C, Kahn A, Phan DTF: CC Ar GG boxes, cis-acting elements with a dual specificity. Muscle-specific transcriptional activation and serum responsiveness. *J Mol Biol* 1990;213:677–686
164. Sartorelli V, Webster KA, Kedes L: Muscle-specific expression of the cardiac alpha-actin gene requires MyoD1, CArG-box binding factor, and Sp1. *Genes Dev* 1990;4:1811–1822
165. Treisman R: Identification of a protein-binding site that mediates transcriptional response of the c-*fos* gene to serum factors. *Cell* 1986; 46:567–574
166. Treisman R: Identification and purification of a polypeptide that binds the c-fos serum response element. *EMBO J* 1987;6:2711–2717
167. Boxer LM, Prywes R, Roeder RG, Kedes L: The sarcomeric actin CArG-binding factor is indistinguishable from the c-fos serum response factor. *Mol Cell Biol* 1989;9:515–522
168. Gustafson TA, Taylor A, Kedes L: DNA bending is induced by a transcription factor that interacts with the human c-FOS and alpha-actin promoters. *Proc Natl Acad Sci USA* 1989;86:2162–2166
169. Lee TC, Chow KL, Fang P, Schwartz RJ: Activation of skeletal alpha-actin gene transcription: the cooperative formation of serum response factor-binding complexes over positive cis-acting promoter serum response elements displaces a negative-acting nuclear factor enriched in replicating myoblasts and nonmyogenic cells. *Mol Cell Biol* 1991;11:5090–5100
170. Santoro IM, Walsh K: Natural and synthetic DNA elements with the CArG motif differ in expression and protein-binding properties. *Mol Cell Biol* 1991;11:6296–6305
171. Lee TC, Shi Y, Schwartz RJ: Displacement of BrdU-induced YY1 by serum response factor activates skeletal alpha-actin transcription in embryonic myoblasts. *Proc Natl Acad Sci USA* 1992;89:9814–9818
172. Gualberto A, Lepage D, Pons G, et al: Functional antagonism between YY1 and the serum response factor. *Mol Cell Biol* 1992;12:4209–4214
173. Ueno H, Colbert H, Escobedo JA, Mader SL, Park KS, Atchison ML,

Walsh K: Inhibition of PDGF beta-receptor signal transduction by coexpression of a truncated receptor. *Science* 1991;252:844–848

174. Kashles O, Yarden Y, Fischer R, Ullrich A, Schlessinger J: A dominant negative mutation suppresses the function of normal epidermal growth factor receptors by heterodimerization. *Mol Cell Biol* 1991;11:1454–1463

175. Ueno H, Gunn M, Dell K, Tserg A, Williams L: A truncated form of fibroblast growth factor receptor-1 inhibits signal transduction by multiple types of fibroblast growth factor receptor. *J Biol Chem* 1992;267:1470–1476

176. Cantley LC, Auger KR, Carpenter C, Duckworth B, Graziani A, Kapeller R, Soltoff S: Oncogenes and signal transduction. *Cell* 1991;64:281–302

177. Koch CA, Anderson D, Moran MF, Ellis C. Pawson T: SH2 and SH3 domains: Elements that control interactions of cytoplasmic signaling proteins. *Science* 1991;252:668–674

178. Fantl WJ, Escobedo JA, Martin GA, Turck CW, Deirosario M, McCormick F, Williams LT: Distinct phosphotyrosines on a growth factor receptor bind to specific molecules that mediate different signaling pathways. *Cell* 1992;69:413–423

179. Wennstroem S, Landgren E, Blume-Jensen P, Claesson-Welsh L: The platelet-derived growth factor β-receptor kinase insert confers specific signaling properties to a chimeric fibroblast growth factor receptor. *J Biol Chem* 1992;267:13749–13756

180. Mulcahy LS, Smith MR, Stacey DW: Requirement for ras proto-oncogene function during serum stimulated growth of NIH 3T3 cells. *Nature* 1985;313:241–243

181. Feig LA, Cooper GM: Inhibition of NIH 3T3 cell proliferation by a mutant ras protein with preferential affinity for GDP. *Mol Cell Biol* 1988;8:3235–3243

182. Cai H, Szeberenyi J, Cooper GM: Effect of a dominant inhibitory Ha-ras mutation on mitogenic signal transduction in NIH 3T3 cells. *Mol Cell Biol* 1990;10:5314–5323

183. Medema RH, Wubbolts R, Bos JL: Two dominant inhibitory mutants of p21(ras) interfere with insuin-induced gene expression. *Mol Cell Biol* 1991;11:5963–5967

184. Han M, Sternberg PW: Analysis of dominant-negative mutations of the caenorhabditis-elegans let-60 ras gene. *Genes Dev* 1991;5:2188–2198

185. Whitman M, Melton DA: Involvement of p21*ras* in *Xenopus* mesoderm induction. *Nature* 1992;357:252–254

186. Bowtell D, Fu P, Simon M, Senior P: Identification of murine homologues of the Drosophila son of sevenless gene: potential activators of ras. *Proc Natl Acad Sci USA* 1992;89:6511–6515

187. Martin GA, Yatani A, Clark R, Polakis P, Brown AM, McCormick F: GAP domains responsible for *ras* p21-dependent inhibition of muscarinic atrial K⁺ channel currents. *Science* 1992;255:192–194

188. Medema RH, Delaat WL, Martin GA, McCormick F, Bos JL: GTPase-activating protein SH2-SH3 domains induce gene expression in a ras-dependent fashion. *Mol Cell Biol* 1992;12:3425–3430

189. Yatani A, Okabe K, Polakis P, Halenbeck R, McCormick F, Brown AM: Ras p21 and GAP inhibit coupling of muscarinic receptors to atrial K$^+$ channels. *Cell* 1990;61:769–776

190. Wong G, Muller O, Clark R, Conroy L, Moran MF, Polakis P, McCormick F: Molecular cloning and nucleic acid binding properties of the GAP-associated tyrosine phosphoprotein p62. *Cell* 1992;69:551–558

191. Settleman J, Narasimhan V, Foster LC, Weinberg RA: Molecular cloning of cDNAs encoding the GAP-associated protein p190: implications for a signaling pathway from Ras to the nucleus. *Cell* 1992;69:539–549

192. deVries Smits AM, Burgering BM, Leevers SJ, Marshall CJ, Bos JL: Involvement of p21ras in activation of extracellular signal-regulated kinase 2. *Nature* 1992;357:602–604

193. Chen R-H, Sarnecki C, Blenis J: Nuclear localization and regulation of erk- and rsk-encoded protein kinases. *Mol Cell Biol* 1992;12:915–927

194. Hunter T, Karin M: The regulation of transcription by phosphorylation. *Cell* 1992;70:375–387

195. James G, Olson EN: Deletion of the regulatory domain of protein kinase Cα exposes regions in the hinge and catalytic domains that mediate nuclear targeting. *J Cell Biol* 1992;116:863–874

196. Szeberenyi J, Cai H, Cooper GM: Effect of a dominant inhibitory Ha-ras mutation on neuronal differentiation of PC12 cells. *Mol Cell Biol* 1990;10:5324–5332

197. Mulder KM, Morris SL: Activation of p21ras by transforming growth factor-beta in epithelial cells. *J Biol Chem* 1992;267:5029–5031

198. Schneider MD, Payne PA, Ueno H, Perryman MB, Roberts R: Dissociated expression of c-myc and a fos-related competence gene during cardiac myogenesis. *Mol Cell Biol* 1986;6:4140–4143

199. Starksen NF, Simpson PC, Bishopric N, Coughlin SR, Lee WMI, Escobedo J, Williams LT: Cardiac myocyte hypertrophy is associated with c-myc protooncogene expression. *Proc Natl Acad Sci USA* 1986;83:8348–8350

200. Iwaki K, Sukhatme VP, Shubeita HE, Chien KR: Alpha- and beta-adrenergic stimulation induces distinct patterns of immediate early gene expression in neonatal rat myocardial cells. Fos/jun expression is associated with sarcomere assembly; Egr-1 induction is primarily an alpha 1-mediated response. *J Biol Chem* 1990;265:13809–13817

201. Black FM, Parker TG, Michael LH, Roberts R, Schneider MD: The c-*jun* and *jun*B proto-oncogenes are induced in myocardium by a hemodynamic load in vivo and fibroblast growth factors in vitro (abstract). *J Cell Biochem* 1991;15C:176

202. Brand T, Rohmann S, Sharma HS, Schaper W: Expression of proto-oncogenes after stimulation of β-adrenergic receptors in rat heart. *J Mol Cell Cardiol* 1989;21(suppl III):3

203. Brand T, Sharma HS, Fleischmann KE, Duncker DJ, McFalls E, Verdouw PD, Schaper W: Molecular response of porcine myocardium to ischemia and reperfusion. *Circ Res* 1992;71:1351–1360

204. Caffrey JM, Brown AM, Schneider MD: Mitogens and transfected

oncogenes can selectively block the expression of voltage-gated ion channels. *Science* 1987;236:570–574

205. Schneider MD, Perryman MB, Payne PA, Spizz G, Roberts R, Olsen EN: Autonomous expression of c-myc in BC_3H_1 cells partially inhibits but does not prevent myogenic differentiation. *Mol Cell Biol* 1987;7:1973–1977

206. Miner JH, Wold BJ: C-myc inhibition of myoD and myogenin-initiated myogenic differentiation. *Mol Cell Biol* 1991;11:2842–2851

207. Lassar AB, Thayer MJ, Overell RW, Weintraub H: Transformation by activated ras or fos prevents myogenesis by inhibiting expression of MyoD1. *Cell* 1989;58:659–67

208. Li L, Chambard JC, Karin M, Olson EN: Fos and Jun repress transcriptional activation by myogenin and MyoD: the amino terminus of Jun can mediate repression. *Genes Dev* 1992;6:676–689

209. Bengal E, Ransone L, Scharfmann R, Dwarki VJ, Tapscott SJ, Weintraub H, Verma IM: Functional antagonism between c-Jun and MyoD proteins: a direct physical association. *Cell* 1992;68:507–519

210. Olson EN: MyoD family: a paradigm for development? *Genes Dev* 1990;4:1454–1461

211. Weintraub H, Davis R, Tapscott S, Thayer M, Krause M, Benezra R, Blackwell TK, Turner D, Rupp R, Hollenberg S, Zhuang V, Lassar A: The myoD gene family: nodal point during specification of the muscle cell lineage. *Science* 1991;251:761–766

212. Rosenzweig A, Halazonetis TD, Seidman JG, Seidman CE: Proximal regulatory domains of rat atrial natriuretic factor gene. *Circulation* 1991;84:1256–1265

213. Kovacic-Milivojevic B, Gardner DG: Divergent regulation of the human atrial natriuretic peptide gene by c-jun and c-fos. *Mol Cell Biol* 1992;12:292–301

214. Bishopric NH, Webster KA: Fos and Jun regulate preferential induction of the skeletal α-actin gene in neonatal rat heart cells (abstract). *Circulation* 1991;84:II–87

215. Neyses L, Nouskas J, Vetter H: Inhibition of endothelin-1 induced myocardial protein synthesis by an antisense oligonucleotide against the early growth response gene-1. *Biochem Biophys Res Commun* 1991;181:22–27

216. Kupfer JM, Rubin SA: Differential regulation of insulin like growth factor I by growth hormone and thyroid hormone in the heart of juvenile hypophysectomized rat. *J Mol Cell Cardiol* 1992;24:631–639

217. Kurihara H, Yoshizumi M, Sugiyama T, Takaku F, Yanasigawa M, Masaki T, Hamaoki M, Kato H, Yazaki Y: Transforming growth factor-β stimulates the expression of endothelin mRNA by vascular endothelial cells. *Biochem Biophys Res Commun* 1989;159:1435–1440

218. Bhambi B, Eghbali M: Effect of norepinephrine on myocardial collagen gene expression and response of cardiac fibroblasts after norepinephrine treatment. *Am J Pathol* 1991;139:1131–1142

219. Long CS, Hartogensis W, Corry M, Simpson PC: β-adrenergic stimulation of cardiac non-myocytes increases non-myocyte growth factor production. *J Mol Cell Cardiol* 1992;24:I–S.245

220. Long CS, Henrich CJ, Simpson PC: A growth factor for cardiac myocytes is produced by cardiac nonmyocytes. *Cell Reg* 1991;2:1081–1095
221. Long CS, Ordahl CP, Simpson PC: α_1-Adrenergic receptor stimulation of sarcomeric actin isogene transcription in hypertrophy of cultured rat heart muscle cells. *J Clin Invest* 1989;83:1078–1082
222. Brown KD, Littlewood CJ: Endothelin stimulates DNA synthesis in Swiss 3T3 cell: synergy with polypeptide growth factors. *Biochem J* 1989;263:977–980
223. Appel RG: Growth-regulatory properties of atrial natriuretic factor. *Am J Physiol* 1992;262:F911–F918
224. Clemo HF, Baumgarten CM: Atrial natriuretic factor decreases cell volume of rabbit atrial and ventricular myocytes. *Am J Physiol* 1991;260:C681–C690
225. Bishopric NH, Kedes L: Adrenergic regulation of the skeletal α-actin gene promoter during myocardial cell hypertrophy. *Proc Natl Acad Sci USA* 1991;88:2132–2136
226. Collie E, Muscat G: The human skeletal α-actin promoter is regulated by thyroid hormone: identification of a thyroid hormone response element. *Cell Growth Differ* 1992;3:31–42
227. Clark WA, Decker RS, Borg TK (ed): *Biology of Isolated Adult Cardiac Myocytes.* New York: Elsevier, 1988
228. Volz A, Piper HM, Siegmund B, Schwartz P: Longevity of adult ventricular rat heart muscle cells in serum-free primary culture. *J Mol Cell Cardiol* 1991;23:161–173
229. Kitsis RN, Buttrick PM, Mcnally EM, Kaplan ML, Leinwand LA: Hormonal modulation of a gene injected into rat heart in vivo. *Proc Natl Acad Sci USA* 1991;88:4138–4142
230. Rossant J, Hopkins N: Of fin and fur: mutational analysis of vertebrate embryonic development. *Genes Dev* 1992;6:1–13

Chapter 6

Role of Hemodynamic Load in the Genesis of Cardiac Hypertrophy

Peter M. Buttrick, MD

One of the most exciting revelations in cardiology in the past 10 to 20 years has been an appreciation of the complexity inherent in the ability of the heart to adapt to an imposed load. In contrast to the dogma articulated in the first half of the century, which maintained that cardiac hypertrophy was pathological (and that all athletes were consequently destined to die young), we now appreciate that cardiac hypertrophy is not a single monochromatic response but rather a complex family of adaptations whereby the heart is able to alter not only its size and shape but also both its contractile properties and its biochemical and molecular genetic make-up.[1] Nowhere is this more evident than in the study of the cardiac responses to chronic exercise conditioning.[2] Isotonically trained athletes and experimental animals are able to increase their left ventricular mass by approximately 20%, over a relatively short period of time, and critically they also are able to restructure their sarcomeric organization. The heart of a dynamically conditioned individual has an increased number of sarcomeric units arrayed in series, which results in a heart with an increased end-diastolic dimension and that manifests enhanced pump and muscle performance. This remodeling is not limited to the overall architecture of the left ventricle and, in fact, is reflected by the altered biochemical and molecular genetic make-up of the hypertrophied myocardium.

A paradigm of this type of biochemical and molecular genetic adaptation is the contractile protein myosin. Myosin is a hetero-dimer consisting of two heavy chains (MHC) and two pairs of light

Work on this chapter was supported by NIH HL-46034.

From Fletcher GF, (ed): *Cardiovascular Response to Exercise.* Mount Kisco, NY, Futura Publishing Company, Inc., © 1994.

chains. The heavy chain contains both the actin-binding sites and the adenosine triphosphatase (ATPase) sites, which participate in the energetics of contraction.[3] In adult cardiac muscle, two myosin heavy chains are expressed that are encoded by two separate genes, α and β.[4] The former is characterized by a high ATPase activity and the latter by a lower ATPase activity. In response to chronic dynamic conditioning in the rodent, the percent of α-MHC increases, resulting in a cardiac muscle with overall increased ATPase activity and enhanced pump and muscle performance.[5,6] This genetic response is striking and provides a link between molecular genetics, biochemical enzymology, and physiology, but it is by no means unique. A spectrum of other genes encoding contractile proteins and other components in excitation-contraction coupling also have been shown to have altered patterns of expression in the chronically conditioned heart, including α-actin, troponin, and the sarcoplasmic reticular calcium ATPase.[1]

The architectural and genetic remodeling seen in the hypertrophied heart of a chronically isotonically conditioned person should of course be contrasted with that seen in an isometrically conditioned athlete or in a patient with hypertension.[7] In these conditions the heart also is hypertrophied, but the sarcomeres are replicated in parallel so as to increase wall thickness and not end-diastolic dimension. Directionally opposite changes are seen both in contractile performance and in the expression of a number of gene products, including MHC, troponin, and the sarcoplasmic reticular calcium ATPase.

A potential link between the cardiac remodeling at both the macroscopic and the molecular genetic levels is hemodynamic load. The hemodynamic load in acute dynamic exercise is reflected most prominently by a decrease in peripheral vascular resistance (associated with a shunting of blood to the relatively low resistance vascular bed of skeletal muscle); an increase in venous return; and a subsequent marked increase in both stroke volume and cardiac output. The net effect has been described as a diastolic or volume load. Of course, during periods of rest, the trained individual also manifests a resting bradycardia, which enhances this characteristic load. This should be contrasted with the hemodynamics to which the heart is subjected during bouts of isotonic exercise or in hypertension in which the load is predominantly systolic or a pressure load. It is not surprising that the architecture of the remodeled ventricle would reflect the nature of these discordant loads and, in fact, the heart of a chronically conditioned athlete, with an increase in end-diastolic volume and in rates of fractional shortening, seems both shaped by and well adapted to accommodate this load just as the concentrically hypertrophied heart of a hypertensive individual seems adapted to maintain stroke volume in the face of a chronically elevated afterload.

How, and indeed whether, hemodynamic load influences changes in gene and protein expression is not well established, although a number of studies dating back 20 years would seem to support this contention. The first of these, from Peterson and Lesch,[8] examined the effect of both active and passive isotonic stretch on protein synthesis and amino acid incorporation in isolated rabbit papillary muscles and demonstrated quite clearly that these anabolic processes were remarkably enhanced by the load, with passive stretch being the predominant contributor. Of course, this artificial system does not allow a distinction between systolic or diastolic loading but it does establish a link between a mechanical stimulus, stretch, and a cellular adaptation, increased protein synthesis.

A somewhat more elegant but still limited recapitulation of this message came from the work of Morgan's laboratory and others in the early and mid-1980s.[9–11] This group used an isolated perfused working heart preparation, in which load was modulated by increasing aortic impedance. At high systolic loads, they were able to demonstrate increases in total protein synthesis that were similar to those reported earlier. Furthermore, the increase in protein synthesis was seen regardless of whether the ventricle was vented, ruling out intraventricular pressure development or accelerated oxygen consumption as obligatory components in the process. In fact, ventricular stretch alone appeared to be necessarily related to the acceleration of protein synthesis. The nature of the biochemical mediator responsible was not addressed. Also, in these studies the stretch imposed was systolic so that whereas the link between a mechanical signal and a biochemical adaptation appears irrefutable, the relevance to isotonic exercise in which the load is predominantly diastolic and not systolic is unclear. Studies by others in which end-diastolic pressure was elevated[12] were done under such extreme circumstances that the endocardium was ischemic and unable to participate in normal cellular processes. Another study using the isolated perfused heart as a model system was published recently by Schunkert et al.[13] This group used an isovolumic preparation in which coronary flow and heart rate were held constant but left ventricular volume and systolic pressure were increased by inflating a latex balloon inside the ventricular chamber. They noted that increasing both systolic and diastolic wall stress in this fashion resulted in increased transcription (by three- to four-fold) of two proto-oncogenes, c-*myc* and c-*fos*, by cardiac myocytes. This induction was prevented if the hearts were concomitantly treated with monoxime, an agent that prevents systolic cross-bridge cycling, and was reduced in the presence of established pressure overload hypertrophy. These proto-oncogenes have been implicated as transcriptional factors in many cell types in association with both hyperplasia and hypertrophy[14–16] and their induction in association with a systolic load in this model of isovolumic stress is of interest. However, an important caveat is that the exact role of these presumed transcription factors in the development of cellular hyperplasia and hypertrophy has not been established and it is conceivable that their induction is only epiphenomenal and not etiologic.

One other model that uses the intact heart is the rat heterotopic isograft. In this model, a heart from a donor animal is transplanted into the abdomen of a recipient animal via an end-to-side anastomosis between its ascending aorta and the subdiaphragmatic aorta of the recipient. The coronary effluent of the isograft is drained via the pulmonary circulation into the inferior vena cava. In this model, the isograft is perfused normally but its intrinsic heart rate slows (unlike transplanted hearts in humans in which heart rate increases) and the amount of external work that it performs is markedly reduced. The isograft undergoes prompt atrophy and within approximately 1 week has reduced its weight, probably in large part by increasing protein degradation rates, by 50%. Korecky and Masika[17] were able to induce graded amounts of aortic insufficiency in this system, thus allowing the ventricular chamber to fill and eject, and showed that with the increase in end-diastolic pressure and volume associated with this valvular lesion the cardiac atrophy was attenuated and in more severe cases it did not develop at all. A similar result also was obtained by Klein et al.,[18] who were able to load the heterotopic isograft isovolumically and show that under these circumstances it did not atrophy.

A more elegant and mechanistic understanding of the relationship between mechanical loads and cellular adaptations has come from recent cell culture studies. Although these studies are spectacular in their ability to isolate and implicate various intracellular phenomena, they too can be criticized at the outset in that they do not realistically replicate a physiological process. First, cell culture studies cannot reproduce specific features of hemodynamic loading in the intact heart; second, the cell morphology of attached myocytes in culture dishes, with interdigitating pseudopods and inconsistent intercellular connections, does not reflect the organization of the intact organ. Nonetheless, cell culture studies have provided a great deal of intriguing information and certainly offer potentially testable hypotheses linking mechanical signals to cellular adaptations.

The work of two groups of investigators, directed by Yazaki and Cooper, warrants review.[19–22] These imaginative investigators plated primary neonatal[19,20] or adult cardiocytes[21,22] on a silicone/elastic matrix that was slightly distensible so that the cells in culture could be subjected to stretch after they had attached. The cells were stretched by approximately 10%; this load was imposed for up to 24 to 48 hours, at which times the cells were isolated and compared with an unstretched population plated under otherwise identical conditions. Sarcomere structure was not obviously altered by the load.[21] This stimulus was associated with an increase in amino acid incorporation into myocytes[21] and also with induction of the specific proto-oncogenes c-*myc* and c-*fos*.[19,20] In addition, stretch was associated with an increase in total RNA content concordant with increased activity of generalized anabolic processes and with the induction of at least one specific sarcomeric messenger RNA, skeletal actin, a fetal isoform associated with pressure overload hypertrophy.[20] Using this cell culture system, Komuro et al.[20] have further explicated possible mechanisms by which stretch might induce patterns of gene expression. They first transfected myocytes with promoter/reporter gene constructs containing various 5' flanking regions of the c-*fos* promoter and showed that the so-called serum response element (SRE) appeared to be required for increased transcription of this gene. Further, they demonstrated that stretch increased inositol phosphate (IP) turnover (and presumably protein kinase C activity) and that conditions that result in suppression of protein kinase C activity, such as treatment with staurosporin and/or desensitization with phorbol acetate, blocked the specific stretch-associated induction in c-*fos*. Thus, this work begins to suggest proximal mechanisms by which the mechanical signals of stretch might be transduced into an altered cellular phenotype: stretch increases IP turnover and protein kinase C activity, which in turn are involved in the activation of specific transcription factors and of specific sarcomeric genes. Of course, as noted above, the relevance of this artificial mechanical load to exercise is at best inferential.

A final component in this cascade of cellular processes comes from the work of Cooper and associates[21,22] and from the recent description of stretch-activated ion channels by Sachs, Morris, and others.[23-25] These workers implicate a proximal molecular signal in the cellular response to a mechanical load that is particularly satisfying in that the signal is a mechanochemical one, namely stretch-activated ion channels. These comprise a group of channels whose gating is pressure dependent. That is, traction on a cell results in increased channel activity (mostly resulting in increased inward sodium currents) in a dose-dependent manner. In light of this finding, this group explored the role both of stretch and of inhibition of inward sodium currents on anabolic cellular processes. They, as others, have demonstrated a tension-related induction of both protein and RNA synthesis in isolated adult cardiocytes. In addition, they have demonstrated that contractile protein synthesis is specifically enhanced and, using autoradiographic techniques, they have clearly identified stretched myocytes as the responsive cell type.[21] Finally, and quite strikingly, they have shown that sodium influx is increased in stretched cells and that a variety of agents, such as streptomycin, which block inward sodium currents, can attenuate the increased protein synthesis seen with cell stretching.

To recapitulate the data presented thus far, it seems clear that stretch of cells, isolated muscle, or the intact heart is a sufficient stimulus to increase generalized transcriptional activity and protein synthesis as well as to induce expression of unique genes, such as skeletal actin, which might alter cellular phenotype. Attractive biochemical mediators of this process include stretch-activated sodium channels and/or protein kinase C. Model systems employed that involve intact muscle and heart have more closely approximated systolic but not diastolic overload and their relevance to exercise-induced cardiac hypertrophy is therefore conjectural. Cell culture systems, although remarkable in their ability to provide information on cellular regulation, probably are inadequate to model complex hemodynamic loads that might modulate gene expression in vivo. Consequently, a number of fundamental questions remain unanswered: Is the hemodynamic load associated with exercise sufficient to induce this cascade of anabolic processes? If so, why is a different pattern of gene and protein expression evoked by exercise than the more conventionally studied pressure overload? Are different cellular regulators involved?

The answers to these questions likely will come from an understanding of the regulatory elements of the various genes that are induced by a specific hemodynamic load. Two approaches that are currently being used to address these issues are the development of transgenic mice[26] and direct in vivo gene transfer.[27–29a] Using these techniques, it is possible to transfect permanently (transgenics) or transiently (in vivo gene transfer) recombinant genes consisting of cellular promoter sequences coupled to reporter genes selectively into cardiac myocytes within the intact beating adult mammalian heart. This allows the mapping of regulatory regions of the cellular promoters in vivo. One such promoter of interest in the study of exercise-induced adaptations is α-MHC, a gene that appears to be induced selectively by isotonic exercise in the rat. This gene also is induced by thyroid hormone and we have used the technique of in vivo gene transfer to describe the hormonal regulation of the α-MHC gene in vivo. Using a group of 5′ promoter deletions and mutations, we have shown that the *cis*-acting thyroid response element (TRE) located approximately 150 bp upstream from the transcription start site is necessary but not sufficient for thyroid hormone induction.[29b] This result differs from tissue culture data that demonstrate that the TRE is both necessary and sufficient for thyroid hormone responsiveness of the gene[30,31] and suggests that multiple *cis*-acting elements are responsible for regulated gene expression in vivo, some of which may well be responsive to hemodynamic loads. A similar result has been obtained by Subramaniam et al. using a transgenic mouse model.[32] We also have shown that 613 bp of 5′ flanking sequence of α-MHC is sufficient to impart exercise-induced responsiveness to a reporter gene (unpublished data).

Using these techniques, it should be possible to establish which sequences in the promoter regions of individual genes (such as α-MHC) are responsive to exercise and whether these are similar to those responsive to hypertension or other types of pressure overload. For example, is the SRE that is contained upstream of c-*fos* as important in the response of this gene to diastolic as it is to systolic loading? Further, these techniques can be combined with the isolated perfused heart approach to identify regions of genes that respond to carefully defined hemodynamic loads, such as increased end-diastolic volume with decreased afterload, or to establish whether treatments that interfere with protein kinase C or stretch-activated sodium channels are important to all or only selective transcriptional processes.

References

1. Nadal-Ginard B, Mahdavi VJ: Molecular basis of cardiac performance. *J Clin Invest* 1989;84:1693–1700
2. Schaible TF, Scheuer J: Response of the heart to exercise training. *Prog Cardiovasc Dis* 1985;27:297–324
3. Swynghedauw B: Developmental and functional adaptation of contractile proteins in cardiac and skeletal muscle. *Physiol Rev* 1986;66:710–754
4. Leinwand LA, Fournier EK, Nadal-Ginard B, Shows TB: Multigene family for sarcomeric myosin heavy chain in mouse and human DNA: localization on a single chromosome. *Science* 1983;221:766–769
5. Scheuer J, Malhotra A, Hirsch C, Capasso J, Schaible T: Physiologic cardiac hypertrophy corrects contractile protein abnormalities associated with pathologic cardiac hypertrophy in rats. *J Clin Invest* 1982;70:1300–1305
6. Schaible TF, Ciambrone GJ, Capasso JM, Scheuer J: Cardiac conditioning ameliorates cardiac dysfunction associated with renal hypertension in rats. *J Clin Invest* 1984;73:1086–1094
7. Scheuer J, Buttrick PM: The cardiac hypertrophic response to physiologic and pathologic loads. *Circulation* 1987;75:I63–I68
8. Peterson MB, Lesch M: Protein synthesis and amino acid transport in the isolated rabbit right ventricular papillary muscle. Effect of isometric tension development. *Circ Res* 1972;31:317–327
9. Morgan HE, Chua BHL, Fuller EO, Siehl DL: Regulation of protein synthesis and degradation during *in vitro* cardiac work. *Am J Physiol* 1980;238:E431–E442
10. Kira Y, Kochel PJ, Gordon EE, Morgan HE: Aortic perfusion pressure as a determinant of cardiac protein synthesis. *Am J Physiol* 1984;246:C247–258
11. Xenophontos XP, Morgan HE: Effect of intraventricular pressure on protein synthesis in arrested rat hearts. *Am J Physiol* 1986;251:C95–C98
12. Takala T: Protein synthesis in the isolated perfused rat heart. Effects of mechanical workload, diastolic ventricular pressure, and coronary flow on amino acid incorporation and its transmural distribution into left ventricular protein. *Basic Res Cardiol* 1981;76:44–61
13. Schunkert H, Jahn L, Isumo S, Apstein CS, Lorell BH: Localization and regulation of c-fos and c-jun protooncogene induction by systolic wall stress in normal and hypertrophied rat hearts. *Proc Natl Acad Sci USA* 1991;88:11480–11484
14. Izumo S, Nadal-Ginard B, Mahdavi V: Protooncogene induction and

reprogramming of cardiac gene expression produced by pressure overload. *Proc Natl Acad Sci USA* 1988;85:339–343

15. Simpson PC: Role of protooncogenes in cardiac hypertrophy. *Am J Cardiol* 1988;62:13G–19G

16. Starksen NF, Simpson PC, Bishopric N, Coughlin SR, Lee WMF, Escobedo JA, Williams LT: Cardiac myocyte hypertrophy is associated with c-myc protooncogene expression. *Proc Natl Acad Sci USA* 1986;83:8348–8350

17. Korecky B, Masika M: Direct effects of increased hemodynamic load on cardiac mass. *Circ Res* 1991;68:1174–1178

18. Klein I, Hong C, Schreiber SS: Isovolumic loading prevents atrophy of the heterotopically transplanted rat heart. *Circ Res* 1991;69:1421–1425

19. Komuro I, Kaida T, Shibazaki Y, Kurabayashi M, Katoh Y, Hoh E, Takaku F, Yazaki Y: Stretching cardiac myocytes stimulates protooncogene expression. *J Biol Chem* 1990;265:3595–3598

20. Komuro I, Katoh K, Kaida T, Shibazaki Y, Kurabayashi M, Hoh E, Takaku F, Yazaki Y: Mechanical loading stimulates cell hypertrophy and specific gene expression in cultured rat cardiac myocytes. *J Biol Chem* 1991;266:1265–1268

21. Mann DL, Kent RL, Cooper G: Load regulation of the properties of adult feline cardiocytes: growth induction by cellular deformation. *Circ Res* 1989;64:1079–1090

22. Kent RL, Hoober KJ, Cooper G: Load responsiveness of protein synthesis in adult myocardium: role of cardiac deformation linked to sodium influx. *Circ Res* 1989;64:74–85

23. Guharay F, Sachs F: Stretch-activated single ion channel currents in tissue-cultured embryonic chick skeletal muscle. *J Physiol (Lond)* 1984;352:685–701

24. Morris CE: Mechanosensitive ion channels. *J Membrane Biol* 1990;113:93–107

25. Bustamante JO, Ruknudin A, Sachs F: Stretch-activated channels in heart cells: relevance to cardiac hypertrophy. *J Cardiovasc Pharm* 1991;17(suppl 2):S110–S113

26. Ross RS, O'Brien TX: The mouse that roared: cardiogenic applications of transgenic technology. *Heart Failure* 1992;8:109–120

27. Ascadi G, Jiao S, Duke D, Williams P, Chong W, Wolff JA: Direct gene transfer and expression into rat heart *in vivo*. *New Biol* 1991;3:71–81

28. Kitsis R, Buttrick P, McNally E, Kaplan ML, Leinwand LA: Hormonal modulation of a gene injected into rat heart in vivo. *Proc Natl Acad Sci USA* 1991;88:4138–4142

29a. Lin H, Parmacek MS, Morle G, Bolling S, Leiden JM: Expression of recombinant genes in myocardium in vivo after direct injection of DNA. *Circulation* 1990;82:2217–2221

29b. Buttrick PM, Kaplan ML, Kitsis RN, Leinwand LA: Distinct behavior of cardiac myosin heavy chain gene constructs in vivo. Discordance with in vitro results. *Circ Res* 1993;72:1211–1217

30. Tsika RW, Bahl JJ, Leinwand LA, Morkin E: Thyroid hormone regulates expression of a transfected human α myosin heavy chain fusion gene in fetal rat heart cells. *Proc Natl Acad Sci USA* 1990;87:379–383

31. Izumo SB, Nadal-Ginard B, Mahdavi V: All members of the MHC multigene family respond to thyroid hormone in a highly tissue-specific manner. *Science* 1986;231:597–600
32. Subramaniam A, Jones WK, Gulick J, Wert S, Neumann J, Robbins J: Tissue specific regulation of the α myosin heavy chain gene promoter in transgenic mice. *J Biol Chem* 1991;266:24613–24620

Chapter 7

Effects of Chronic Tachycardia on the Myocardium

C. David Ianuzzo, PhD, Peter J. O'Brien DVM, PhD, DVSc, Tomas A. Salerno, MD, and M. Harold Laughlin, PhD

This chapter provides some basic insights into the biochemical strategies of myocardial adaptations to chronic tachycardia; the underlying purpose is to provide the clinician with some basic information that he or she ultimately will apply to patient treatment. The use of data from mammals with inherently different resting heart rates but with the same stroke work index, wall stress, and arterial pressures provides a unique opportunity to view how the myocardium may adapt to tachycardia.[1-3] We have attempted to confirm the hypotheses put forth from the comparative tachycardia found in different-sized mammalian hearts[4,5] by using several experimental models. The findings from these experimental models support the hypotheses generated from the myocardial biochemical differences observed in the natural tachycardia found in different-sized mammalian myocardia.

Muscle cells contain three subcellular systems that are the underlying basis for muscle performance (Figure 1). In cardiac muscle the metabolic system is well developed, with the mitochondrial volume occupying 20–45% of the total cell volume. The metabolic pathways transduce substrate-derived bond energy into adenosine triphosphate (ATP), which is used primarily for regulating sarcoplasmic reticulum-cytosolic calcium cycling and for myosin cross-bridge cycling in highly active muscle. The

These studies were supported by NIH HL 36531, HL 36088, NSERC 0404 and Ontario Heart and Stroke Foundation Grants.

From Fletcher GF, (ed): *Cardiovascular Response to Exercise.* Mount Kisco, NY, Futura Publishing Company, Inc., © 1994.

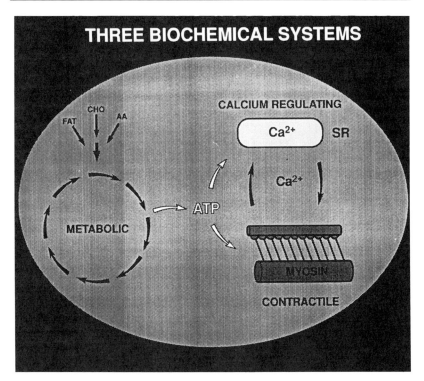

FIGURE 1. *The three primary subcellular systems that determine the physiological expression of the myocardium. The metabolic system transduces substrate-derived energy into ATP. The calcium-regulating and contractile systems use ATP to perform their respective functions in the cardiac myocyte. These three systems have the property of adapting to chronic alternations in myocardial function.*

adaptive strategies of these three systems are discussed in this chapter.

Heart rate is the prime determinant of cardiac minute work (*ie,* cardiac power output) and myocardial metabolism when other hemodynamic variables remain constant. We have used some experimental paradigms in which heart rate has been the independent variable with the purpose of studying the biochemical metabolic correlates associated with this hemodynamic parameter. Specific capacities for the enzymatic pathways of intermediary metabolism are essential to provide an adequate rate of substrate conversion for ATP production to support cardiac minute work. The extent to which these pathways and the associated mitochondrial organelle can expand to support myocardial energetic demands has some definite upper limits.[6] These enzyme pathways adapt by replicating copies of the same metabolic units and not by switching expression to a different protein isoform.[6] It was of interest to determine the extent to which these pathways adapt to accommodate tachycardiac demands.

The cyclical pumping of blood through the cardiovascular system by the heart is timed precisely by the cyclical pumping of Ca^{2+} from the myocardial sarcoplasm into the lumen of the sarcoplasmic reticulum (SR) by Ca^{2+}-ATPase.[7] During systole, Ca^{2+} rapidly diffuses through a Ca^{2+} release channel from the SR into the sarcoplasm and activates contraction as well as other cellular events. The Ca^{2+}-release channel is activated by entry into the cell of a small amount of "trigger" Ca^{2+} during a similar, but smaller, cyclical Ca^{2+} pumping mechanism situated at the cell surface membrane. The four major components of the SR Ca^{2+} cycle have been identified, cloned, and sequenced. There is only one cardiac isoform for each of these SR proteins: the Ca^{2+}-ATPase pump; calsequestrin, the Ca^{2+} storage protein; the ligand-gated Ca^{2+} release channel; and phospholamban, the Ca^{2+}-ATPase regulatory protein.[8-10] The components of the Ca^{2+} cycle of the surface membrane are a distinctive Ca^{2+}-ATPase, a Na^{+}-Ca^{2+} antiport, and voltage-gated Ca^{2+} channels. However, since this surface Ca^{2+} cycle plays a much less important role in adult mammalian ventricular myocytes than the SR Ca^{2+} cycle,[7] it is not reviewed in this chapter.

The SR has marked plasticity, that is, its amount and activity changes in response to altered functional demand or hormonal stimulation. The most plastic components of the Ca^{2+} cycle are the Ca^{2+}-ATPase pump and the Ca^{2+} release channel. Calsequestrin and phospholamban appear to be much less responsive, although muscle calsequestrin content may change in response to altered sarcoplasmic Ca^{2+} dynamics.[8-10] Therefore, in the series of studies described in this chapter, we have focused on the Ca^{2+} pump and channel.

The contractile protein system, which determines the contractile speed and energetic economy of the myocardium,[11] has fewer adaptive options to altered functional demands in comparison with the richness of options available to the skeletal muscle contractile system.[12] The main adaptive maneuver for the cardiac myocyte is to switch expression of its myosin isoform to either a V_1 (fast catalytic type) or V_3 (slow catalytic type). Other possibilities are phosphorylation of several of the contractile proteins.[13] Little is known at present about the adaptive role of phosphorylation of the cardiac contractile proteins. The contractile adaptations will focus on the possible myosin isoform switches with tachycardia.

Methods

Several different experimental models were used to study the effects of tachycardia on myocardial biochemical adaptations. A brief summary of the models and methodology is provided. The detailed methods are contained in the original papers, which are given in the references in this chapter.

Experimental Models

In the *comparative heart studies*, seven to nine different orders of mammals were used including the mouse, rat, guinea pig, white rabbit, mongrel dog, swine, sheep, and cattle.[4,5,14] These mammals were used because they had a 10-fold range in resting heart rates (RHR)[15,16] In the calcium regulation studies the seal, horse, and turkey also were used.

In one of our *chronic tachycardia studies,*[17] cardiac pacemakers (Medtronic, Inc., Minneapolis, MN) were implanted in nine Yorkshire pigs. The pacemaker lead was attached to the left atrium and the pulse generator set at 180 pulses/min. Control pigs were sham operated and had a suture placed in the left atrium. The duration of the tachycardial period was 35 to 42 days, after which the pigs were anesthetized and selected hemodynamic parameters measured at different pacing rates. In another study[18] mongrel dogs had cardiac pacemakers implanted with a unipolar lead placed in the apex of the right ventricle. One week after the surgical implantation procedure the pacemakers were activated and set at 250 beats per minute until the clinical symptoms of congestive heart failure developed. The average time period until the onset of failure was 4.4 ± 1.7 (SD) weeks.

Primary *cultures of neonatal rat cardiac myocytes* were prepared as previously described[19,20] and cultured for 14 days, 12 of which were in a serum-free defined medium. Flasks containing cultured cells were divided randomly into a spontaneously contracting group and into a group in which cells were arrested by 50 mM KCl or 10 μM verapamil (VER). Some flasks also were treated with 10 nM T_3 to determine the response of myosin expression.

In the *exercise-training study*, female Yucatan miniature swine were exercised for 85 minutes at running intensities ranging from 50–100% VO_2 max, 5 days/week for 16 to 22 weeks.[21] The trained pigs had an increased exercise tolerance, lower heart rates during submaximal exercise, moderate cardiac hypertrophy, increased coronary blood flow, and increased mitochondrial oxidative capacity in the exercised skeletal muscle.

Biochemical Procedures

Maximal enzyme activities were used as markers to estimate the maximal capacity of the common pathways of intermediary metabolism. The metabolic enzymes presented in this chapter are glycogen phosphorylase, 6-phosphofructokinase, hexokinase, lactate dehydrogenase, citrate synthase, and 3-hydroxyacyl-Co-A dehydrogenase. The ^{14}C-glucose and ^{14}C-palmitate oxidation rates were determined from the rate of production of radioactively labeled $^{14}CO_2$ from fresh whole heart homogenates. Detailed descriptions of these assays can be found in refs 4,17–19.

Tissue specimens used for Ca^{2+} transport studies were excised and flash frozen in liquid N_2 immediately after removing the beating hearts from the animals. The Ca^{2+}-transport activities by SR were estimated by directly monitoring Ca^{2+}-sequestration and Ca^{2+}-release activities of homogenates,[22] and by determining Ca^{2+}-dependent ATP hydrolytic activities of isolated SR membranes.[23,24] Mitochondrial ATPase activity, which represents the F1-ATP synthetase of the respiratory chain working in reverse, was determined as azide-inhibitable ATPase activity.[25] Total ATP cycling activity was defined as the sum of activities of the ATP-synthetase and all other ATPases. The Ca^{2+}-sequestration activity of myocardial homogenates was determined using radiometric emission spectrofluorometry and the fluorescent Ca^{2+} binding dye indo-1.[22,26]

The capacity of the contractile system was estimated from the following assays: Myofibrillar (MF) ATPase and myosin (M) ATPase activities were determined at pH 7.0 using isolated myofibrils as previously described by others.[5,14,21] M-ATPase activity was determined using purified myofibrils and calculated using 42% as the myosin portion of the total myofibrillar protein.[5] The percentages of cardiac ventricular myosin isoforms were determined by densitometric scanning after electrophoretic separation.[5]

Results

Metabolic System and Tachycardia

Tachycardia in Nature

Tachycardia was studied as it occurs in nature.[4,5] Different-sized mammals were used in these comparative heart studies that had a 25,000-fold difference in heart mass and a 10-fold difference in resting heart rates ranging from approximately 50 to 475 beats per minute.[15,16] The hemodynamic determinants of cardiac minute work rate among these different-sized mammals are constant, namely, stroke work index, mean arterial pressure, and ventricular wall stress,[1–3] with the only exception being heart rate. Therefore, heart rate could be isolated as the main determinant of cardiac power output and myocardial metabolic rate. The metabolic capacities of these hearts to transduce substrate-derived energy into ATP production was estimated using maximal activities of selected enzymes as the dependent variable and RHR as the independent variable. Correlation and regression analysis were accomplished. The regression equations derived from the comparative data were used for the prediction of data obtained from the other experimental models.[5] The coefficient of determination (R^2) has been presented as an estimate of the percent association between the independent RHR and dependent variables.

The capacity of the glycolytic pathway was estimated using several enzymes that represent the anaerobic and aerobic components of this enzyme pathway. Glycogen phosphorylase activity, the rate-limiting enzyme of glycogenolysis, remained relatively constant among these different mammalian hearts (Figure 2).[4,5] The average maximal activity of this enzyme for these mammals was approximately 18 U/g at 30°C. Extrapolating this activity to normal body temperature of 37°C, assuming a $Q_{10} = 2$, the reaction rate of glycogenolysis would allow for the complete catabolism of cardiac glycogen (40 µmol/g) within 2 minutes. The activity of phosphofructokinase, the rate-limiting enzyme of glycolysis, also was similar across these hearts that had a 10-fold difference in heart rates (Figure 2). The average maximal phosphofructokinase (PFK) activity was 39 U/g at 30°C. This activity level would provide for the anaerobic synthesis of 120 µmol ATP/min, which would provide the energetic support for about 570 heartbeats, assuming 0.21 µmol of ATP is used/beat/g.[27] In the case of the large mammal hearts, with 50 beats per minute, this substrate would provide ATP for about 10 minutes, whereas in the small hearts with rapid beating rates of 475 beats per minute the glycogen concentration would be depleted within about 1 minute in a totally anaerobic condition. The enzymes of glycolysis that are involved with aerobic carbohydrate metabolism (hexokinase and H-form of the lactate dehydrogenase enzyme) showed a positive correlation ($R^2 = 0.89$) with RHR.[4]

The mitochondrial capacities for aerobic metabolism and fatty acid oxidation were estimated by the activities of citrate synthase (CS) and 3-hydroxyacyl-CoA dehydrogenase (HADH), respectively. There was nearly a threefold difference in CS activity among these hearts, ranging from 73 U/g in the cattle hearts to 181 U/g in the mouse hearts. The coefficient of determination for CS versus RHR was $R^2 = 0.94$ (Figure 2). The correlative relationship between CS, a marker of myocardial oxidative capacity, and cardiac minute work rate (cardiac power output) was $R^2 = 0.98$ (Figure 2). HADH also had a threefold difference in activity ranging from 13 to 42 U/g from the cattle to the mouse, respectively ($R^2 = 0.86$) (Figure 2). The ^{14}C-glucose ($R^2 = 0.77$ vs. RHR) and ^{14}C-palmitate ($R^2 = 0.88$ vs. RHR) oxidation rates in whole heart homogenates were consistent with the positive correlations of these enzyme activities with RHR (Figure 2D).[4] Myofibrillar and myosin ATPase activities are discussed below.

In summary, the results from the comparative tachycardia study indicate that the anaerobic capacity of heart muscle did not correspond with differences with a range of 10-fold in cardiac power output, whereas the mitochondrial capacities for oxygen consumption and fat oxidation were highly associated with the RHR and power output of the myocardium.

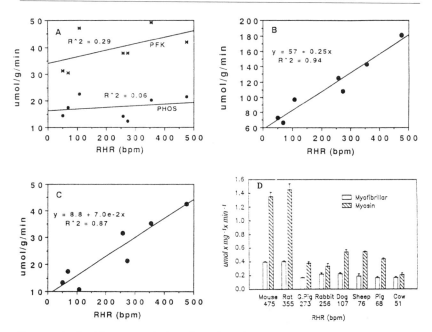

FIGURE 2. **A:** *Glycogenolytic [phosphorylase (PHOS) activity] and glyco-lytic [phosphofructokinase (PFK) activity] capacities of the myocardia from mammals with different resting heart rates (RHR).* **B:** *Mitochondrial aerobic capacity [citrate synthase (CS) activity] of hearts from different mammals.* **C:** *Fatty acid oxidative capacity [3-hydroxyacyl-Co-A dehydro-genase (HADA) activity] of hearts from different mammals.* **D:** *The myosin and myofibrillar ATPase activities of different mammal hearts.*

Chronic Experimental Tachycardia

Experimental tachycardia was imposed on the heart of a large mammal, the Yorkshire pig, to determine the possible causal relation-ship of cellular metabolic capacity to the hemodynamic parameter of heart rate.[17] The general hypothesis was that by imposing chronic tachycardia on the heart of a large mammal it would adapt its metabolic capacities in proportion to the imposed heart rate and, therefore, the metabolic character of the large mammal's heart would become more like that of a small mammal.

The glycolytic capacity (PFK activity) was unchanged after 5 to 6 weeks of chronic tachycardia at 180 beats per minute (Figure 3). This

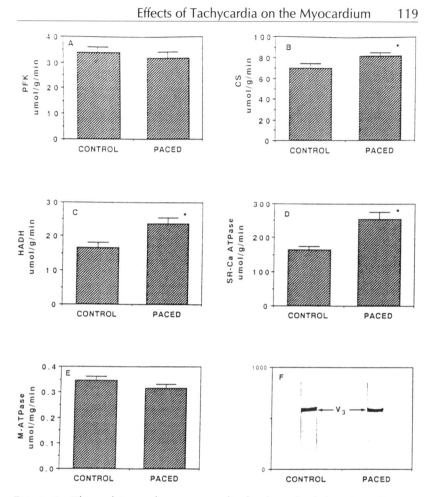

FIGURE 3. These data are from myocardia that have had chronic tachycardia imposed for a period of 5 to 6 weeks at double the normal resting heart rate (see text for explanation).

finding is consistent with the prediction from the comparative heart data indicating that glycolytic capacity is constant and not mutable by contractile frequency. The mitochondrial oxidative capacity (CS activity) was increased 20% by chronic pacing (Figure 3). The predicted percent increase using the linear regression equation also was 20%, although the actual predicted activity was 102 U/g, compared with the actual of 82 U/g. The fatty acid oxidative capacity increased 42% with tachycardia, with the predicted increase being 57% (Figure 3). From these findings it appears that heart rate is a hemodynamic correlate of mitochondrial capacity and not glycolytic potential. This would be predicted from the comparative data.

Chronic tachycardia also was studied in a canine model in collaboration with Armstrong's group at the University of Toronto (St. Michael's Hospital).[18] Chronic rapid ventricular pacing has been shown to be an effective method for producing congestive heart failure. After ventricular pacing at 250 beats per minute severe clinical congestive heart failure occurred at 4.4 ± 1.7 (SD) weeks. PFK activity was reduced by 30% compared with the sham-operated animals. This decline in glycolytic capacity would not have been predicted from the comparative data. Mitochondrial oxidative capacity (CS activity) was predicted to increase by about 40%. In contrast to this prediction, there was no significant change observed in the failing hearts compared with those from the control sham-operated animals. Another TCA cycle enzyme, oxoglutarate dehydrogenase, did, however, show a 60% increase in activity, but in the judgment of these authors CS activity is a more reliable mitochondrial marker. HADH activity increased in the failing paced hearts by 30%, whereas the predicted percentage change was 75%. The differential changes between CS and HADH are difficult to interpret since the TCA cycle and fatty acid oxidative capacities usually covary.

In summary, the level of chronic tachycardia imposed on the canine hearts, which ultimately results in failure, did not result in predictable adaptive metabolic changes in the canine myocardium. However, predictable adaptations may have occurred at an earlier time before cardiac failure ensued. This lack of predictability with excessive tachycardia may be an indicator of heart failure. The disproportionate adaptations of these three essential subcellular systems may be implicated as the cause of failure resulting from chronic tachycardia.

Cultured Cardiac Myocytes

In another attempt to test whether contractile frequency was a determinant of the level of myocardial metabolic capacity, neonatal cardiac myocytes were cultured and maintained in defined medium for 12 days.[20] Some of the cultured cells were allowed to beat

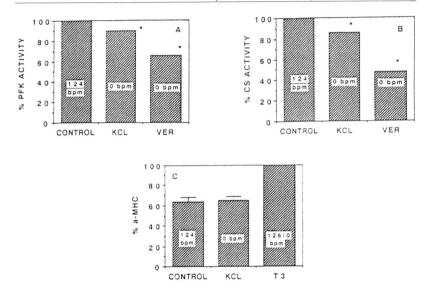

FIGURE 4. These figures summarize the data from cultured cardiac myocytes that were beating spontaneously compared with those that were arrested by KC1 or verapamil (VER). (See text for a further description.)

spontaneously (average rate was 124 beats per minute), whereas others were arrested by adding KCl or verapamil (VER) to the culture medium (Figure 4). PFK activity was not affected by contractile arrest from membrane depolarization, which was consistent with the comparative data. Contractile arrest using the Ca^{2+} channel blocker, VER, resulted in a 50% lower PFK activity, suggesting the level of cytosolic Ca^{2+} may be involved in maintaining myocardial glycolytic enzyme levels. CS activity was reduced by 15% in the KCl arrested cells and by 50% in the VER cells. The predicted percentage decline in CS activity as a result of the reduction in contractile frequency was 35%. The metabolic changes observed in the arrested cultured myocytes were predictable from the comparative data, with the exception of the VER-treated cultures.

Exercise-training Study

In the studies described, chronic myocardial contractile frequency was found to be highly correlated with mitochondrial oxidative and fatty metabolic capacities. The purpose of this study was to use daily exercise to determine whether or not a daily pulse dose of tachycardia was an adequate stimulus to induce the changes that were predicted from the comparative data.[21] A daily pulse of tachycardia was administrated to porcine hearts by daily treadmill exercise for 85 minutes at differing intensities that required a heart rate of between 200 and 300 beats per minute for a period of 16 to 22 weeks. The findings showed PFK activity was unchanged after exercise training (Figure 5). This was consistent with the prediction from the comparative data. Furthermore, neither CS nor HADH

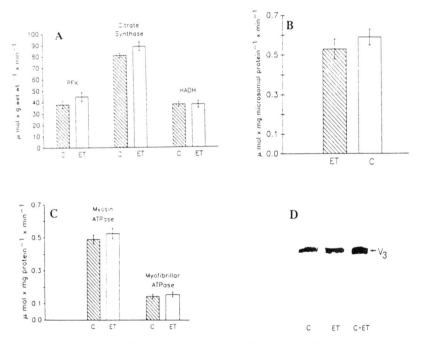

FIGURE 5. A: *Metabolic enzyme activities from control (c) and exercise-trained (ET) pig hearts.* B: *Sarcoplasmic reticulum ATPase activity in the microsomal fraction of control (C) and exercise-trained (ET) pig hearts.* C: *Myosin and myofibrillar ATPase activities of control (C) and exercise-trained (ET) pig hearts.* D: *Polyacrylamide gel electrophoretograms of native myosin from control (C), exercise-trained (ET), and co-electrophoresed C and ET myosin. (See text for a further explanation.) Reproduced with permission from Reference 21.*

activities were altered by this training program (Figure 5). If this pulsed dose of tachycardia associated with daily exercise provided a stimulus equivalent to chronic tachycardia, a 30–50% increase in mitochondrial capacity would have been expected.

In summary, it appears that endurance training resulting from daily exercise does not provide an adequate enough stimulus to induce changes in the glycolytic or mitochondrial capacities of the trained porcine myocardium. It is possible, however, that the tachycardia during exercise is counterbalanced by the bradycardia that occurs in the trained pig heart for the remainder of a normal day (*ie*, 80% of the day of nonexercise); thus, adaptations are not evident.

Ca^{2+} Regulatory System

Tachycardia in Nature

In Figure 6, the inter-relationships between Ca^{2+} cycling activities, ATP cycling activity (as defined above), and RHR are indicated for various species of animals with widely varying RHR. These animals included cow, calf, seal, sheep, pig, dog, horse, rat, rabbit, guinea pig, turkey, and mouse. To compare graphs more easily, all values are expressed as a percentage of the mean value for dogs. There was a strong log-linear relationship between heart rate and both of the cycling activities (Figures 6C and D), each of which was linearly correlated with the other. The largest differences in Ca^{2+}-ATPase activities were observed in the comparative study of mammals, where activity was 10-fold greater for the mouse than for the cow.[5,14,25] Differences across species of mammals in SR Ca^{2+}-ATPase activities were not attributable to differences in specific activity but rather to differences in the amount of membrane yields.

Using the comparative mammal model, Ca^{2+} sequestration and Ca^{2+} release activities of myocardial homogenates also were determined (Figures 6B and C). The Ca^{2+}-uptake activity was only threefold greater in the mouse than the cow. Ca^{2+}-release activity when corrected for the influence of Ca^{2+}-uptake activity[28] (by dividing by Ca^{2+}-pump activity), also was threefold higher in the mouse compared with the cow.

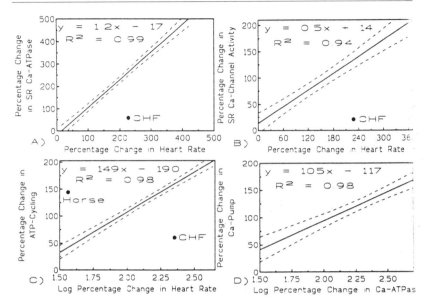

FIGURE 6. *Inter-relationships of Ca cycle, ATP cycle, and cardiac cycle. Correlations between the Ca and ATP cycling (as defined in text) activity and resting heart rate are indicated for various species of animals with widely varying resting heart rates, including cow, calf, seal, sheep, pig, dog, horse, rat, rabbit, guinea pig, turkey, and mouse. Lines of regression are plotted with the 95% confidence intervals. To compare graphs more easily, all values are expressed as a percentage of the mean value for dogs. For* **A,** *values for the various models of tachy- or bradycardia are also plotted: moderate chronic pacing, severe pacing leading to heart failure, cardiac transplantation, and dysthyroidism. In* **A, B,** *and* **C,** *the value falling below the 95% confidence interval for the line of regression is for dogs with congestive heart failure due to rapid ventricular pacing. In* **C,** *the value found above the 95% confidence interval for the line of regression is for the horse.*

Chronic Experimental Tachycardia

Chronic, moderate tachycardia produced by 5 to 6 weeks of atrial pacing of 20-kg swine at double the RHR was associated with a 50% greater Ca^{2+}-ATPase specific activity, with no difference in SR yield.[17,24] This increase was in marked contrast to the decrease we observed with severe tachycardia.[18] Rapid ventricular pacing of adult dogs for 5 to 6 weeks at 250% of their RHR resulted in 30–50% decreases in Ca^{2+}-ATPase and Ca^{2+}-uptake activity of isolated SR and homogenates. The pulsed tachycardia from daily exercise resulted in no detectable difference in specific activity of myocardial SR ATPase after chronic treadmill exercise training of swine.[21] However, in the perfused, nonpumping, transplanted heart there was a 20% reduction in the yield, with no change in specific activity, of SR membranes in association with an approximately 25% reduction in heart rate, but this model also had a reduction in stroke work.[29]

Other Models of Tachycardia

In addition to data from the comparative mammal model (Figure 6A), the percentage change (or difference) in isolated SR Ca^{2+}-ATPase activity has been plotted against the percentage change in heart rate for the various models of tachy- or bradycardia: moderate chronic pacing, severe pacing leading to heart failure, cardiac transplantation, and dysthyroidism. With the exception of dogs with heart failure produced by excessive pacing, all values fell within the 95% confidence interval of the least-squares regression line.

Chronic electrical stimulation of canine latissimus dorsi muscle at the same frequency as the RHR resulted in the SR Ca^{2+}-ATPase activity being reduced by more than 80% to an activity indistinguishable from that of canine myocardium (data not shown).[30,31]

The tachy- or bradycardia produced by dysthyroidism were proportionate in severity to the change in myocardial Ca^{2+}-cycling activity.[24] Moderately hyperthyroid rats, with a 250% increased serum T_3 concentration compared with controls, had approximately a 50% increase in both heart rate and specific activity of the Ca^{2+}-ATPase in isolated SR. In contrast, moderately hypothyroid rats, with a 75% reduced serum T_3 concentration compared wtih controls, produced a 50% decrease in both of these parameters. Comparable findings were made for mildly dysthyroid rabbits. Mildly hyperthyroid rabbits, with a 130% increased serum T_3 concentrations compared with controls, had a 30% decreased SR Ca^{2+}-ATPase, whereas mildly hypothyroid rabbits with a 30% decreased serum T_3 concentration compared with controls had a 30% decreased Ca^{2+}-ATPase.[32]

Contractile System

Myosin is the major contractile protein and is a determinant of the velocity and the energetic efficiency of cardiac muscle contraction.[11] Therefore, the capacity of the contractile system was examined in the following studies by determining the protein isoforms of myosin and the MF-ATPase and myosin M-ATPase activities.

Tachycardia in Nature

In hearts of these different mammals with a 10-fold difference in RHR it was postulated that the capacity of he contractile system would be congruent with the chronotropic rate of the different myocardia. We observed,[5,14] as did Lompre et al.,[33] that large mammals with slow RHR have a slow cardiac myosin isoform (V_3) and a low catalytic activity for both M- and MF-ATPases compared with those of smaller mammals. The most interesting observation was that a switch in the cardiac ventricular myosin isoform occurred between the guinea pig and the rat, which have RHRs of 270 and 350 beats per minute, respectively (Figure 2). From this observation it was hypothesized that there is a "threshold" heart rate of approximately 300 beats per minute that is associated with the switch in myosin isoforms from a V_3 to a V_1.

Chronic Experimental Tachycardia

To test whether chronotropism had a causal relationship on myosin gene expression, the hearts of two different large mammals had cardiac pacemakers implanted and the impulse generator set at 180 beats per minute for the Yorkshire pigs and at 250 beats per minute for the canine hearts. After 5 to 6 weeks of myocardial pacing at 180 beats per minute of the Yorkshire pig hearts, the myosin isoform remained V_3, as indicated by only a single band in the polyacrylamide pyrophosphate gel electrophoretograms (Figure 3). The M-ATPase activity of purified myosin preparations was similar for both the sham-operated and paced hearts (Figure 3). There was no indication of failure in the swine hearts as shown by the hemodynamic measurements.[17]

The canine myocardia were paced at 250 beats per minute until the clinical symptoms of congestive heart failure were evident. There was no evidence of a switch in myosin isoform or in M-ATPase activity in the paced versus sham-operated hearts. However, there was a 25% decline in MF-ATPase activity. In summary, these findings are in agreement with the predicted outcome from the comparative data, namely, that a change in myosin isoform would not be expected until a chronic tachycardia of about 300 beats per minute was achieved. This did not occur in either the swine hearts, which had no evidence of failure, or in the failing canine hearts.

Cultured Cardiac Myocytes

In this study neonatal myocytes were cultured for 12 days in defined medium.[20] Flasks containing cultured cells were randomly selected either to contract spontaneously or to become KCl arrested to determine if contractile activity influenced myosin expression. The percentage of the α-myosin heavy chain (α-MHC) was $64 \pm 4\%$ in cells that were spontaneously beating at 124 beats per minute and $65 \pm 4\%$ in the arrested cells (Figure 4). Both the contracting and quiescent cultured cells were able to alter myosin gene expression, as noted by the 100% expression of α-MHC when treated with T_3 (Figure 4). The lack of change in myosin type at these beating rates was consistent with the hypothesis put forth from the comparative data.

Exercise Training

To determine whether a daily pulsed dose of tachycardia (200–300 beats per minute) produced by moderate-to high-intensity endurance exercise would alter cardiac myosin expression from 100% V_3 toward V_1, exercise-trained pig hearts were examined for myosin changes. The effects of training were confirmed after 16 to 22 weeks of exercise by increased exercise tolerance, bradycardia during exercise, increased coronary blood flow capacity, cardiac hypertrophy, and increased mitochondrial oxidative capacity of the exercised limb muscles.[21] This training protocol resulted in no changes in the percentage of V_3 or V_1 myosin isoform or in M-ATPase or MF-ATPase activities in the trained versus control pig hearts (Figure 5). In summary, a daily pulse of exercise-induced tachycardia, which reached 300 beats per minute during the intermittent sprints portion of the exercise, was found to be an adequate stimulus to induce a switch in ventricular myosin isoforms from V_3 to V_1 in the heart of this large mammal.

Discussion

Metabolic Adaptations to Tachycardia

The metabolic enzyme data from these studies suggest the anaerobic aspect of glycolysis is not mutable by the physiological stimulus of tachycardia when the other hemodynamic factors that determine cardiac minute work are constant. These findings agree with those from the exercise-training studies involving skeletal muscle,[34] but do not agree with the changes that occur in glycolytic capacity in skeletal muscle with continuous contractile activity produced by chronic electrical stimulation.[30] Glycolytic capacity also is altered when stroke work is reduced.[29] Although those studies demonstrate that contractile activity of skeletal muscle and certain hemodynamic factors other than heart rate can influence the glycolytic potential, in studies in which heart rate was the main determinant of cardiac power output, the anaerobic glycolytic capacity remained constant. This was not the case for the aerobic components of the glycolytic pathway. The correlative association of RHR with hexokinase (HK) and heart lactate dehydrogenase (H-LDH) implies that these components of glycolysis do adapt to tachycardia probably to accommodate the added requirements for the transport of plasma glucose and the uptake and use of blood lactate. The studies of experimentally imposed chronic tachycardia, culture myocytes, and exercise training all support the findings from the comparative heart study that the cardiac glycolytic potential is highly resistant to changes in contractile frequency. Thus, the general conclusion drawn from these studies as it relates to the adaptations of glycolysis is that anaerobic glycolysis is not mutable when challenged by chronic tachycardia. The aerobic aspects of glycolysis, on the other hand, are adaptable in what is an apparent attempt to use more exogenous substrates. This constant glycolytic capacity provides the myocardium with a stable energetic reserve capacity when it is challenged by anaerobic conditions. However, the hearts with slower RHRs have a 10-fold greater effective reserve during anaerobic types of myocardial stresses (eg, during ischemia) than do hearts with high beating rates.

The capacities of the metabolic systems associated with the mitochondrion are highly correlated with the frequency of myocardial contractions. These data suggest that the energetic strategy of the myocardium when adapting to tachycardia is to expand its mitochondrial aerobic and fatty acid oxidation capcities to correspond with the increase in cardiac power output. This principle has been observed for a wide variety of vertebrates.[35] The increase in the mitochondrial volume density required to accommodate this increase in aerobic metabolism ranges from a mitochondrial volume of about 20% in the cow to 40% in the mouse.[5,36,37] It is interesting, but in conflict with the tachycardiac studies, that experimentally imposed bradycardia also has been reported to increase oxidative capacity.[38]

Since the combined mitochondrial and myofibrillar volumes occupy 90% of the cell volume, there must be a reciprocal change in these two cellular systems when adaptation occurs by the expansion of the volume density of either of these two subcellular systems. Therefore, as mitochondrial volume increases, the contractile system must undergo a reciprocal decrease accompanied by a commensurate loss in force-generating capacity. Thus, there must be an upper limit in the amount of mitochondrial expansion that can occur and still retain the required level of force-generating capacity to maintain adequate hemodynamics. Hochachka[6] has indicated that the shrew heart with 45% mitochondrial volume and with an equivalent myofibrillar volume may have reached the upper limit for a mammalian heart.

The adaptive strategy of increasing mitochondrial enzyme activities is to increase fatty acid oxidation rates without increasing the fatty acid concentration. Based on Michaelis-Menten kinetics, an increase in enzyme activity would result in a proportional increase in the reaction rate without a change in substrate concentration.[34] In cardiac muscle with metabolic rates that correspond with RHR, it seems logical to increase fat metabolism in proportion to total aerobic myocardial metabolism in order to conserve the limited source of cardiac glycogen.

The metabolic findings from the experimentally imposed tachycardia studies are consistent with the assumption that the biochemical differences in the hearts among different orders of mammals results from adaptations to the different heart rates and not from intrinsic phylogenic characteristics.[35] The findings from experimentally paced hearts along with those from the cultured cardiac myocyte study[20] indicate that the adaptive metabolic strategy of the myocardium to tachycardia is to increase its mitochondrial capacity while maintaining a constant anaerobic glycolysis capacity. This is analogous to the metabolic adaptations that occur in skeletal muscle with endurance training.[34] The extent of these metabolic adaptations can be reasonably well predicted from the linear regression equations based on heart rates. However, in the experimental condition in which a contractile frequency overload was imposed, congestive heart failure occurred[18] and the biochemical changes were either maladaptations or undertook a different adaptive strategy that was not predictable from the regression equations.

The clinical insights provided by these findings indicate that the myocardium has the capability to up-regulate its mitochondrial aerobic capacity when exposed to chronic tachycardia, thus demonstrating that mitochondrial capacity is not at its upper limit in the heart of a large mammal such as a human. Therefore, the inability to up-regulate mitochondrial biogenesis is not the apparent cause of failure caused by tachycardiac overload. These findings suggest further that the reduced myocardial ATP concentration found in congestive heart failure produced by rapid ventricular pacing was not the cause of the failure but was possibly an adaptive maneuver to increase free adenosine diphosphate (ATP) to drive mitochondrial respiration at a higher rate in order to maintain ATP turnover without increasing mitochondrial cell volume, which would require a commensurate reduction in myofibrillar volume and force-generating capacity per unit tissue cross-section.[39] The failure induced by chronic tachycardia does not appear to be associated etiologically with limitations in mitochondrial capacity. Furthermore, it is unlike ischemia-induced failure since it is not vascular in origin and has a different energy status profile.[39]

Adaptations of Calcium Regulation to Tachycardia

Data presented and reviewed in this chapter indicate that in the normofunctioning state, heart rate is a hemodynamic correlate of myocardial Ca^{2+}-cycling activity. There is an approximately 1:1 relationship between the cardiac cycling of blood in and out of the ventricles and the cycling of Ca^{2+} in and out of the myocardial SR. The chronotropic effects on the heart found in all of the animal models used in the series of studies described herein were associated with similar percentage changes in myocardial Ca^{2+}-cycling activity. Tachycardia, whether due to thyroid hormone,[24,32] moderately rapid pacing,[17,24] or increased basal metabolic rate,[5,14,25] was associated with proportionately increased Ca^{2+} cycling. Bradycardia, whether due to lack of thyroid hormone,[24,32] heterotopic transplantation,[29] or decreased basal metabolic rate,[5,14,25] was associated with proportionately decreased Ca^{2+} cycling.

β-Adrenergic stimulation of the heart has chronotropic and inotropic effects because of increased rate and magnitude of cardiac relaxation and contraction. The biochemcal basis for the enhanced activity lies in the increased rate and magnitude of Ca^{2+} cyclying.[40] In addition, decreased Ca^{2+} sensitivity of myofibrils facilitates relaxation and shortens the contraction–relaxation cycle.[41] These changes are effected by phosphorylation of key regulatory proteins, including the voltage-gated Ca^{2+} channel and Ca^{2+}-ATPase of the surface membrane, phospholamban, which is the endogenous inhibitor of the SR Ca^{2+}-ATPase, and troponin-I, which mediates the Ca^{2+} sensitivity of myofibrils. Furthermore, the level of phosphorylation is enhanced by phosphorylation of a cytoplasmic inhibitor-1, which inhibits protein phosphatases. Phosphorylation of surface Ca^{2+} channels increases their activity, and consequently the activity of the SR Ca^{2+} release channel, by admission of more "trigger" Ca^{2+} at a faster rate. Phosphorylation of the surface membrane Ca^{2+}-ATPase accelerates the extrusion of the additional trigger Ca^{2+} during relaxation.[42] Phosphorylated phospholamban dissociates from and disinhibits the SR Ca^{2+}-ATPase, resulting in its increased activity and affinity for Ca^{2+}. Phosphorylation of troponin-I decreases its sensitivity to Ca^{2+}.

The hypothesis that heart rate is a hemodynamic correlate of SR Ca^{2+}-cycling activity is supported further by reports that with acute, short-term tachycardia due to β-adrenergic stimulation, there is increased protein phosphorylation and consequently increased SR activity.[43]

With excessive chronotropic stimulation of the canine heart, produced by rapid ventricular pacing, there was apparent dissociation of heart rate, which was increased, and SR Ca^{2+}-pumping activity, which was decreased. The excessive activity produced myocardial fatigue and failure.[18] The biochemical, physiological, and clinical features of this heart failure state were similar to those arising from excessive stimulation by thyroid hormone, exhaustive exercise, and chronic volume or pressure overload. The basis for this apparent dissociation may lie in the adaptive strategy of the heart in compensating for excessive overload. We have determined recently that in the development of heart failure, the apparent strategy of the myocardium is not only to mildly down-regulate SR Ca^{2+}-ATPase but to markedly down-regulate its SR Ca^{2+} channel.[28] Furthermore, Ca^{2+} channel activity is inhibited in heart failure.[28] These changes reduce by 50% the total amount of Ca^{2+} cycled and, therefore, conserve energy. Thus, the Ca^{2+}-ATPase pumping activity need not be increased to produce tachycardia since the amount of Ca^{2+} transported per beat is 50% reduced.

The horse was found not to be consistent with the other animals studied with respect to ATP cycling, but was substantially higher compared with other mammals. This may result from the horse having an unusually high vagal tone at rest, and therefore an unusually low RHR.[44] Alternatively, it may reflect that the horse is an elite athlete among mammals, with a higher heart-to-body weight ratio, higher maximum heart rate, and higher maximal oxygen uptake per body mass than other mammals of similar size.[45]

The range of homogenate Ca^{2+} uptake and release activities across species was approximately threefold smaller than the range for isolated SR Ca^{2+}-ATPase activities. However, Ca^{2+} flux activities are expressed per volume of entire myocardium and not per volume of Ca^{2+}-diffusible space, resulting in the homogenate method underestimating the in vivo activity. The volume fraction of sarcoplasm, the intracellular Ca^{2+}-diffusing space, apparently is reduced substantially in species with more rapid heart rates, in order to accommodate proliferation of organelles. In these species, compared with animals with slower hearts, the volume fraction of mitochondria and SR is increased substantially, moreso than the volume fraction of myofibrils is decreased. For example, the mitochondria, SR, and myofibril volume fractions in the mouse are 33, 7, and 48%, whereas in the cow they are 19, 1, and 57%, resulting in a net loss of 11% cell volume for sarcoplasm in the smaller mammal.[46,47] There are only mild differnces in nuclear volume fractions (1–3%) for myocytes of different species.[46,48] Furthermore, the volume fraction for the interstitial space of myocardium is relatively constant across species.[46,48,49] These differences in organelle volume fractions across species would result in the sarcoplasmic volume fraction, which in the mouse is estimated to be 5–6%,[43] being approximately two- to threefold less in the mouse than the cow. Furthermore, since the rate of lowering the homogenate Ca^{2+} is linearly related to he Ca^{2+}-ATPase, when sarcoplasmic volume fraction is constant, but is logarithmically related to Ca^{2+}-ATPase activity across mammals with different sarcoplasmic volumes, the relationship of sarcoplasmic volume and heart rate is log-linear.

The direct relationship between Ca^{2+}-cycling rates and heart rates has important clinical implications. In heart disease, the reduction in the maximal rate of Ca^{2+} cycling by myocardial sarcoplasmic reticulum that occurs[18,22,28,50] must be reflected in a comparable reduction in the maximal rate of blood cycling by the heart. This relationship provides a rationale for understanding the basis for alterations in clinical cardiologic measurements of heart rate, including maximal heart rate, and heart rate variability,[28] both of which must be limited by Ca^{2+} cycling capacity. We have shown recently that in dogs with congestive heart failure, occurring either spontaneously or because of rapid ventricular pacing, both heart rate variability and Ca^{2+} channel release activity (the most sensitive indicator of impaired Ca^{2+}-cycling activity) are reduced by approximately 80%.[50] This reduction of heart rate variability may be the most important and accessible clinical predictor of cardiac patients who are at risk of sudden death or serious ventricular arrhythmia.[51]

Adaptations of the Contractile System to Tachycardia

The type of myosin protein isoform expressed is a primary determinant of the contractile characteristics of muscle. Myosin types with fast catalytic rate result in a rapid velocity of shortening and contractile power, whereas slow myosin isoforms provide added energetic economy.[11] In skeletal muscle, fast and slow myosin types are associated with high-intensity power movements and fatigue-resistant endurance activities, respectively. In cardiac ventricles two myosin types (fast—V_1, slow—V_3) exist. There are several factors that can cause a switch in gene expression of the two myosin heavy chain genes (α and β), which are the basis of the three myosin protein isoforms (V_1, V_2, V_3).[52] These factors include hormonal, nutritional, developmental, and physiological demands. Altered physiological demands such as pressure overload of the rat myocardium resulting in hypertrophy and a switch in myosin from the V_1 toward the V_3 and exercise-training studies using rodents have shown small percentage increases in the already predominant V_1 myosin isoform.[53] The physiological demand of chronic tachycardia does not appear to induce a switch in the myosin type from a V_3 to a V_1 in the various experimental approaches used by us. The hypothesis put forth from the comparative findings is that if heart rate is the hemodynamic signal for switching myosin expression the rate must be in the 300-beats per minute range.[5] This hypothesis was supported by a recent study[54] in which heterotopically transplanted rat hearts were paced experimentally to prevent the usual decline in rate to determine whether the shift in myosin isoforms would be prevented. The paced hearts retained the same percentage of V_1 myosin as the native hearts, whereas the nonpaced transplanted hearts switched to increasing the expression of the β-type of myosin.

The effects of exercise training on cardiac myosin expression have been of considerable interest to diverse research groups. The findings have been both conflicting and controversial. The question of whether exercise training causes a rebalancing of the percent of myosin types in the cardiac ventricles has not been definitively answered. It appears that training by submaximal running of large mammals does not result in myosin changes.[21,53] The effects of training on the hearts of small rodents is not clear. Swim training has been shown to result in the increase of the already predominant V_1 myosin type and the ATPase activities of the contractile proteins.[53] The change in the myosin protein and its ATPases recently have been shown by the clever use of the heterotopic heart transplant procedure to be induced by humoral and hormonal changes that are specific to the stress associated with swimming.[55,56] In contrast to swim training, training by submaximal treadmill exercise has, for the most part, been reported to result in little or no change in myosin.[53] If an up-regulation of myosin were to occur with exercise training, it would be expected to result from training of large mammals that have a 100% V_3 myosin type, which allows for the full range of up-regulation to occur. In a recent study by us,[21] high level, long-term, endurance treadmill training of a large mammal gave no indication that there was a change in the myosin isoform or in the activities of its ATPases. Our findings in combination with those of others[53] provide convicing evidence that the daily pulsed hemodynamic overload associated with moderate to high intensity endurance exercise is not adequate to induce myosin changes in the heart of a large mammal, which has a myosin type similar to that of humans.

Chronic tachycardia within the range allowed by the human heart does not result in re-expression of myosin from a V_3(slow) to a V_1(fast). Thus, a shift to a less energetically efficient myosin isoform cannot be implicated as the cause of myocardial failure. Although one could suggest that the V_3 isoform is not as efficient in this chronic tachycardiac condition and a myosin shift would be beneficial, the comparative findings argue against that viewpoint. There has been a considerable amount of investigation into the possible involvement of the contractile proteins in cardiac failure. Congestive failure induced by rapid ventricular pacing has been reported to have a reduced myofibrillar ATPase activity[18] without a change in myosin isoforms. This suggests possible alterations in the regulatory proteins, isoforms, or covalent phosphorylation parameters, which have not been investigated in this heart failure model.

Summary

Several different experimental models have been studied with the purpose of determining the biochemical adaptive strategy of the myocardium when it is challenged by chronic tachycardia. The comparative differences observed in the capacities of the three major subcellular systems that are the basis of myocardial performance between different mammalian hearts with a 10-fold range in resting heart rates has provided considerable insight into tachycardial adaptations. The regression equations derived from the data from tachycardia found in nature were shown to have good predictive capabilities when used on other experimental models. The fundamental adaptive strategy of the myocardium when exposed to chronic tachycardia is to increase its aerobic, glycolytic, and mitochondrial capacities while retaining a constant anaerobic glycoltyic reserve. The calcium regulating system increases both its calcium uptake and release capacities in proportion to the imposed chronotropism. This system appears to be the most responsive and closely associated with tachycardia. The major contractile protein, myosin, is relatively immutable to levels of tachycardia below the hypothesized "threshold" heart rate of 300 beats per minute, at which the switch in myosin expression may occur.

The adaptations predicted from the comparative and chronic tachycardia data of these three systems to endurance types of exercise training are minor. The empirical data confirm these predictions showing that no major metabolic, calcium, or contractile adaptations are commonly observed in the myocardia of large mammals after training. The subcellular and biochemical basis for the changes in myocardial performance with training remains unanswered.

The three subcellular systems in the hearts of the different-sized mammals studied showed that a proportional relationship exists between the capacities of aerobic energy transducing of the mitochondria and the two major energy-using systems (Ca^{2+} regulation and contraction). It has been estimated that one third of the ATP production is used for calcium cycling and two thirds for cross-bridge cycling and that more than 90% of the ATP is synthesized by aerobic metabolism located within the mitochondria. Therefore, we calculated a cellular capacity quotient (CCQ) as shown below. Since all but 10% of the ATP production is used in the processes of excitation-contraction coupling and cross-bridge cycling, the small amount used in other cellular processes was not included in this CCQ formula.

$$CCQ = \frac{\frac{1}{3} \text{ Ca}^{2+} \text{ Regulatory System Capacity} + \frac{2}{3} \text{ Contractile System Capacity}}{\text{Mitochondrial Aerobic Capacity}}$$

SR-ATPase and MF-ATPase activities are used to represent the calcium and contractile systems, respectively, and citrate synthase as the aerobic metabolic indicator, the CCQ is relatively constant (5×10^{-3}) across a wide range of mammal hearts with significantly different capacities for each of these three systems. It may be necessary to retain this proportionality to maintain normal myocardial function. For example, when this proportionally was reduced by about 30%, congestive heart failure was evident.[18] This quotient in normal heart muscle (a muscle with nonfatiguable properties) is different by 10- and 30-fold from fatiguable skeletal muscle of sheep and dog, respectively.[14,30,31] When skeletal muscle is transformed electrically for use in cardiac assist devices, the CCQ changes from about 150×10^{-3} in sheep and from 50×10^{-3} in dog latissimus dorsi muscles, respectively, to 17×10^{-3} for the muscles of both of these animals, which is approaching the value for heart muscle. This concept may prove useful as an index to evaluate the cellular status of the myocardium in pathological conditions.

Acknowledgment

The authors wish to thank Loretta D'Costa for proofreading this chapter.

References

1. Coulson R, Hernandez T, Herbert J: Metabolic rate, enzyme kinetics *in vivo*. *Comp Biochem Physiol* 1977;56A:251–262
2. Henderson A, Craig R, Sonnenblick E, Urschel CW: Species differences in intrinsic myocardial contractility. *Proc Soc Exp Biol Med* 1970;134: 930–932
3. Holt J, Rhode E, Kines H: Ventricular volumes and body weights in mammals. *Am J Physiol* 1968;215:704–715
4. Blank S, Chen V, Hamilton H, Salerno TA, Ianuzzo CD: Biochemical characteristics of mammalian myocardia. *J Mol Cell Cardiol* 1989;21:367–373
5. Ianuzzo CD, Blank S, Hamilton N, O'Brien PJ, Chen V: The relationship of myocardial chronotropism to the biochemical capacities of mammalian hearts. *Inter Series Sport Sci* 1990;21:145–163
6. Hochachka P: The biochemical limits of muscle work. *Int Series Sport Sci* 1990;21:1–9
7. Carafoli E: The homeostatis of calcium in heart cells. *J Mol Cell Cardiol* 1985;17:203–212
8. Arai M, Otsu K, MacLennan DH, Alpert NR, Periasmy M: Effect of thyroid hormone on the expression of mRNA encoding sarcoplasmic reticulum proteins. *Circ Res* 1991;69:266–276
9. Arai M, Otsu K, MacLennan DH, Periasmy M: Regulation of sarcoplasmic reticulum gene expression during cardiac and skeletal muscle development. *Am J Physiol* 1992;262:C614–C620
10. Nagai R, Zarain-Herxberg A, Brandl CJ, Fujü J, Tada M, MacLennan DH, Alpert NR, Periasmy M: Regulation of the myocardial Ca-ATPase and phospholamban mRNA expression in response to pressure overload and thyroid hormone. *Proc Natl Acad Sci* 1989;86:2966–2970

11. Alpert NR, Mulieri LA: Functional consequences of altered cardiac myosin isoenzymes. *Med Sci Sports Exerc* 1986;18:309–313
12. Pette D, Staron RS: Cellular and molecular diversities of mammalian skeletal muscle fibers. *Rev Physiol Biochem Pharmacol* 1990;116:2–76
13. Pagani ED, Silver PJ: Physiological and pharmacological modulation of cardiac contractile proteins. *Drug Dev Res* 1989;18:279–293
14. Hamilton N, Ianuzzo CD: Contractile and calcium regulating capacities of myocardia of different sized mammals scale with resting heart rate. *Mol Cell Biochem* 1991;106:133–141
15. Altman PL, Dittmer DS: *Biology Data Book.* Bethesda: Federal Society of Experimental Biology, 1979, pp 1688–1692
16. *Guide to the Care and Use of Experimental Animals.* Canadian Council on Animal Care. Ottawa, 1980
17. Ianuzzo CD, Brotherton S, O'Brien PJ, Salerno TA, Laughlin MH: Myocardial biochemical and hemodynamic adaptations to chronic tachycardia. *J Appl Physiol* 1991;70:907–913
18. O'Brien PJ, Ianuzzo CD, Moe GW, Howard R, Stopps T, Armstrong PW: Rapid ventricular pacing in the dog: biochemical and physiological studies of heart failure. *Can J Physiol Pharm* 1990;68:34–39
19. Williams H, Ianuzzo CD: The effects of triiodothyronine on cultured neonatal rat cardiac myocytes. *J Mol Cell Cardiol* 1988;20:689–699
20. Li B, Ianuzzo CD: Effects of contractile activity and thyroid hormone on the biochemical character of cultured cardiac myocytes. *Basic Res Cardiol* (in review)
21. Laughlin MH, Hale CC, Novela L, Gute D, Hamilton N, Ianuzzo CD: Biochemical characterization of exercise-trained porcine myocardium. *J Appl Physiol* 1991;71:229–235
22. O'Brien PJ, Shen H, Weiler JE, Mirsalimi SM, Julian RJ: Myocardial Ca cycling defect in furazolidone cardiomyopathy. *Can J Physiol Pharm* 1991;69:1833–1840
23. O'Brien PJ: Porcine malignant hyperthermia susceptibility: increased calcium-sequestering activity of skeletal muscle sarcoplasmic reticulum. *Can J Vet Res* 1986;50:329–337
24. O'Brien PJ, Ling E, Williams H, Salerno TA, Ianuzzo CD: Compensatory increase of myocardial sarcoplasmic reticulum Ca-ATPase activity in response to chronic metabolic overload. *Can J Cardiol* 1988;4:243–306
25. Martin V, McCutcheon LJ, Poon L, *et al:* Comparative mammal model of chronic rate overload: relationship of myocardial Ca-cycling to heart, metabolic and lipoperoxidation rates. *Comp Biochem Physiol* (in press)
26. O'Brien PJ: Calcium sequestration by isolated SR: real-time monitoring using radiometric dual-emission spectrofluorometry and the fluorescent calcium-binding dye indo-1. *Mol Cell Biochem* 1990;94:113–119
27. Wilson D, Nishiki K, Erecinska M: Energy metabolism in muscle and its regulation during individual contraction-relaxation cycles. *TIBS* 1981;6:16–19
28. Cory CR, Shen H, O'Brien P: Compensatory asymmetry in down-regulation and inhibition of the Ca-cycle in congestive heart failure produced by idiopathic dilated cardiomyopathy and rapid ventricular pacing in dogs. *J Mol Cell Cardiol* 1992: in press

29. Hornby L, Hamilton N, Marshall D, Salerno TA, Laughlin MH, Ianuzzo CD: Role of cardiac work in regulating myocardial biochemical characteristics. *Am J Physiol* 1990;258:H1482–H1490

30. Ianuzzo CD, Hamilton N, O'Brien PJ, Desrosiers C, Chiu R: Biochemical transformation of canine skeletal muscle for use in cardiac-assist devices. *J Appl Physiol* 1990;68:1481–1485

31. Ianuzzo CD, Hamilton N, O'Brien PJ, Dionisopoulos T, Salerno TA, Chiu RC-J: Biochemical character of cardiac and transformed canine skeletal muscle, in Chiu R, Bourgeois I (eds): *Transformed Muscle for Cardiac Assist and Repair*. New York: Futura Publishing Co, Inc, 1990, pp 25–40

32. Ling PJ, O'Brien PJ, Salerno T, Ianuzzo CD: The effects of altered thyroid status on the myocardium. *Can J Cardiol* 1988;4:301–306

33. Lompre AM, Mercadier J, Wesnewsky C, Bouveret P, Pantaloni C, D'Albis A, Schwartz: Species- and age-dependent changes in the relative amounts of cardiac myosin isoenzymes in mammals. *Dev Biol* 1981;84:286–290

34. Saltin B, Gollnick PD: Skeletal muscle adaptability: significance for metabolism and performance. *Handbook of Physiology Section 10: Skeletal Muscle*. Bethesda: American Physiological Society, 1983, pp 555–631

35. Driedzic WR, Sidell BD, Stowe D, Branscombe R: Matching of vertebrate cardiac energy demand to energy metabolism. *Am J Physiol* 1987;252:R930–R937

36. Hoppeler H, Lindstedt S, Classen H, Taylor CR, Mathien C: Scaling mitochondrial volumes in heart to body mass. *Respir Physiol* 1984;55:131–137

37. Eisenberg BR: Quantitiative ultrastructure of mammalian skeletal muscle. *Handbook of Physiology Section 10: Skeletal Muscle*. Bethesda: American Physiological Society, 1983, pp 73–112

38. Hudlicka O, Wright AJA, Hoppeler H, Uhlmann E: The effect of chronic bradycardial pacing on the oxidative capacity in rabbit hearts. *Respir Physiol* 1988;72:1–12

39. Montgomery C, Hamilton N, Ianuzzo CD: Energy status of the rapidly paced canine myocardium in congestive heart failure. *J Appl Physiol* 1992;73:2363–2367

40. Akera T: Pharmacologic agents and myocardial calcium, in Langer GA (ed): *Calcium and the Heart*. New York: Raven Press, Publishers, 1990, pp 299–331

41. Thompson RB, Warber KD, Potter JD: Calcium at they myofilaments, in Langer GA (ed): *Calcium and the Heart*. New York: Raven Press, Publishers, 1990, pp 127–185

42. Carafoli E: Sarcolemmal calcium pump, in Langer GA (ed): *Calcium and the Heart*. New York: Raven Press, Publishers, 1990, pp 299–331

43. Panagia V, Pierce GN, Dhalla KS, Ganguly PI, Beamish H: Adaptive changes in subcellular calcium transport during catecholamine-induced cardiomyopathy. *J Mol Cell Cardiol* 1985;17:411–420

44. Bayly WM, Gabel AA, Barr SA: Cardiovascular effects of submaximal

aerobic training on a treadmill in standard bred horses using a standardized exercise test. *Am J Vet Res* 1983;44:544–553

45. Snow DH: The horse and dog, elite athletes—why and how? *Proc Nutr Soc* 1985;44:267–272

46. Forbes MS, Hawkey LA, Jirge SK, Sperelaki SN: the sarcoplasmic reticulum of mouse heart: its divisions, configurations, and distribution. *J Ultrastruct Res* 1985;93:1–16

47. Hamilton N, Ashton ML, Ianuzzo CD: Cell size of mammalian myocardia is not related to physiological demand. *Experentia* 1991;47:1070–1072

48. O'Brien PJ, Fletcher TF, Metz AL, Kurtz HJ, Redd BK, Rempel WE, Clark EG, Louis CF: Malignant hyperthermia susceptibility: cardiac histomorphometry of dogs and young and market-weight swine. *Can J Vet Res* 1987;51:50–55

49. Anversa P, Loud AV, Giacomelli F, Wiener J: Absolute morphometric study of myocardial hypertrophy in experimental hypertension, II. Ultrastructure of myocytes and interstitium. *Lab Invest* 1978;38:597–608

50. Cory CR, McCutcheon LJ, O'Grady M, Pang AW, Geiger JD, O'Brien PJ: Compensatory down-regulation of myocardial ryanodine-binding Ca-release channel in isolated terminal cisternae of sarcoplasmic reticulum from dogs with spontaneous and experimental congestive heart failure. *Am J Physiol* 1993;264:H926–H937

51. Malik M, Camm AJ: Electrophsiology pacing and arrhythmia. Heart rate variability. *Clin Cardiol* 1990;13:570–576

52. Swynghedauw B: Developmental and functional adaptations of contractile proteins in cardiac and skeletal muscles. *Physiol Rev* 1986;66:710–771

53. Baldwin KM: Effects of chronic exercise on biochemical and functional properties of the heart. *Med Sci Sports Exerc* 1985;17:522–528

54. Geenen DL, Malhtra A, Buttrick PM, Scheuer J: Increased heart rate prevents the isomyosin shift after cardiac transplantation in the rat. *Circ Res* 1992;70:554–558

55. Advani SV, Geenen D, Malhotra A, Factor SM, Scheuer J: Swimming causes myosin adaptations in the rat cardiac isograft. *Circ Res* 1990;67:780–783

56. Geenen D, Buttrick P, Scheuer J: Cardiovascular and hormonal responses to swimming and running in the rat. *J Appl Physiol* 1988;65:116–123

Chapter 8

Factors Contributing to the Myocardial Adaptations of Long-Term Physical Exercise

James Scheuer, MD

The heart and the myocardium respond to long-term physical training programs with several characteristic adaptations. End-diastolic volume and myocardial mass increase, the latter mainly by elongation of the myocytes.[1] This results in cardiac hypertrophy similar to that found with volume overload of the heart. The myocardial microvasculature adapts so that myocardial perfusion can reach levels greater than in normal hearts.[2–4] This results from both neovascularization and enhanced vasodilatory capacities.[1,5] The myocardial mechanics associated with chronic training also differ from those observed in hypertrophy due to systolic overload. Whereas in the former, contraction and relaxation rates are diminished,[6] in the hypertrophy associated with chronic physical exercise contraction and relaxation velocities are either enhanced, as in rats, or preserved, as in larger animals,[7,8] thus permitting greater ventricular filling and emptying during exercise. In rodent hearts these changes relate to increased enzymatic activities of contractile proteins and to functional up-regulation of the sarcoplasmic reticulum, other membranes, and enzymatic systems.[9]

This chapter describes studies that elucidate the mechanisms that may be responsible for these adaptive alterations. Contrasts are drawn between large and small animals. The effects of volume overload tachycardia and bradycardia, and relationships to serum and myocardial catecholamines and angiotensin II are described.

Work reported in this chapter was supported by U.S. Public Health Grant HL 15498 and a Grant-In-Aid from the American Heart Association.

From Fletcher GF, (ed): *Cardiovascular Response to Exercise.* Mount Kisco, NY, Futura Publishing Company, Inc., © 1994.

Experiments are cited using the heterotopic transplant heart model in which the heart from a donor rat is transplanted into the abdomen of a recipient rat, and is chronically perfused through its arterial tree. The effect of a long-term swimming program, of pacing-induced tachycardia, and of repeated infusion of subhypertensive doses of angiotensin II are all described in order to isolate the factors of heart rate, growth factor, and catecholamines in this model of cardiac denervation.

Animal Models

When reviewing animal investigations, it is important to define the animal model and the special characteristics that model might confer on the experimental results. For instance, if one compares training effects on rat and pig hearts, there are certain important differences. Resting and submaximal heart rates in trained animals are diminished in both species,[10,11] and the heart-to-body weight ratios are increased, suggesting that cardiac hypertrophy has resulted from the vigorous training programs. Maximal coronary flow also is increased in both species. However, myocardial mechanical alterations such as enhanced rates of contraction and relaxation, and biochemical factors such as myosin or sarcoplasmic reticular adaptations, which are quite prominent in hearts of trained rats, do not occur in pigs.[9,10] The increased myosin adenosine triphosphatase (ATPase) observed in rodents appears to result from the greater proportion of α-myosin heavy chain present in hearts of physically trained rats, a system unaffected in the pig heart. Thus, the main biochemical mechanisms responsible for enhanced velocities of myocardial contraction and relaxation are increased in rats, but not effected in pigs. These kinds of results suggest that the cardiovascular adaptations found in the trained pig heart, which probably are more like those in trained humans, relate more to neurohumoral and structural alterations (the relative bradycardia, and the increased diastolic volume and myocardial mass), whereas adaptations in the rat relate not only to the these factors but also to intrinsic myocardial biochemical alterations.

Different modes of exercise also may result in qualitative and quantitative variations of cardiovascular effects. For instance, in the rat, swimming causes more profound increases in cardiac mass and in enzymatic activity than running,[7,11,12] even though an intense run causes a greater tachycardia and perhaps higher levels of circulating catecholamines.[13] On the other hand, swimming is associated with a greater accumulation of endogenous myocardial norepinephrine than running. The hearts of female rats also appear to respond more dramatically to training programs than do the hearts of male rats.[14]

Diastolic Loading

One of the factors that may influence cardiac adaptation in long-term exercise programs is the repeated diastolic loading secondary to increased venous return and the cardiac dilatation that takes place acutely during exercise. This can lead to chronic ventricular dilatation as the myocytes lengthen. In experimental animals, chronic volume overloading induced by surgically created arterial venous fistulae or mitral regurgitation may result in myocardial adaptations that are similar to those seen in long-term physical training[15] at a time when ventricular function is either normal or enhanced.[16] During the compensated state in rabbits, the myosin ATPase system, myosin isoenzymes, and sarcoplasmic reticulum activities are all normal.[17] However, as hypertrophy progresses, myocardial mechanical responses and isoenzymes in rats become more characteristic of those observed in systolic overload hypertrophy rather than in exercise-induced hypertrophy.[18] With extremes of hypertrophy in dogs with arterial venous fistulas, depressed ventricular and myocellular function occur.[19,20] In the rat heart, volume overload results in alterations of capillary structure reminiscent of those seen with physical training.[21,22] Thus, some of the cardiac changes found with physical training are mimicked by diastolic overload alone in its early phases, and therefore, during exercise increased venous return and intermittent dilatation of the ventricle may be a stimulus to some of these adaptations.

Heart Rate

Intense exercise causes tachycardia. Prolonged tachycardia by itself may be associated with up-regulation of several components of heart function.[23] Training results in bradycardia at rest and during submaximal exercise and, therefore, it is important to consider both tachycardia and bradycardia as factors in the myocardial effects of long-term physical exercise.

To address the issue of tachycardia, studies have been conducted using the heterotopic heart transplant model mentioned previously.[24] In this model the aorta of the donor heart is anastomosed end-to-side to the descending aorta of the recipient rat so that blood perfuses the coronary vessels and myocardium. The coronary sinus effluent drains into the right atrium and through the pulmonary artery, which is anastomosed to the recipient's vena cava. This provides a chronic denervated heart that is perfused normally through its myocardial bed, where the left ventricle is performing isovolumically but without external work, and that is not affected by alterations in blood pressure or heart rate of the donor rat. Hearts transplanted in this manner become relatively bradycardic and undergo rapid atrophy because they perform reduced internal ventricular work per beat and have lower levels of wall stress per beat and per minute.

By placing a pacemaker on the right ventricle, it has been possible to pace these hearts chronically and determine the effect of controlled tachycardia.[24] In experiments where hearts were paced at 420 beats per minute, as opposed to the nonpaced rate of 300 beats per minute heart rate and the rate-pressure product were the only variables. Pacing had no effect on either left ventricular pressure or dp/dt in the transplanted heart. The transplanted hearts were paced for 1 week after surgery.[24] Cardiac mass was 15% greater in paced transplanted hearts than in hearts not subjected to pacing. The paced transplanted hearts also had myosin ATPase activities 30% higher than the nonpaced hearts and identical with the ATPase activities observed in the native hearts. The percent of myosin heavy chain present as α-myosin averaged 27% higher in the paced than the nonpaced transplanted hearts (all differences $p < 0.05$). Thus, the effect of increased heart rate or rate pressure product in the absence of neural innervation, endogenous catecholamines, or external cardiac work resulted in shifts in heart mass and of the myosin type in the same direction as observed with a physical training program. Although this study demonstrates that increased heart rate and/or rate-pressure product can mimic some of the effects of exercise training, in a swimming exercise training program tachycardia is not profound,[13] and other factors must be responsible for the myocardial alterations. Among possibilities to consider in the intact heart, besides diastolic loading, are circulating and endogenous catecholamines or other circulating humoral substances.

As mentioned previously, bradycardia also is a prominent component of the adaptation to physical conditioning. Chronic pacing-induced bradycardia results in increased stroke volume and stroke work and enhanced ventricular responses to norepinephrine administration.[25] Increased capillary density also has been observed in these hearts similar to that observed in the trained heart. Thus, chronic bradycardia with its increased stroke volume may mimic the diastolic loading mentioned previously, and result in certain myocardial alterations similar to those observed with long-term physical training. Similar improvement in capillary growth also has been observed, even in hearts with hypertrophy secondary to volume overload hypertrophy.[26] This should be useful in pathological cardiac hypertrophy because in that state, coronary reserve frequently is diminished.

Plasma Catecholamines

Plasma catecholamines rise abruptly during intense exercise and, thus, repeated surges of these hormones might be responsible for some of the cardiac adaptations found in physical training.[27] In rats, serum catecholamines rise during both running and swimming sessions, but myocardial catecholamines are increased only in the swimming model of exercise.[13] Dobutamine administration causes cardiac resoponses similar to running (*ie*, an acute rise in serum catecholamines associated with significant tachycardia).[28] When this agent was injected intermittently in rats using the same time schedule as exercise bouts for long-term conditioning, the cardiac effects were more similar to running than to swimming. That is, there were modest increases in heart mass and concomitant alterations in myosin isoenzymes.

When rats with heterotopic transplants were made to swim intensely, their transplanted heart rates and blood pressures did not change significantly. Their hearts were exposed only to changes in blood constituents during the exercise. When such rats were subjected to a swimming program for 8 weeks, their native hearts underwent the expected hypertrophy induced by this protocol, but the transplanted hearts did not demonstrate the expected increase in mass.[29] Since endogenous myocardial catecholamines were absent and there were no acute increases in heart rate or rate-pressure product, one of these factors or other unmeasured blood-borne substances must be required for the hypertrophic response to the swimming program. Since myosin isoenzymes showed the expected shift of a swimming protocol (ie, an increase in α-MHC), this is compatible with surges of plasma catecholamines during the bouts of swimming, and similar to the significant alterations of this contractile protein observed with infusions of dobutamine.

Angiotensin II

The renin-angiotensin system is activated during acute exercise, causing increases in plasma levels of angiotensin II.[27,30] Angiotensin II is a growth-promoting substance that enhances protein synthesis in cultured neonatal myocytes[31] and, therefore, might be a direct growth factor in adult hearts. Several studies show that inhibition of angiotensin-converting enzyme in hypertensive states dissociates the hypertension from cardiac mass, suggesting indirectly that such a growth factor relationship exists.[32,33] This question has been explored in rats with heterotopically transplanted hearts in which angiotensin II was infused by alzet pumps in minute doses (3 μg/kg per hour) for 1 week after the heart transplant.[34] These doses were not associated with any change in blood pressure in the recipient or in left ventricular pressure or dp/dt in the transplanted heart. Weights of transplanted hearts were 12% greater in animals exposed to the angiotensin II than in controls, and when protein synthesis was measured using radioactive leucine, there was a 39% greater fractional synthesis of protein and a 55% increase in total protein synthesis per day in the hearts exposed to angiotensin II (all $p < 0.05$). Although the heart weight differences in these short experiments were modest, increases in protein synthesis were substantial. Thus, this study demonstrates a direct effect on adult hearts in vivo of very small doses of angiotensin II that cannot be attributed to any change in mechanical load. On the other hand, angiotensin II administration had no effect on the ratio of α- to β-MHC. Thus, it appears that cardiac growth can be dissociated from the control of myosin isoenzyme balance and that a growth factor like angiotensin can have a direct effect on heart mass.

Summary

The cardiac effects of isotonic exercise are summarized and modeled in Figure 1. Intense exercise causes increases in cardiac output and venous return, tachycardia, and rate-pressure product, activation of sympathetic neural pathways, and increases in plasma catecholamines, angiotensin II, and perhaps other important blood-borne substances. The increased venous return results in acute ventricular dilatation, and this plus the tachycardia results in increased myocardial wall stress per minute. The rate-pressure product and the increased wall stress above can augment protein synthesis and myocyte growth and cause myosin isoenzyme down-regulation in the rodent heart. However, the down-regulation of myosin isoenzymes may be countered by increased plasma or myocardial catecholamines in running or swimming, or to tachycardia alone in pacing. The increased protein synthesis caused by rate × pressure may be augmented by the repeated exposures to elevated angiotensin II levels. Thus, plasma and myocardial catecholamines may have direct effects on protein synthesis and isoenzyme balance and probably on other selective protein synthetic systems, and growth factors such as angiotensin II also can influence these processes. In combination with other factors, they probably serve to facilitate mechanical effects of load and heart rate. Chronic bradycardia, which develops during the conditioning process, exaggerates the diastolic load on the ventricle, perpetuating the remodeling effect.

The final common pathways of these various influences are through a series of growth and genetic factors that can activate different genetic components of the myocyte, resulting in enhancement of overall protein synthesis and cell growth or selective protein synthesis for enhanced mechanisms of contraction and relaxation. The selective protein synthetic processes that augment myocyte contraction and relaxation rates appear to be significant in the rat heart, but are much less important in hearts of larger animals like pigs and humans. Thus, in larger mammals, the heart's adaptation

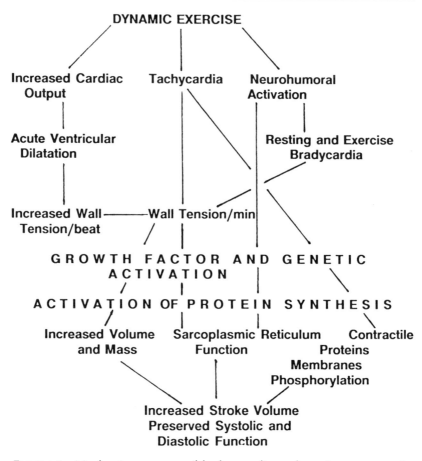

FIGURE 1. Mechanisms responsible for cardiac adaptations to exercise training programs.

to long-term physical exercise probably depends much more on global remodeling and myocyte growth, and on the relative bradycardia characteristic of the training effect. In rodents, in addition to those effects observed in larger mammals, biochemical and myocardial mechanical alterations permit greater inotropic and lusotropic responses to exercise. These cellular responses also may be significant but less obvious in the larger animals since the slowing of contraction and relaxation observed in hypertrophied hearts due to severe overloads is not observed in hearts with training-induced hypertrophy.

Acknowledgment

I thank Ms. Eileen Doherty for expert secretarial assistance.

References

1. Anversa P, Beghi C, Levicky V, McDonald SL, Kikkawa Y: Morphometry of right ventricular hypertrophy induced by strenuous exercise in rat. *Am J Physiol* 1982;243:H856–H861
2. Tomanek RJ: Effects of age and exercise on the extent of the myocardial capillary bed. *Anat Rec* 1970;167:55–62
3. Wyatt HL, Mitchell J: Influence of physical training and deconditioning on coronary vasculature of dogs. *J Appl Physiol* 1978;45:619–625
4. Yipintsoi T, Rosenkrantz J, Codini M, Scheuer J: Myocardial blood flow responses to acute hypoxia and volume loading in physically trained rats. *Cardiovasc Res* 1980;14:50–57
5. Laughlin M H, Overholser KA, Bhatte MJ: Exercise training increases coronary transport reserve in miniature swine. *J Appl Physiol* 1989;67:1140–1149
6. Capasso JM, Strobeck JE, Malhotra A, Scheuer J, Sonnenblick EH: Contractile behavior of rat myocardium after reversal of hypertensive hypertrophy. *Am J Physiol (Heart Circ Physiol)* 1982;242:H882–H889
7. Bersohn MM, Scheuer J: Effect of ischemia on the performance of hearts from physically trained rats. *Am J Physiol* 1978;234:H215–H218
8. White FC, McKirnan MD, Breisch EA, Guth BD, Liu Y, Bloor CM: Adaptation of the left ventricle to exercise-induced hypertrophy. *J Appl Physiol* 1987;62:1097–1110
9. Scheuer J, Buttrick PM: The cardiac hypertrophic responses to pathologic and physiologic loads. *Circulation* 1987;75:I63–I68
10. Laughlin MH, Hale CC, Novela L, Gute D, Hamilton N, Ianuzzo CD: Biochemical characterization of exercise-trained porcine myocardium. *J Appl Physiol* 1991;71:229–235
11. Schaible TF, Scheuer J: Cardiac adaptations to chronic exercise. *Prog Cardiovasc Dis* 1985;27:297–324
12. Penpargkul S, Malhotra A, Schaible T, Scheuer J: Cardiac contractile proteins and sarcoplasmic reticulum in hearts of rats trained by running. *J Appl Physiol: Respir Environm Exerc Physiol* 1980;48:409–413
13. Geenen D, Buttrick P, Scheuer J: Cardiovascular and hormonal re-

sponses to swimming and running in the rat. *J Appl Physiol* 1988;65: 116–123

14. Schaible TF, Penpargkul S, Scheuer J: Cardiac responses to exercise training in male and female rats. *J Appl Physiol: Respir Environm Exerc Physiol* 1981;50:112–117

15. Liu Z, Hilbelink DR, Gerdes AM: Regional changes in hemodynamics and cardiac myocyte size in rats with aortocaval fistulas—2. Long-term effects. *Circ Res* 1991;69:59–65

16. Gerdes AM, Campbell SE, Hilbelink DR: Structural remodeling of cardiac myocytes in rats with arteriovenous fistulas. *Lab Invest* 1988; 59:857–861

17. Gibbs CL, Wendt IR, Kotsanas G, Young IR: Mechanical, energetic, and biochemical changes in long-term volume overload of rabbit heart. *Am J Physiol (Heart Circ Physiol* 31) 1992;262:H819–H827

18. Takeda N, Ohkubo T, Hatanaka T, Takeda A, Nakamura I, Nagano M: Myocardial contractility and left ventricular myosin isoenzyme pattern in cardiac hypertrophy due to chronic volume overload. *Basic Res Cardiol* 1987;82(suppl 2):215–221

19. Malik AB, Tomio A, O'Kane HO, Geha AS: Cardiac performance in ventricular hypertrophy induced by pressure and volume overloading. *J Appl Physiol* 1974;37:867–874

20. Urabe Y, Mann DL, Kent RL, Nakano K, Tomanek RJ, Carabello BA, Cooper IV G: Cellular and ventricular contractile dysfunction in experimental canine mitral regurgitation. *Circ Res* 1992;70:131–147

21. Batra S, Rakusan K: Geometry of capillary networks in volume overloaded rat heart. *Microvasc Res* 1991;42:39–50

22. Kawamura, K, Tohda K, Kobayashi M, Masuda H, Shozawa T: Fine structure of capillary proliferation in myocardium of volume overloaded rats. *Adv Exp Med Biol* 1990;227:387–394

23. Ianuzzo CD, Brotherton S, O'Brien P, Salerno T, Laughlin MH: Myocardial biochemical and hemodynamic adaptations to chronic tachycardia. *J Appl Physiol* 1991;70:907–913

24. Geenen DL, Malhotra A, Buttrick PM, Scheuer J: Increased heart rate prevents the isomyosin shift after cardiac transplantation in the rat. *Circ Res* 1992;70:554–558

25. Wright AJA, Hudlicka O: Capillary growth and changes in heart performance induced by chronic bradycardial pacing in the rabbit. *Circ Res* 1981;49:469–478

26. Wright AJA, Hudlicka O, Brown MD: Beneficial effect of chronic bradycardial pacing on capillary growth and heart performance in volume overload heart hypertrophy. *Circ Res* 1989;64:1205–1212

27. Tidgren B, Hjemdahl P, Theodorsson E, Nussberger J: Renal neurohormonal and vascular responses to dynamic exercise in humans. *J Appl Physiol* 1991;70:2279–2286

28. Buttrick P, Malhotra A, Factor S, Geenen D, Scheuer J: Effects of chronic dobutamine administration on hearts of normal and hypertensive rats. *Circ Res* 1988;63:173–181

29. Advani SV, Geenen D, Malhotra A, Factor SM, Scheuer J: Swimming

causes myosin adaptations in the rat cardiac isograft. *Circ Res* 1990;67: 780–783
30. Staessen J, Fagard R, Hespel P, Lijnen P, Vanhees L, Amery A: Plasma renin system during exercise in normal men. *J Appl Physiol* 1987;63:188–194
31. Baker KM, Aceto JF: Angiotensin II stimulation of protein synthesis and cell growth in chick heart cells. *Am J Physiol* 1990;259 (*Heart Circ Physiol* 28):H610–H618
32. Linz W, Scholkens BA, Ganten D: Converting enzyme inhibition specifically prevents the development and induces regression of cardiac hypertrophy in rats. *Clin Exp Hyper—Theory Practice* 1989;All:1325–1350
33. Baker KM, Chernin MI, Wixson SK, Aceto JF: Renin-angiotensin system involvement in pressure-overload cardiac hypertrophy in rats. *Am J Physiol* 1990;259 (*Heart Circ Physiol* 28):H324–H332
34. Geenen DL, Malhotra A, Liang D, Yarlaggada A, Scheuer J: Angiotensin II increases protein synthesis in the rat heart. *J Mol Cell Cardiol* 1992; 24(suppl III):P74:S.29

Part 3

Systemic Responses to Exercise and Results of Training

Chapter 9

Blood Pressure Responses to Resistive, Static, and Dynamic Exercise

J. D. Macdougall, PhD

Increases in cardiac output and blood pressure and regional redistribution of blood flow parallel the increase in muscle metabolism that occurs with exercise, so that muscle blood flow is generally tightly coupled to its metabolism. During *dynamic* (eg, locomotory) exercise, contractions are rhythmic, so that muscles are active during a portion of the movement cycle and relaxed during the remainder. As the speed of the movement increases, the actual duration of each phase decreases, but the proportion of time spent in contraction or relaxation remains relatively constant.[1] *Static* or isometric exercise involves sustained force production with muscles remaining at a constant length; thus, there is no cycling or muscle pumping effect between an active and relaxed state. *Resistive* exercise such as weightlifting can be considered as a combination of static and dynamic exercise in that each movement begins with a static contraction (until force production exceeds the weight of the object to be lifted) followed by a forceful concentric contraction (while the weight is being raised), an eccentric "contraction" (while the weight is being lowered), and finally a brief relative relaxation before the initiation of the next repetition. This chapter summarizes the arterial blood pressure response to these three types of exercise, the effects of physical training on this response, and briefly discusses some of the mechanisms involved.

From Fletcher GF, (ed): *Cardiovascular Response to Exercise.* Mount Kisco, NY, Futura Publishing Company, Inc., © 1994.

Dynamic Exercise

The typical blood pressure response to progressive dynamic exercise such as treadmill walking or cycle ergometry is summarized in Figure 1. Systolic pressure increases almost linearly with exercise intensity to values of 200 mm Hg or more at maximum exercise. Although during this time cardiac output may have increased four- to sixfold, the rise in systolic pressure is to a large extent buffered by the concomitant decrease in peripheral resistance caused by the progressive vasodilation that occurs in the vessels of the exercising muscles. Because of this decrease in peripheral resistance, diastolic pressure shows little or no increase, and in normotensive persons generally decreases slightly at higher workloads. Mean blood pressure during this type of exercise seldomly exceeds 120 mm Hg.

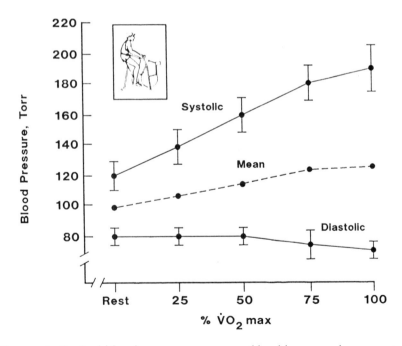

FIGURE 1. Typical blood pressure response of healthy normal persons to progressive dynamic exercise. $\dot{V}O_2max$ = maximal oxygen consumption in $ml/kg/min$.

Arm Vs. Leg Exercise

It is well known that with exercise primarily involving the upper body muscles, both systolic and diastolic pressures are higher than when the same absolute work is performed with the legs (Figure 2). Several explanations have been suggested for the apparently higher peripheral resistance during arm exercise compared with leg exercise requiring the same cardiac output. One possibility is that because of the relatively smaller active muscle mass involved in arm exercise, the total size of the vascular bed is such that even when maximally dilated it effects a smaller drop in peripheral resistance than that with comparable exercise involving the leg muscles. A second possibility is that the exercise pressor response is most

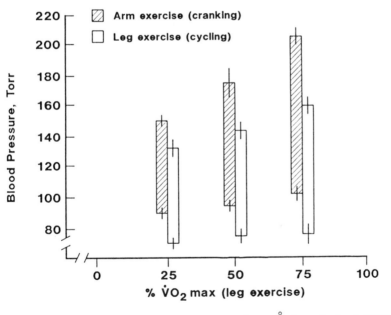

from Åstrand et al, 1965

FIGURE 2. *Blood pressure response of persons performing arm exercise and leg exercise at the same absolute power output ($\dot{V}O_2$). Adapted from Reference 22 with permission.*

tightly coupled to the *relative* exercise intensity, and thus would be greater at a given absolute power output with arm exercise since this would represent a higher relative intensity than when performing the same exercise with the legs. A third possibility may relate to a greater relative involvement of the Valsalva or partial Valsalva maneuver with upper-body exercise, as discussed later in this chapter. Whatever the explanation, the greater blood pressure response with upper body work may have important implications for individuals whose exercise patterns involve such activities as shoveling, digging, or carpentry work.

Effects of Training

Endurance training attenuates the blood pressure response to exercise so that at the same absolute power output, post-training systolic and mean pressures are lower than their pretraining values.[2–5] In normotensive individuals, resting systolic and diastolic pressures are generally unaffected by training, although mean pressure may decrease as a result of the acquired resting bradycardia. Maximum systolic pressure remains unchanged but it occurs at a higher power output (Figure 3). With hypertensive persons, several investigations,[2,3,6] although not all,[7,8] also have noted significant decreases in resting systolic and diastolic pressures after a period of endurance training (Figure 4). For a detailed review of this topic see Tipton[4] and Hagberg.[9]

Static Exercise

Force production during the rhythmic contraction cycles in dynamic exercise, such as locomotion, is relatively low compared with that which normally occurs during static exercise (*eg*, even during maximum sprinting, peak concentric force production of the quadriceps would rarely exceed 50% of its maximum isometric strength). When static contractions are performed at increasing percentages of maximum voluntary contraction force (MVC) there is a proportional increase in intramuscular compression that eventually will exceed muscle perfusion pressure and occlude local blood

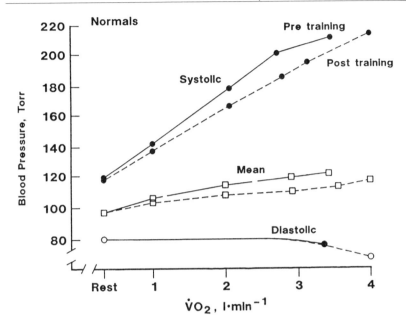

FIGURE 3. *Typical effects of endurance training on the blood pressure response to progressive exercise.* $\dot{V}O_2$ = *oxygen consumption. Compiled from References 2–5.*

flow. Measurements of the intensity at which blood flow becomes impeded by the contraction range from approximately 40%–60% MVC and varies considerably among muscle groups.[10,11] Up to this point, blood flow is maintained by a marked pressor response that serves to adjust perfusion pressure in relation to the increasing intramuscular pressure, although the mechanisms that activate and control this response are not fully understood. This increase in blood pressure is largely the result of an increase in cardiac output and to a lesser extent a reflex vasoconstriction in vascular beds other than those of the exercising muscles.[12,13] In addition, if the desired force production is sufficient to elicit a Valsalva maneuver, the elevation in intrathoracic pressure also will be transmitted directly to the arterial tree.[14]

Because of the mechanical compression of the blood vessels in the contracting muscles, peripheral resistance does not decrease as in dynamic exercise and diastolic pressure increases in proportion to the increase in systolic pressure resulting in large increases in mean blood

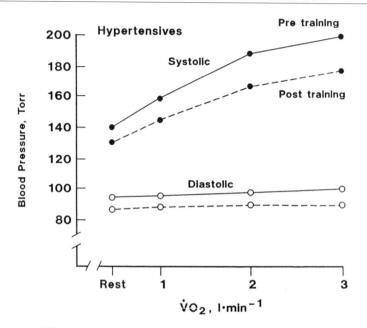

FIGURE 4. *Effects of endurance training on the blood pressure response to progressive exercise in hypertensive and borderline hypertensive persons. Note decrease in resting systolic and diastolic pressure in addition to the attenuated exercise response. $\dot{V}O_2$ = oxygen consumption. Compiled from References 3 and 6.*

pressure (Figure 5). The increase in systolic and diastolic pressure is almost directly proportional to the relative intensity of the contraction,[14,15] affected by the size of the muscle mass actuated[5,14] and the duration over which the contraction is sustained[5] (Figure 6).

Resistive Exercise: Weightlifting

Intra-arterial recordings from the brachial artery during heavy dynamic weightlifting indicate that extreme increases in systolic and diastolic pressure occur with the exertional phase of each lift (Figure 7). During maximum efforts that involve a large muscle mass, pressures >350/250 mm Hg are not uncommon in healthy young individuals.[16] The increase in pressure is the sum of the effects of a potent pressure response, mechanical compression of

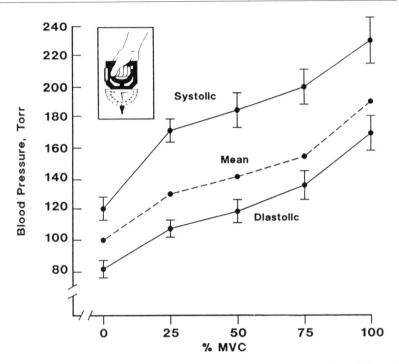

FIGURE 5. *Typical blood pressure response to progressive intensities of isometric contraction. Data from References 14 and 15. MVC = maximal voluntary contractile force.*

blood vessels in the contracting muscles, and the Valsalva maneuver. The magnitude of the increase in pressure is almost directly related to the relative intensity of the contraction, and within each person, also is affected by the size of the active muscle mass, although this is not a direct relationship (*ie*, peak blood pressure is only slightly higher during a double leg press compared with a single leg press at the same relative intensity).[16]

Typical mean pressure and heart rate response during a set of maximum leg press exercises is illustrated in Figure 8. Peak pressures tend to increase with each repetition so that the highest pressure usually is evident during the last repetition before failure. Over this time heart rate may increase to 165–170 beats per minute. Immediately after the last repetition, blood pressure falls below pre-exercise values before increasing again after approximately 10 seconds. The rapid drop in pressure after exercise probably is the

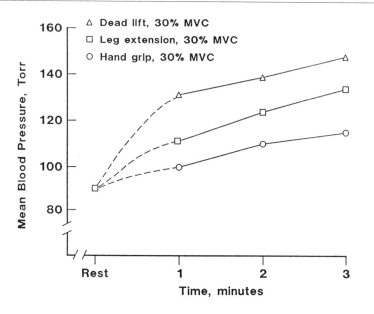

from Seals et al, 1983

FIGURE 6. *The effects of active muscle size and duration of contraction on the blood pressure response to static exercise. Note mean pressure is highest during the dead lift exercise (requiring the greatest muscle mass) and lowest during the hand grip exercise (requiring the smallest muscle mass). Data from Reference 5. MVC = maximal voluntary contractile force.*

result of a sudden perfusion of a large vasodilated muscle mass that was previously mechanically occluded, as well as a transient pressure undershoot initiated by baroreceptor and cardiopulmonary reflex tone activated during the lifting. This temporary drop in pressure is the probable cause of the feelings of faintness or dizziness that persons often experience immediately after heavy lifting.

In healthy young individuals, weightlifting can be considered a relatively safe activity with a low incidence of vascular injury despite the extreme elevations in blood pressure. In instances in which a large muscle mass is involved in maximum lifts to failure, however, intradermal hemorrhages or petechiae are not uncommon, and some instances of brainstem ischemia and subarachnoid hemorrhage have been documented in apparently healthy young persons

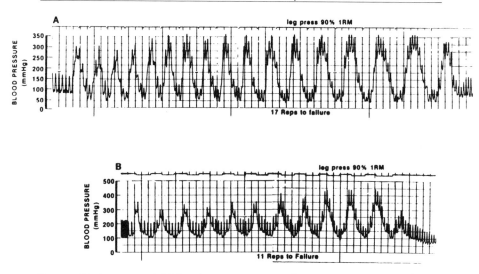

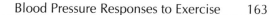

FIGURE 7. *Intra-arterial blood pressure traces from two persons performing double-leg presses to failure at 90% of their single maximum repetition. RM = maximal repetition. Data from Reference 16.*

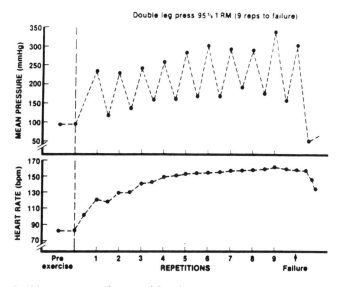

FIGURE 8. *Heart rate and mean blood pressure response for one person performing leg-presses at 95% of the single maximum repetition. Data from Reference 16.*

during weightlifting. (see ref. 16) Although most fitness instructors and coaches counsel persons to avoid a Valsalva maneuver during lifting, as discussed later in the chapter a brief Valsalva may serve an important protective function for the heart and vessels of the brain.

The Pressor Response to Weightlifting

The mechanisms that regulate the pressor response to exercise are thought to include both a central (feedforward) component that originates in the motor cortex and a reflex (feedback) neural component that originates in the active muscles and is transmitted along group III and IV afferents to cardiovascular control centers.[17] By manipulation of such factors as muscle size and strength in our subjects and the type of contraction, joint angle, and presence of fatigue during weightlifting, we have recently[14] uncoupled the normal relationship between the intensity of the effort (central component) and force production (neural component) to determine which has the greatest effect on the pressor response. In all instances it was found that it was the degree of voluntary effort or central feedforward mechanism that dominated in determining the magnitude of the pressor response to weightlifting and isometric exercise. For example, when a group of persons representing a wide range in muscle size and strength performed double leg presses to failure at the same *relative* intensity, similar peak blood pressures occurred that were independent of the absolute weight lifted[14] (Figure 9).

The Valsalva Maneuver

When a person performs a Valsalva maneuver (forced expiration against a closed or partially closed glotis) there is an abrupt increase in intrathoracic pressure that is transmitted to the arterial tree causing an immediate increase in systolic and diastolic blood pressure (Figure 10). Initially this is an almost direct response (*ie*, for each rise of 1 mm Hg in intrathoracic pressure there is an approximate 1 mm Hg rise in systolic and diastolic pressure). If, however, the maneuver is maintained, after approximately 3 seconds systolic, diastolic and pulse pressures begin to decline rapidly because of reduced diastolic filling caused by impaired venous return (Figure 10).

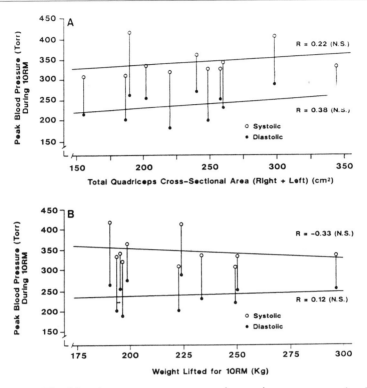

FIGURE 9. *The blood pressure response to heavy leg press exercise in a group of healthy young persons representing a wide range in muscle size and strength. Peak systolic (open circles) and diastolic (closed circles) pressure has been graphed against total muscle size (**A**) and absolute weight lifted (**B**). The regression lines for systolic and diastolic pressure indicate a nonsignificant relationship (N = 11). RM = maximal repetition. Data from Reference 14.*

During weightlifting, the Valsalva maneuver provides a mechanical advantage of stabilizing the trunk and thus becomes an integral component of the lifting process during maximum or near maximum efforts. The threshold, above which it is necessary to perform the Valsalva maneuver, varies somewhat for different muscle groups and between individuals, but occurs at approximately 80–85% MVC.[14] Similarly, when a resistance that initially may not require a Valsalva maneuver is lifted repeatedly until failure, it becomes necessary to invoke an increasingly forceful

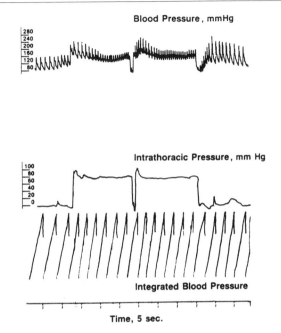

FIGURE 10. *Actual trace for blood pressure and intrathoracic pressure while a person, seated at rest, maintains a target intrathoracic pressure at 60% of his maximum Valsalva maneuver. The sudden drop in intrathoracic pressure indicates a breath. Data from Reference 14.*

Valsalva maneuver as motor units progressively fatigue (Figure 11). During maximum dynamic lifting to failure, intrathoracic pressures may reach as much as 100 mm Hg, or up to 70% of that which occurs during a maximum voluntary Valsalva maneuver.

A major portion of the increase in blood pressure that occurs during very heavy lifting can thus be attributed directly to the Valsalva maneuver. It has been shown, however, that in addition to elevating blood pressure, the increase in intrathoracic pressure with the Valsalva maneuver also is transmitted to the cerebrospinal fluid (CSF) so that CSF pressure increases in proportion to that in the thorax and abdomen.[18] This would cause a *decrease* in transmural pressures in cerebral vessels and thus reduce the risk of vascular damage under the extremes in pressure that are generated by heavy weightlifting. Similarly, the compressive effect of the elevated intrathoracic pressure on the heart reduces myocardial transmural

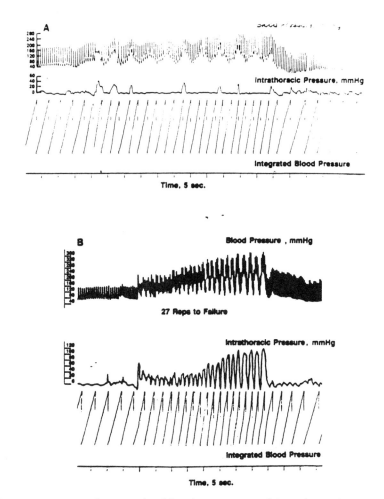

FIGURE 11. *Actual traces for blood pressure and intrathoracic pressure while a person performs dynamic leg presses. The weight represents ~75% MVC and the person only occasionally performs a Valsalva maneuver. The weight represents ~85% MVC performed to failure and the person finds it necessary to enlist a Valsalva maneuver with each repetition. Note that the intensity of the Valsalva maneuver increases as the subject approaches failure. Data from Reference 14.*

pressure at the time of peak peripheral resistance. Thus, the performance of a brief Valsalva maneuver (the natural response to lifting) may constitute an important protective function during lifting that should not be discouraged in healthy young persons.

Effects of Training

The normal adaptation to heavy resistance training is an increase in the size (cross-sectional area) and strength of the motor units that were active in training. As a result, the same absolute weight as before training now represents a lower relative resistance since the lift can be performed by recruiting fewer motor units and thus requiring less effort or central command. The blood pressure response to the same absolute load is thus attenuated after training. This is illustrated in Figure 12, which summarizes the blood pressure response of six young men lifting the same absolute weight after five months of heavy resistance training during which they increased their leg strength by 26%.[19] Systolic, diastolic, and mean pressure was reduced by approxi-

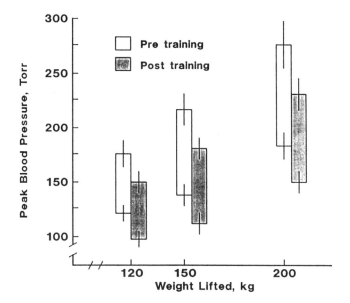

FIGURE 12. *Pre- and post-training blood pressure response of six persons lifting the same absolute weight. The resistance training program resulted in an increase of 26% in leg press strength. Note the attenuation of the pressor response after training. Data from Reference 19.*

mately 17% at similar points in the lift and heart rate was approximately 15% lower.

This attenuation of blood pressure response to the same load after training is not confined to healthy young individuals. We recently have completed a study in which 15 older men (x age 66 ± 1 year) underwent 12 weeks of resistance training that resulted in a 24% increase in leg press strength.[20] Intra-arterial recordings of blood pressure during 10 repetitions of leg press exercise at the same absolute load (80% of their original single maximum repetition) indicated significant 17% and 25% reductions in systolic and diastolic pressure, respectively, after training. There was an even greater (27%) reduction in rate-pressure product (Figure 13).

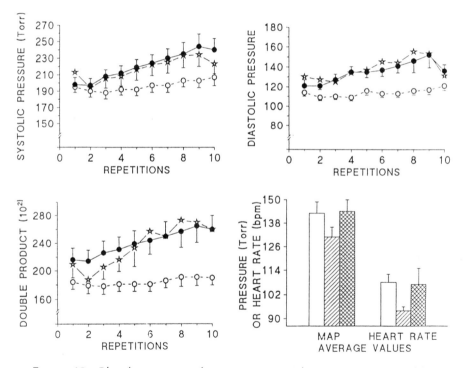

Figure 13. *Blood pressure and rate pressure product response in 15 older men (x̄ age 67 yr) after a 12-week resistance training program that resulted in an increase of 24% in leg press strength. Peak pressures are presented before (closed circles) and after (open circles) training while lifting the same absolute weight (80% of pretraining MVC) 10 times. The starts indicate the response at 80% of the post-training MVC. Note the attenuation of the pressor response after training. Data from Reference 20.*

Cardiac Dynamics During Weightlifting

We also have recently examined cardiac volume responses during weightlifting in healthy young men.[21] Simultaneous measurements of cardiac volume (by two-dimensional echocardiography), intrabrachial arterial pressure, and intrathoracic pressure (esophageal catheter tip transducer) were made in five experienced weightlifters performing leg press exercise to failure at 95% of their single maximum repetition. Data were analyzed at rest and at a point during the lifting (concentric) phase, the lockout phase (knee fully extended), and the lowering (eccentric) phase of a typical lift.

For the repetition studied, mean group arterial pressure was 160/91 mm Hg pre-exercise, increased to 270/183 mm Hg, decreased to 176/116 mm Hg at lockout, and increased again to 207/116 mm Hg during the lowering phase of the lift. Esophageal pressure increased to 58 mm Hg at the initiation of the lifting phase, declined to − 13 mm Hg at lockout, and increased again to 16 mm Hg during the lowering phase (Figure 14). In one person, an arterial pressure of

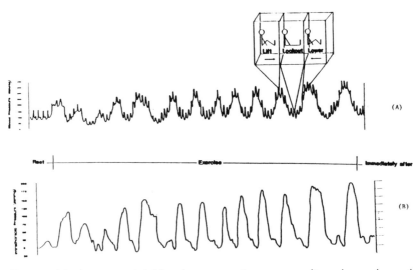

FIGURE 14. *Intra-arterial blood pressure (upper panel) and esophageal pressure (lower panel) while a person performs double leg press exercise to failure at 95% 1 RM. The inset indicates the person's knee angle and direction of movement during lifting, lock out and lowering phases of each repetition. Data from Reference 21.*

390/290 mm Hg and an esophageal pressure of 185 mm Hg were recorded during the lifting phase.

Compared with pre-exercise, end-diastolic volume decreased significantly during the lifting phase, increased to pre-exercise values at lockout, and decreased again during lowering. End-systolic volumes also decreased during lifting, increased at lockout, and decreased during lowering (Figure 15). Stroke volume changed from a mean value of 94 ml at rest to 77 ml during lifting, 103 at lockout, and 79 ml during the lowering phase. Ejection fraction thus continued to increase throughout the lift. Changes in cardiac transmural pressures were to a large extent buffered by the increased intrathoracic pressure caused by the Valsalva maneuver.

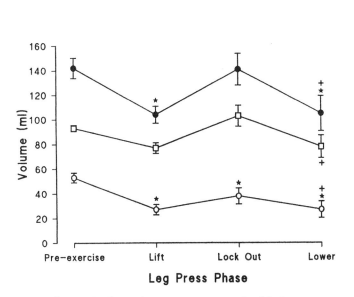

FIGURE 15. *Left ventricular volume response to double leg press exercise at different phases (pre-exercise, lifting, lock out, and lowering) of the repetition. The closed circles represent end-diastolic volume, the open squares stroke volume, and the open circles end-diastolic volume (n = 5). Data from Reference 21.*

Summary

The increase in cardiac output and blood pressure that occurs in response to exercise results in a coupling of muscle blood flow to muscle metabolism. The magnitude of the increase in blood pressure thus depends on the exercise intensity and the size of the active muscle mass and also is affected by the mode of exercise. During progressive dynamic exercise, systolic pressure increases almost linearly with exercise intensity whereas diastolic pressure changes little or decreases slightly. During static contractions both systolic and diastolic pressures increase in proportion to exercise intensity. Heavy weightlifting exercise results in extreme increases in systolic and diastolic pressures with the exertional phase of each lift. The pressor response to static and weightlifting exercise is controlled primarily by central command (feedforward mechanisms) and thus relates directly to the relative intensity or effort of the contraction(s).

During forceful static contractions and weightlifting exercise, it becomes necessary to perform a brief Valsalva maneuver to achieve the desired force production. The increase in intrathoracic pressure from the Valsalva is transmitted directly to the arterial tree and thus exaggerates the blood pressure response with this form of exercise. The general effect of physical training is an attenuation of the blood pressure response to a given absolute level of exercise or force production.

References

1. Laughlin MH: Skeletal muscle blood flow capacity: Role of muscle pump in exercise hyperemia. *Am J Physiol* 1987;253:H993–H1004
2. Clausen JP: Physical training in management of coronary artery disease. *Circulation* 1969;30:143–154
3. Choquette G, Ferguson RJ: Blood pressure reduction in borderline hypertensives following physical training. *Can Med Assoc J* 1973;108:699–703
4. Hagberg JM: Exercise, fitness and hypertension, in Bouchard C, Shephard RJ, Stephens T, et al, (eds): *Exercise Fitness and Health.* Champaign, IL, Human Kinetics Press, 1990, pp 455–465
5. Seals DR, Hagberg JM: The effect of exercise training on human hypertension: A review. *Med Sci Sports Exerc* 1984;16:207–215
6. Hanson JS, Nedde WH: Preliminary observations on physical training

for hypertensive males. *Circ Res* 1970;(suppl 1):49–53

7. Gilders RM, Voner C, Dudley GA: Endurance training and blood pressure in normotensive and hypertensive adults. *Med Sci Sports Exerc* 1989;21:629–636

8. Cleroux J, Peronnett F, DeChamplain J: Effects of exercise training on plasma catecholamines and blood pressure in labile hypertensive subjects. *Eur J Appl Physiol* 1987;56:550–554

9. Tipton CM: Exercise training and hypertension. *Exerc Sport Sci Rev* 1984;12:245–306

10. Mitchell JH, Payne FC, Saltin B, Schibye B: The role of muscle mass in the cardiovascular response to static contractions. *J Physiol* (Lond) 1980;309:45–54

11. Bonde-Petersen F, Mørk AL, Nielsen E: Local muscle blood flow and sustained contractions of human arms and back muscles. *Eur J Appl Physiol* 1975;34:43–50

12. Nutter DO, Wickliffe CW: Regional vasomotor responses to the somatopressor reflex from muscle. *Circ Res* 1981;48 (suppl I):98–103

13. Shepherd JT, Blomquist CG, Lind AR, Mitchell JH, Saltin B: Static (isometric) exercise. Retrospection and introspection. *Circ Res* 1981;48 (suppl I):179–188

14. MacDougall JD, McKelvie RS, Moroz DE, Sale DG, McCartney N, Buick F: Factors affecting blood pressure during heavy weightlifting and static contractions. *J Appl Physiol* 1992;73:1590–1597

15. McArdle WD, Katch FI, Katch VL: *Exercise Physiology, Energy Nutrition and Human Performance.* Philadelphia, Lea and Febiger, 1991

16. MacDougall JD, Tuxen D, Sale DG, Moroz JR, Sutton JR: Arterial blood pressure response to heavy resistance exercise. *J Appl Physiol* 1985;58:785–790

17. Mitchell JH: Neural control of the circulation during exercise. *Med Sci Sport Exerc* 1990;22:141–154

18. Hamilton WF, Woodbury RA, Harper HT, Jr: Arterial, cerebrospinal, and venous pressures in man during cough and strain. *Am J Physiol* 1944;141:42–50

19. Sale DG, Moroz DE, McKelvie RS, MacDougall JD, McCartney N: Effect of training on the blood pressure response to weightlifting. (submitted)

20. McCartney N, McKelvie RS, Martin J, Sale DG, MacDougall JD: Weight-training induced attenuation of the circulatory response to weightlifting in older males. *J Appl Physiol* 1993;74:1056–1060.

21. Lentini AC, McKelvie RS, McCartney N, Tomlinson CW, MacDougall JD: Assessment of left ventricular response of strength trained atheltes during weightlifting exercise. *J Appl Physiol* (in press)

22. Åstrand P-O, Ekblom B, Messin R. Saltin B, Stenberg J: Intra-arterial blood pressure during exercise with different muscle groups. *J Appl Physiol* 1965;20:253–258

Chapter 10

Adaptation of Coronary Circulation to Exercise Training

M. Harold Laughlin, PhD, Christine L. Oltman, PhD, Judy M. Muller, PhD, P. Robert Myers, MD, PhD, and Janet L. Parker, PhD

As discussed in detail in other chapters of this monograph, there is substantial evidence to support the notion that regular physical activity is associated with a reduced risk of coronary heart disease. Powell et al. in 1987[1] and Blair in 1992[2] concluded that the available literature indicates that not only is physical activity inversely related to the incidence of coronary heart disease, but that low levels of physical activity are causal to coronary heart disease. The mechanisms responsible for the beneficial effects of exercise training have not been established.

Ekelund et al.[3] reported that the protective effects of exercise must act by mechanisms independent of age, smoking status, systolic blood pressure, low-density liproprotein (LDL) level, and high-density liproprotein (HDL) level because adding these covariates to an age-adjusted risk model decreased relative risk by only 10%. Their analysis indicated that it is possible that the beneficial effects of training are the result of adaptations localized in the coronary circulation. There is evidence to support the hypothesis that exercise training causes alterations in the coronary vascular bed that result in an improved capacity of this vascular bed to transport nutrients and waste products. For example, Ehsani et al.[4] reported that, after an exercise training program, patients had less evidence

This work was supported by NIH grant # HL 36531 and HL 47812, by the American Heart Association–Missouri Affiliate, and by a Veterans Administration Career Development Award to P. R. Myers.

From Fletcher GF, (ed): *Cardiovascular Response to Exercise.* Mount Kisco, NY, Futura Publishing Company, Inc., © 1994.

of myocardial ischemia during exercise stress tests (ie, less ST-segment depression). The trained patients were capable of sustaining a greater cardiac double product at the same time the reduced maximal ST-segment depression was observed. These results suggest that the ability of the coronary circulation to provide blood flow was increased in these patients after exercise training.[4] There also is evidence that exercise training results in increases in coronary blood flow capacity in animals.[5,6] For example, we have found that exercise training induces an increase in coronary vascular transport capacity in dogs[7] and miniature swine.[8] The increase in transport capacity involves increases in both coronary blood flow capacity and coronary capillary diffusion capacity.

There appear to be two major types of modifications operative in the vascular adaptation induced in the coronary circulation by exercise training: *structural vascular modifications* and *modifications in the control of vascular resistance*.[5] Structural vascular adaptation generally involves both growth of vessels such as increased length and/or diameters of existing vessels, as well as increases in the number of vessels per unit of myocardium (ie, angiogenesis). Both types of structural vascular adaptation occur in response to exercise training.[5,6,9,10] For example, training has been reported to result in increases in the cross-sectional area of the proximal coronary arteries (see Chapter 19),[11,12] and training-induced angiogenesis has been demonstrated in that training causes moderate cardiac hypertrophy while maintaining or increasing capillary density[13–17] and increasing arteriolar density.[18] Structural remodeling of the coronary vasculature may occur independently or in concert with adaptations in the control of coronary vascular resistance. Adaptive changes in vascular control can be the result of alterations in neural-humoral control of the vascular bed, alterations in local vascular control mechanisms, and/or alterations of intrinsic vasomotor function of coronary arteries.[5]

In support of this hypothesis is experimental evidence demonstrating that exercise training produces alterations in systemic cardiovascular control systems,[19] neurohumoral control of the coronary circulation,[9,20] and local control of the coronary circulation.[5] In addition, there is evidence of training-induced changes in intrinsic vasomotor function of coronary arteries,[21–23] including exercise training–induced alterations in the cellular-molecular control of intracellular free Ca^{2+} in vascular smooth muscle cells isolated from coronary arteries of exercise trained animals.[24,25]

This chapter summarizes the results of a series of studies designed to test the hypothesis that exercise training induces modifications in endothelium-mediated vasoregulation.[8,21,26,27-29] Vasodilator mechanisms were examined in the intact coronary circulation in vivo, and in isolated vessel segments in vitro. To allow comparison of training effects on vasomotor control among arterial vessels throughout the coronary vascular tree, experiments were conducted on vessel segments from proximal coronary arteries (2 mm diameter),[21] near-resistance arteries (150–240 μm in diameter,[29] and in resistance arteries (<100 μm in diameter)[26-28] of sedentary control and exercise-trained miniature swine. In vitro techniques were used because they provide a focused evaluation of the intrinsic contractile properties of coronary arteries independent of confounding nonvascular influences present in the intact animal.

Materials and Methods

Experimental Animals

Adult female miniature swine weighing 25–40 kg were obtained from the breeder (Charles River) in batches of eight animals each. Upon arrival, the pigs were familiarized with treadmill exercise over a 1 to 2 week period. Treadmill performance tests were administered to each animal. Each batch of eight pigs was randomly divided into two groups of four pigs. One group (exercise trained, ET) underwent a progressive treadmill training program[8] similar to that described by Tipton et al.[30] for dogs. The second group of pigs (sedentary control, SED) was restricted to their pens (6 × 12 feet) for 16 to 22 weeks.

Training Procedures

During the first week, the ET pigs ran on the treadmill at 3 mph, 0% grade for 20 to 30 minutes (endurance), and at 5 mph for 15 minutes (sprint). The speed and duration of running were increased progressively at a rate that depended on the tolerance of each pig.

During the 12th week of training a typical training session consisted of the following 85-minute workout: 1) 5-minute warm-up run at 2.5 mph; 2) 15-minute sprint at speeds of 5 to 8 mph; 3) 60-minute endurance run at 4 to 5 mph; and 4) 5-minute warm-down run at 2 mph. Ranges of running speed are presented because the ET program is customized to each pig's exercise ability. The ET pigs were given positive reinforcement for exercise by feeding them after each training bout. Treadmill performance tests were administered again to the SED and ET pigs at the completion of the training or pen-confinement periods.

Treadmill Performance Test

The performance test used consisted of four stages of exercise: 1) 3.1 mph, 0% grade for 5 minutes; 2) 3.1 mph, 10% grade for 10 minutes; 3) 4.3 mph, 10% grade for 10 minutes (some pigs were unable to sustain 4.3 mph up a 10% grade for 10 minutes); and 4) 6 mph, 10% grade until exhaustion.[8] Heart rates were measured throughout the treadmill performance test and total duration of exercise at stage 4 was recorded.

Oxidative Enzyme Activity

After killing the pigs, samples were taken from the middle of the long head of triceps brachii muscles, frozen in liquid N_2, and stored at $-70°C$ until processed. Citrate synthase activity was measured from whole-muscle homogenate using the spectrophotometric method of Sere.[31]

In Vivo Measurements of Coronary Hemodynamics

In initial experiments we examined vasomotor reactivity of coronary arteries isolated from hearts in which we had documented training-induced vascular adaptation in the form of increased coronary transport capacity measured in situ.[8] This experimental approach allowed us to conduct coronary transport experiments and coronary arterial vasomotor experiments from the same animals. Coronary blood flow capacity and capillary diffusion capacity were measured by cannulating the left anterior descending coronary artery and perfusing the myocardium with a pump withdrawing blood from the pigs' femoral artery. Blood flow was measured with a cannulating electromagnetic flow probe in the perfusion tubing.

A set of preliminary in vivo experiments was conducted to examine bradykinin-induced vasodilator response in the coronary circulation after in vitro experiments indicated that endothelium-mediated vasodilator mechanisms are altered by exercise training. In these experiments, pigs were instrumented to measure arterial, coronary arterial, coronary venous, and left ventricular pressures and coronary blood flow with a narcometic flow probe placed around the left anterior descending coronary artery via a thoracotomy in the fourth left intercostal space.

Coronary Artery Isolation Procedures

In most experiments, pigs were anesthetized with ketamine (30 mg/kg) and pentobarbital sodium (35 mg/kg; Fort Dodge Labs, Fort Dodge, IA); hearts were rapidly removed and placed in cold Krebs bicarbonate buffer. In experiments in which in vivo measurements were made, hearts were removed and placed in iced (4°C) Krebs bicarbonate buffer solution after completion of the in vivo experiments. Hearts were maintained in iced Krebs buffer (0–4°C) during isolation of all coronary vessels. Portions of cardiac muscle from the left ventricular free wall were removed for dissection of near-resistance and resistance arteries and maintained in smaller dissection chambers. The proximal coronary arteries were then dissected as described.

Proximal Coronary Artery Preparation

Segments of the left coronary artery of approximately 2.0 mm outer diameter were dissected carefully from the myocardium. Arteries were trimmed of fat and connective tissue in iced Krebs solution. Vessel samples were taken from similar sites in hearts from SED and ET pigs. Arteries were cut into cross-sectional rings 3.5 to 4 mm axial length; a filar calibrated micrometer eyepiece was used to measure outside diameter (OD), inside diameter (ID), and length of each vessel ring. Vascular rings were mounted on two stainless steel wires: one attached to a force transducer (Grass FT03, Grass Instrument Company, Quincy, MA) and the other to a micrometer microdrive (Stoelting/Prior Microdrive, Stoelting Company, Quincy, MA). Each vessel apparatus was placed in a 20-ml tissue bath containing Krebs bicarbonate buffer equilibrated at $37 \pm 0.5°C$ with 95% O_2:5% CO_2. Isometric contractions and relaxations were recorded on a Grass polygraph recorder. Rings were stretched individually to the maximum of the length-developed tension relationship (L_{max}) by repeated test exposures to KCl (30 mM) at increasing vessel diameters.[21]

Near-resistance Artery Preparation

Segments of the left circumflex coronary artery (LCCA) (1.5-mm axial length) were excised from the heart tissue. Coronary rings (150–250 μm diameter) were prepared and mounted in an isometric microvessel myograph system (Living Systems Instrumentation, Burlington, VT). This system allows direct determination of vessel wall force while internal circumference is controlled (A). A Zeiss S7 stereomicroscope was used for vessel dissection and preparation; vessel measurements and wire dimensions were obtained using a filar eyepiece adaptation. Vessels were superfused continuously with aerated bicarbonate buffer warmed to 37°C and allowed to equilibrate for at least 30 minutes. Internal diameter was set to yield a resting tension of approximately 0.1 to 0.2 mN/mm. After initial equilibration, the resting tension/internal circumference relationship was determined using progressive vessel stretches and measurements of passive tension and interval vessel circumference (L) at each level of stretch. L was calculated as $L = 2f + 4\,d/2 + 2(\pi/2)$, where d = wire diameter and f = distance between the wires. Coronary rings were set at I_{80}, where $L_{80} = 0.8L_{100}$. L_{100} = internal circumference of the vessel under a transmural pressure of 100 mm Hg.

Resistance Artery Preparation

With the aid of a dissecting microscope (Zeiss SV8), unbranched microvessels 70 to 150 μm in diameter and 1 mm in length were carefully dissected free from surrounding tissue 1 to 3 mm below the epicardial surface. The artery was transferred to a Plexiglas chamber containing oxygenated Krebs solution. Each end of the vessel was cannulated with a glass micropipette and secured with 10–0 ethilon suture. The artery was then visualized with a Nikon light microscope (Boyce Scientific, St. Louis MO) and intraluminal diameter was monitored with a video tracking device. Arteries were warmed to 37°C and intraluminal pressure was set at 40 mm Hg and allowed 30 minutes to reach equilibrium. In experiments designed to examine vasomotor responses to pharmacological agents with no flow, a Living Systems (Burlington, VT) video tracking device was used to measure vessel diameters. Alternatively, flow-induced vasodilation was studied using methods previously described by Kuo et al.[32]

Experimental Design

The primary purpose of these experiments was to determine if exercise training alters endothelium-dependent vasodilator responses of coronary arteries. We examined the responses to two endothelium-dependent vasodilator stimuli: bradykinin (BK) and flow-induced vasodilation and two endothelium-independent vasodilators: adenosine (ADO) and sodium nitroprusside (SNP). Vasodilator responses to ADO, SNP, and BK were examined in all types of vessel. Flow-induced vasodilation was examined only in resistance arteries. In proximal coronary arteries precontraction was induced with 30 mM KCl, 30 μM prostaglandin F-2 alpha (PGF$_{2\alpha}$), or 6 nM endothelin (EN). In near-resistance arteries precontraction was induced with 30 mM KCl and 6 nM EN. Resistance arteries were preconstricted with endothelin. Since the resistance arteries often developed spontaneous tone, endothelin was given in sufficient doses to produce a 50% constriction. Resistance arteries from SED pigs required an EN dose of 2.1 ± 0.4 nM to produce 50% constriction, whereas resistance arteries from ET pigs required only $1.3 + 0.3$ nM EN. In the presence of steady-state vasoconstriction (because of KCl, PGF$_{2\alpha}$, or EN) vasodilator responses were investigated by cumulative addition of adenosine (10^{-9}–10^{-4} M), sodium nitroprusside (10^{-10}–10^{-4} M), or BK (10^{-13}–10^{-6} M) to the bath surrounding the vessels in half-log increments. Dilation also was expressed as a percent of the relaxation achieved in response to 100 μM SNP.

Flow-induced Vasodilation

To study flow-induced responses independently of luminal pressure changes, a dual-reservoir system was used to maintain a constant intraluminal pressure over a wide range of flow changes.[32] In brief, the micropipettes were connected to independent reservoir systems and intraluminal pressures were measured through side arms of the two reservoir lines by low-volume displacement strain-gauge transducers. Resistance arteries were pressurized without flow by setting both reservoirs at the same level. Flow was initiated by simultaneously moving the reservoirs in equal but opposite directions, generating a pressure gradient. Since the resistance of the pipettes was equivalent, simultaneous movement of the reservoirs in equal and opposite directions does not change midpoint lumenal pressure.[32]

Solutions and Drugs

The Krebs solutions for the proximal coronary arteries and near-resistance arteries consisted of (mM) 131.5 NaCl, 5.0 KCl, 1.2 NaH_2PO_4, 1.2 $MgCl_2$, 2.5 $CaCl_2$, 11.2 glucose, 13.5 $NaHCO_3$, and resistance arteries 118.3 NaCl, 4.7 KCl, 2.5 $CaCl_2$, 1.2 $MgSO_4$, 1.2 KH_2PO_4, 25 $NaHCO_3$, 11.1 glucose. All solutions contained propranolol (3 μM) and 0.025 mM ethylenediamine-tetraacetic acid. Solutions were aerated with 95% O_2:5% CO_2 (pH 7.4) and maintained at $37 \pm 0.05°C$. Concentrated stock solutions of vasocative agents were prepared with distilled water. Vasoconstrictor agents used included $PGF_{2\alpha}$ and EN. Vasodilator agents used included ADO, SNP, and bradykinin. EN and BK were purchased from Cal Biochem (Cal Biochem Corporation, La Jolla, CA). Other drugs were purchased from Sigma Chemical Company (St. Louis, MO).

Statistical Analysis

Contractile responses to drugs are presented as absolute values in grams of tension. Vasodilator responses are presented as percent relaxation from preconstricted values. Concentration-response curves were evaluated using an analysis of variance for repeated measures (ANOVA), and the Bonferroni correction for multiple comparisons. Data are expressed as $\bar{X} \pm SEM$. Data were analyzed with each vascular ring counted as one observation and with each animal counted as one observation. In the analysis with $n =$ numbers of pigs, data from coronary arterial rings from each pig, used in identical protocols, were averaged for comparisons among groups with respect to each vasoactive agent. IC_{50} is the vasodilator concentration that produced 50% of maximal relaxation. Significance of differences between mean values of citrate synthase activity, treadmill performance times, stress-test heart rates, artery resting tension, maximal effect, and IC_{50} values was assessed with the unpaired t test. p values <0.05 were considered significant.

Physiological State of Animals

Adaptation produced by the training program was evident in the treadmill performance tests in that heart rates were significantly reduced by 10% to 15% at stages 2 and 3 in ET pigs after training. Endurance times in ET pigs were increased from 25 minutes to 35 to 40 minutes. Citrate synthase activity of the long head of the triceps brachii muscles of ET pigs was significantly increased (average ET citrate synthase activity was increased 10–40% above SED values), confirming the shift in skeletal muscle oxidative capacity that characterizes effective exercise training.[19] Heart weight/body weight ratio for the sedentary control pigs was significantly less than the corresponding ET value (SED $= 4.53 \pm 0.3$ g/kg; ET $= 5.25 \pm 0.2$ g/kg; $p<0.05$).

Coronary Vessel Characteristics

Proximal Coronary Arteries

Proximal coronary arteries isolated from SED and ET pigs had similar dimensions for outer and luminal diameter and vessel wall thickness at rest. As per experimental design, arterial segments isolated from SED and ET pigs also had similar axial lengths. Water content, calculated as the percent tissue water (wet wt–dry wt/wet wt) also was similar between groups. Length-dependent responses of active tension and passive tension were similar in arteries from SED and ET pigs. Arteries from SED and ET pigs were of the same resting internal and external diameters and were stretched to the same relative length at L_{max} (LCCA: SED = 172 ± 3% vs. ET = 172 ± 2% nonstretched diameter). Resting tension at L_{max} was similar in LCCA vascular segments from SED pigs (6.21 ± 0.42 g) and ET pigs (5.94 ± 0.46 g).[21]

Near-resistance Coronary Arteries

There was no difference between luminal diameter (SED = 180 ± 8 μm, ET = 195 ± 11 μm), vessel wall thickness (SED = 50 ± 2 μm, ET = 56 ± 2 μm), or axial length (SED = 1.46 ± 0.03 mm, ET = 1.43 ± 0.03 mm) of vessels isolated from SED and ET pigs. However, the I_{80} was significantly greater in vessels from ET pigs (SED = 986 ± 47 μm, ET = 1167 ± 74 μm) whereas there was no difference between passive tension at I_{80}.[29]

Resistance Arteries

The passive relationship between intraluminal pressure and diameter in arterioles isolated from SED and ET pigs was similar. Thus, at an intraluminal pressure of 40 mm Hg, passive intraluminal diameters were similar (SED = 114 ± 3 μm, ET = 117 ± 3 μm).

Vasodilator Responses

Adenosine

Adenosine produced concentration-related decreases in contractile tension in all three types of artery[27] (Figures 1 and 2). Adenosine produced nearly 100% relaxation in all three types of

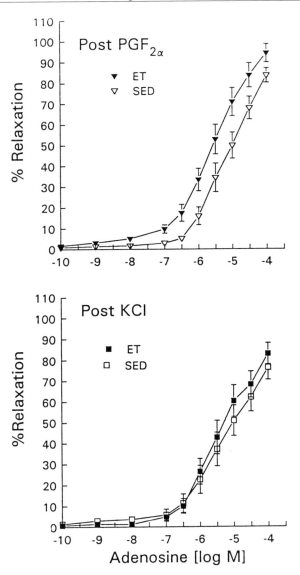

FIGURE 1. *Adenosine-induced relaxation of 30 μM PGF$_{2\alpha}$ (top panel) and 30 mM KCl (lower panel)-induced isometric contractions in proximal coronary artery rings from SED and ET pigs. Values are X̄ ± SEM. SED data represent 47 vessel segments from 15 pigs. ET data represents 50 vessel segments from 16 pigs. Vasorelaxant response curves to adenosine were augmented in the ET group compared with SED after preconstriction with PGF$_{2\alpha}$. Data are from Reference 21.*

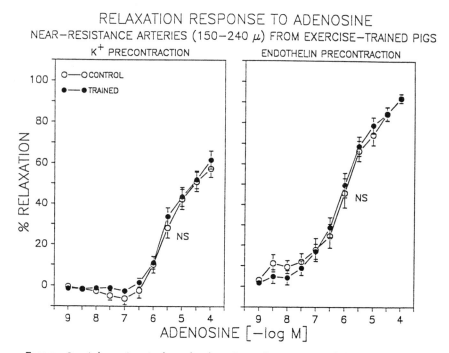

FIGURE 2. *Adenosine-induced relaxation of 30 mM KCl (left panel) and endothelin (right panel) = induced isometric contractions in rings of near resistance coronary arteries from SED and ET pigs. Values are $\bar{X} \pm SEM$. Data are from Reference 29.*

vessel when they were preconstricted with EN or $PGF_{2\alpha}$. In contrast, maximal relaxation averaged only 90% and 60% in KCl-induced precontractions of proximal arteries and near-resistance arteries, respectively. In proximal arteries ADO vasorelaxant response curves of vessel segments from ET pigs were significantly different from the SED curves when the rings were preconstricted with $PGF_{2\alpha}$. When the rings were preconstricted with KCl, the ADO-induced vasorelaxant responses were similar in ET and SED. There were no differences between ADO vasorelaxant responses of near-resistance or resistance arteries isolated from SED and ET pigs (Figure 2). As shown in Figure 3, there was an inverse relationship between artery size and ADO sensitivity in that the IC_{50} values were greatest in proximal coronary arteries and least in resistance arteries.

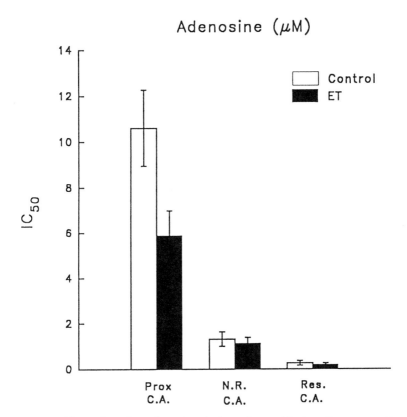

FIGURE 3. *IC_{50} values for adenosine-induced vasodilation. Precontraction was induced with $PGF_{2\alpha}$ in the proximal coronary arteries (Prox C.A.) and endothelin in the near-resistance coronary arteries (N.R.C.A.) and resistance coronary arteries (Res.C.A.). Resistance artery data are from refs. 26 and 27. Clearly definable maximal effects were not always observed with adenosine in the proximal coronary arteries. Therefore, the IC_{50} values represent apparent IC_{50}'s in that they are the concentration of adenosine at which 50% of the contractile force was gone. The difference between sedentary control (Control) and exercise trained (ET) adenosine IC_{50}'s in the proximal coronary artery was significant (p<0.05).*

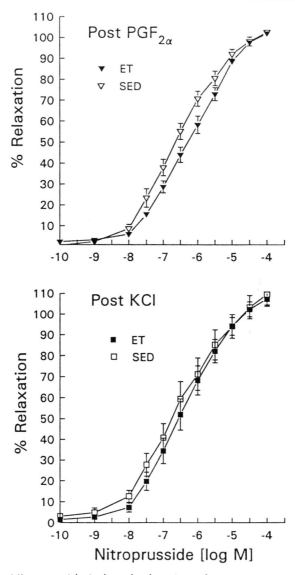

FIGURE 4. *Nitroprusside-induced relaxation of 30 μM PGF$_{2\alpha}$ (top panel) and 30 mM KCl (lower panel)-induced isometric contractions in coronary vascular rings from SED and ET pigs. SED data represent results from 55 vessel segments from 12 animals. ET data represent results from 54 vessel segments from 12 animals. Data are from Reference 21.*

Nitroprusside

Nitroprusside produced concentration-dependent decreases in contractile force and induced complete relaxation in proximal, near-resistance, and resistance coronary arteries from both groups (Figures 4 and 5). The vasorelaxant effects of SNP were similar between groups in all three sizes of coronary artery. The IC_{50} values were similar between groups and among the three sizes of artery (Figure 6).

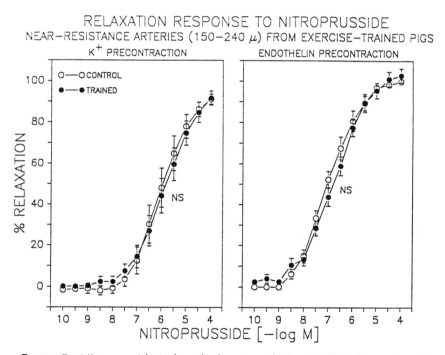

RELAXATION RESPONSE TO NITROPRUSSIDE
NEAR–RESISTANCE ARTERIES (150–240 μ) FROM EXERCISE–TRAINED PIGS

FIGURE 5. *Nitroprusside-induced relaxation of 30 mM KCl (left panel) and endothelin (right panel)-induced isometric contractions in rings of near resistance coronary arteries from SED and ET pigs. Values are $\bar{X} \pm SEM$. Data are from Reference 29.*

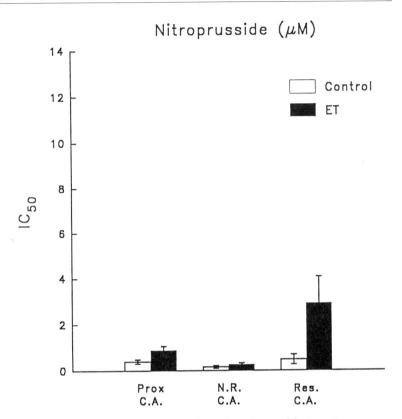

FIGURE 6. *IC_{50} values for nitroprusside-induced vasodilation. Precontraction was induced with $PGF_{2\alpha}$ in the proximal coronary arteries (Prox C.A.) and endothelin in the near-resistance coronary arteries (N.R.C.A.) and resistance coronary arteries (Res.C.A.). Resistance artery data are from References 26 and 27. There were no significant differences between sedentary control (Control) and exercise trained (ET) IC_{50}'s (p>0.05).*

Bradykinin

Bradykinin produced concentration-dependent decreases in contractile force in proximal, near-resistance, and resistance coronary arteries from both groups (Figures 7,8, and 9). Near complete relaxation was produced by BK in both near-resistance and resistance arteries. Maximal relaxation was generally only 50–60% of

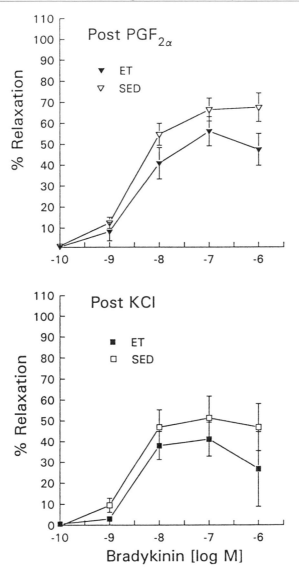

FIGURE 7. *BK-induced relaxation of 30* μ*M PGF$_{2\alpha}$ (top panel) and 30 mM KCl (lower panel)-induced isometric contractions in coronary vascular rings from SED and ET pigs. Post =PGF$_{2\alpha}$ data represent results from 23 vessel segments from 12 pigs in each group. Post-KCl data represent results from 20 vessel segments from 12 pigs in each group. (Unpublished observations.)*

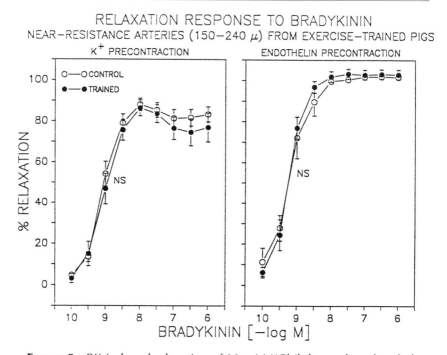

RELAXATION RESPONSE TO BRADYKININ
NEAR–RESISTANCE ARTERIES (150–240 μ) FROM EXERCISE–TRAINED PIGS

FIGURE 8. *BK-induced relaxation of 30 mM KCl (left panel) and endothelin (right panel)-induced isometric contractions in rings of near-resistance coronary arteries from SED and ET pigs. Values are X̄ ± SEM. Data are from Reference 29.*

precontraction force in large arteries. There were no significant differences between BK-induced responses in proximal and near-resistance vessels from ET and SED pigs. In contrast, sensitivity to BK was markedly enhanced in resistance arteries from ET pigs (Figure 10).[26]

Flow-induced Vasodilation in Resistance Arteries

Flow through resistance coronary arteries produced vasodilation in a dose-dependent manner (Figure 11). Dilation tended to be greater in resistance arteries from ET pigs across the range of flows examined. Relaxation was significantly greater in vessels from ET pigs when pressure gradients were 30, 40, and 70 cm H_2O.

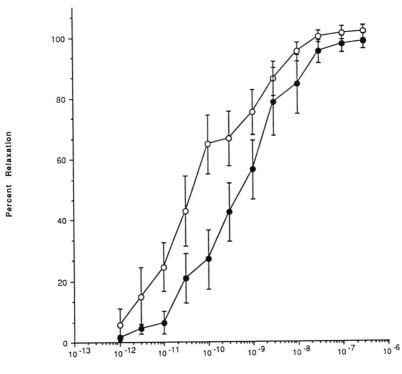

FIGURE 9. *Relaxation responses to bradykinin in resistance arteries. Data are presented as mean ± SEM in eight control (closed circles) and eight trained pigs (open circles). Percent relaxation indicates a percent of the relaxation measured in response to 100 μM SNP after endothelin preconstriction. Data presented previously in abstract form at FASEB 1991.*[26]

Discussion

Aerobic exercise training induces an increase in coronary vascular transport capacity. This increased transport capacity is the result of increases in both blood flow capacity and capillary exchange capacity. These functional changes are the result of two major types of adaptive responses: structural vascular adaptation and altered control of vascular resistance. Training-induced changes

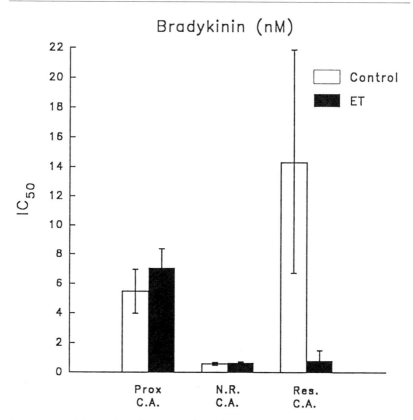

FIGURE 10. IC_{50} values for BK-induced vasodilation. Precontraction was induced with $PGF_{2\alpha}$ in the proximal coronary arteries (Prox C.A.) and endothelin in the near-resistance coronary arteries (N.R.C.A.) and resistance coronary arteries (Res.C.A.). Resistance artery data are from References 26 and 27. The difference between sedentary control (Control) and exercise trained (ET) BK IC_{50}'s in resistance coronary arteries was significant (p<0.05).

in coronary vascular control have been shown to include altered coronary responses to vasoactive substances and alterations in the cellular-molecular control of intracellular free Ca^{2+} in vascular smooth muscle cells isolated from coronary arteries of exercise trained animals. Results presented in this chapter indicate that exercise training also changes endothelium-mediated vasodilator mechanisms in the coronary circulation. It is important to integrate

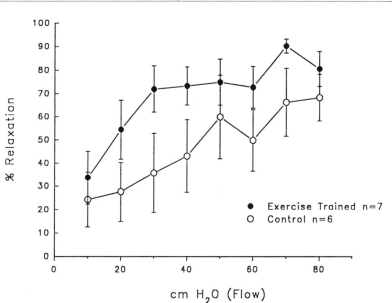

FIGURE 11. *Relaxation responses to increasing intralumenal flow in resistance arteries. Intralumenal flow was generated by establishing a pressure gradient across the vessel. Data are presented as mean ± SEM for a group of seven trained and six control pigs. Percent relaxation indicates a percent of the relaxation measured in response to 100 μM SNP. (Unpublished observations.)*

what is known about the effects of training on coronary vascular control mechanisms if the consequences of these changes in coronary heart disease syndromes are to be fully comprehended.

There is a growing body of evidence that exercise training alters the control of coronary vascular resistance. Gwirtz and Stone[20] and Liang and Stone[33] reported that exercise training alters neural control of the coronary circulation. Also, Bove and Dewey[22] reported diminished phenylephrine-induced vasoconstrictor responses of proximal coronary arteries in intact, anesthetized, exercise-trained dogs. Di-Carlo et al.[9] reported that exercise training for 4 weeks resulted in enhanced coronary resistance vessel sensitivity to both α- and β-adrenergic agents and to adenosine. Finally, blockade of α-adrenergic receptors has been shown to produce greater vasodilation in exercise-trained dogs and pigs than in controls and that adenosine produced greater coronary vasodilation in exercise-trained animals.[7,8] Although the results of these studies support the notion that exercise training alters control of the coronary circulation, they shed little light on mechanisms for these changes. This is important because, as discussed in other chapters in this monograph, it is well known that exercise training alters cardiac function and neural-humoral influences on the heart. As a result, it is difficult to determine whether differences in coronary vascular function observed in exercise-trained subjects in experiments conducted on intact coronary vascular beds are the result of training-induced alterations in neural, humoral, or metabolic influences on the heart or the result of primary alterations in the control of coronary vascular resistance. The vasoregulatory function of blood vessels is the result of the functional characteristics of vascular smooth muscle cells and endothelial cells and the interaction of these functional characteristics with connective tissue elements in the vessels. Therefore, any training-induced changes in vascular control and the intrinsic contractile characteristics of coronary blood vessels are likely the result of alterations in one or more of these components. We did not systematically evaluate the effects of training on connective tissue elements in the coronary arteries. However, the results of this study indicate that the length-dependent passive and active tension relationships of proximal coronary arteries and resistance arterioles do not appear to be altered. In contrast, near-resistance coronary arteries isolated from exercise-trained pigs appear to be more compliant than vessels from sedentary control pigs. These results suggest that the effects of training on connective tissue elements of the coronary vascular bed merit further evaluation.

Effects of Training on Coronary Vascular Smooth Muscle

Active vasomotor control of coronary blood flow and its distribution is accomplished via modulation of total and regional vascular resistances. Coronary vascular resistance is regulated by the level of contractile activity in coronary arterial vascular smooth muscle. Results of previous studies demonstrate that concentration-response relationships for isometric contractions evoked with KCl, prostaglandin F-2-alpha ($PGF_{2\alpha}$), acetylcholine, and endothelin are similar in proximal coronary arteries isolated from sedentary and exercise-trained pigs.[21] In contrast, arteries from trained pigs developed 47% less maximal tension in response to norepinephrine.

Concentration-response vasodilator responses evoked by isoproterenol and forskolin were similar in arteries from sedentary and exercise-trained pigs. However, arteries from exercise-trained animals were less sensitive to the vasodilator actions of sodium nitroprusside and more sensitive to vasodilator actions of adenosine. The alterations in coronary artery responses to norepinephrine and adenosine observed in proximal coronary arteries from exercise-trained animals appeared to be the result of alterations in vascular smooth muscle because they were still apparent after endothelium removal. Oltman et al.[21] concluded that exercise training induced alterations in adenosine and α-adrenergic receptor/signal tranduction events in coronary vascular smooth muscle. These results are consistent with in vivo results reported by DiCarlo et al.[9] and Bove and Dewey,[22] and provide a direct evaluation of contractile responses of vascular smooth muscle of epicardial coronary arteries independent of influences from metabolic and neurohumoral control factors.

Steno-Bittel et al. conducted a study of the effects of exercise training on the cellular-molecular control of contractile activity in coronary vascular smooth muscle.[24,25] Using fura-2 to measure intracellular free Ca^{2+} transients induced by caffeine in isolated vascular smooth muscle cells, they found that the caffeine-releasable pool of sarcoplasmic reticulum (SR) Ca^{2+} was decreased in coronary smooth muscle cells from exercise-trained pigs.[24] The results of subsequent experiments[25] revealed that the training-induced depletion of the caffeine-releasable SR Ca^{2+} store is dependent on the time of recovery of the cells from KCl-induced depolarization. The results further indicated that training resulted in alterations in the functional characteristics and/or distribution of SR Ca^{2+} release channels in coronary vascular smooth muscle cells.

Training does not appear to alter vasoconstrictor responses of near-resistance coronary arteries.[29] In contrast to the effects of training on vasoconstrictor responses of proximal coronary arteries,[21] preliminary results indicate that vasoconstrictor responses may be altered in resistance arterioles.[28] These data indicate that coronary resistance arteries isolated from trained pigs exhibit greater myogenic reactivity.[28] Although sufficient information is not available to allow a complete understanding of the effects of exercise training on coronary vascular smooth muscle, available data indicate that training causes modifications of intrinsic vasomotor control mechanisms in coronary vascular smooth muscle and that the training-induced changes are not uniformly present throughout the coronary arterial tree.

Effects of Training on Endothelium-mediated Vascular Control

Over the past 10 to 15 years, research has shown that the endothelium plays an essential role in the control of vascular tone. It is now known that the endothelium can mediate vasodilator responses, vasoconstrictor responses, and vascular growth (proliferation) in response to several stimuli.[34,35] It appears that the endothelium plays an important role both in the vascular response to physical forces such as shear stress and vessel stretch and neurohumoral agents. The endothelium may be involved in both acute adaptive responses in the form of regulation of vascular resistance as well as chronic responses in the form of adaptations of vascular structure and/or alterations in mechanisms of control of vascular resistance.

Endothelium-dependent vasoregulation is a relatively new area of vascular biology, which is rapidly expanding. However, there is little in the literature about the effects of chronic exercise training on vascular endothelium and endothelium-dependent vasoregulation. The preliminary results presented in this chapter indicate that bradykinin-induced vasodilation is enhanced in coronary resistance arteries (70–100 μM in diameter) isolated from exercise-trained miniature swine.[26] These results do not allow the determination of the mechanisms responsible for this training-induced change. It is known that bradykinin-induced vasodilation is endothelium-dependent in porcine coronary arteries.[36–38] However, the mediators released from the endothelial cells in response to bradykinin are currently being investigated.[38] Thus, training may cause enhanced release of endothelium-derived relaxing factor (EDRF), prostacyclins, endothelium-derived hyperpolarizing factor, or some other substance in coronary resistance arteries. Alternatively, since vasodilation is the result of a net balance between vasorelaxant and vasoconstrictor influences, increased relaxation responses to bradykin could result from a reduced, concomitant release of an endothelium-derived vasoconstrictor substance.

In reference to endothelial function in proximal coronary

arteries from trained animals, the transient increase in intracellular free Ca^{2+} observed in endothelial cells isolated from the proximal coronary artery of trained miniature swine was less, both in magnitude and duration, than in cells isolated from coronary arteries of sedentary control pigs (unpublished observations). Increases in intracellular free Ca^{2+} may serve as a signal for the release of EDRF. It is not clear how to relate these preliminary data with the vasodilator responses that were not altered by training (Figure 7) presented herein.

Flow-induced Vasodilation

Flow-induced vasodilation has been demonstrated in both coronary[39,40] and femoral[41,42] arteries and is believed to be caused by a local (within the blood vessel wall) mechanism. Kuo et al.[32] recently demonstrated flow-induced vasodilation in isolated coronary resistance vessels. Most evidence indicates that flow-induced vasodilation in the coronary resistance arteries depends on the presence of a normal endothelium.[39–43]

To our knowledge, this is the first study of flow-induced vasodilation in coronary arteries of exercise-trained animals. These preliminary data (Figure 11) provide the first indication that exercise training is associated with enhanced flow-induced vasodilation in the coronary circulation. Enhanced flow-induced vasodilation in coronary arterioles may represent an important change in the control of coronary vascular resistance. For example, reports of enhanced sensitivity of the coronary circulation in trained subjects to vasodilator agents[7–9] could be explained on the basis of a training-induced change in flow-induced vasodilation. If exercise training produces an enhancement in flow-induced vasodilation in the coronary microcirculation, then this would be expected to work synergistically with a vasodilator such as adenosine. Thus, for a given dose of adenosine, a greater amount of vasodilation would be produced.

We have not conducted experiments designed to test this prediction. However, in previous studies we determined the effects of maximal adenosine vasodilation under constant flow conditions and constant pressure conditions in the coronary circulation of trained animals.[7,8] If flow-induced vasodilation is in operation during adenosine vasodilation, then coronary resistance will be less during vasodilation with constant pressure (increased flow) than with constant flow. Furthermore, if training enhances flow-induced vasodilation, then coronary vascular resistance with constant pressure will be less in the coronary circulation of exercise-trained animals. Analysis of these data reveals that calculated coronary resistance was indeed less during adenosine vasodilation, under constant pressure conditions in both dogs (1.02 vs. 0.58 PRU/100) and pigs (0.52 vs. 0.32 PRU/100). Further, the difference between minimal coronary resistance under constant flow versus constant pressure conditions tended to be greater in trained animals. Finally, minimal coronary resistance measured during ADO vasodilation with constant pressure was less in trained dogs (SED = 0.58, ET = 0.55) and pigs (SED = 0.32, ET = 0.27). Thus, this analysis of the results of these previous studies supports the hypothesis that exercise training results in enhanced flow-induced vasodilation in the coronary circulation.

Spatial Nonuniformity of Vascular Control

The fact that vasomotor responsiveness of large and small coronary arteries to neurohumoral agents is different has been known for some time.[44] Nonuniformity in the magnitude of response exists for other important vascular control mechanisms as well. Kuo et al.[45] recently proposed a series-coupled model of coronary arterial network that incorporated segmental variations in responsiveness of vessels of different sizes to metabolic, myogenic (pressure), and flow stimuli. In this model, coronary arteries of 100 to 200 μm diameter have the greatest sensitivity to flow-induced vasodilation and the influence of flow stimuli wanes in vessels of larger and smaller diameter. Also, according to the model of Kuo et al.[45] arteries less than 20 μm in diameter are most sensitive to metabolic control and metabolic control factor sensitivity progressively decreases in upstream vessels. If adenosine is considered to be an important component of metabolic control in the coronary circulation, the results of this study are consistent with this model (Figure 3) in that adenosine IC_{50} values progressively increased with increasing diameter. The results of this study also indicate that training-induced alterations in vascular control mechanisms do not occur uniformly throughout the coronary vascular tree. Thus, the fact that proximal coronary arteries from exercise-trained animals exhibited enhanced adenosine sensitivity whereas adenosine responses of near-resistance and resistance coronary arteries were not altered indicates nonuniformity of training-induced changes in vasomotor control of vascular smooth muscle in the coronary circulation. Also, bradykinin-induced vasodilation appears to be unaltered in near-resistance and proximal coronary arteries isolated from exercise-trained pigs but is enhanced in 100-μm diameter coronary arteries. Thus, the bradykinin data obtained in this study also support the notion of nonuniformity of training-induced changes in vasomotor control of the coronary circulation.

Interactions Between Atherosclerosis and Exercise Training

It is of interest to consider the potential impact of exercise training–induced changes in endothelium-mediated vascular control on coronary heart disease. Atherosclerosis has been found to augment vasoconstrictor responses, impair vasodilator responses, and enhance the possibility of coronary artery vasospasm in proximal coronary arteries and other large arteries.[46,47] Similar atherosclerosis-induced alterations in vasomotor control appear to exist in the coronary microcirculation.[48,49] Hypercholesterolemia and elevated levels of circulating lipid, with or without atherosclerosis, also have been shown to result in augmentation of vasoconstriction and blunting of vasodilation of coronary arteries.[50,51] Finally, atherosclerosis has been shown to inhibit flow-induced vasodilation in humans[52] and porcine coronary resistance vessels.[53] These pathological effects of atherosclerosis and hypercholesterolemia on coronary vasomotor function appear to be primarily the result of altered endothelium-mediated events. Exercise training holds the potential for counteracting the effects of atherosclerosis and/or hyperlipidemia. Previous results indicate that training blunts responses of proximal coronary arteries to some vasoconstrictor agents and enhances responses to some vasodilator agents. Also, the results summarized in this chapter indicate that endothelium-mediated vasodilation is enhanced in the coronary microcirculation by exercise training. Therefore, if exercise training alters vasomotor control through alterations in vascular smooth muscle and/or endothelial cells in the presence of atherosclerosis and/or hypercholesterolemia in a manner similar to the alterations observed in normal pigs, such changes could have consequences in relation to incidence of vasospasm in proximal coronary arteries and at the level of the microcirculation as well. We do not currently have enough information to evaluate critically these potentially important effects.

Acknowledgments

The authors wish to thank M. Mattox, P. Thorne, and M. Tanner for their skilled assistance in the completion of the experiments described in this chapter.

References

1. Powell KE, Thompson PD, Caspersen CJ, Kendrick JS: Physical activity and the incidence of coronary heart disease. *Annu Rev Public Health* 1987;8:253–287
2. Blair SN: Physical activity, fitness, and coronary heart disease. *The International Consensus Symposium on Physical Activity, Fitness and Health.* 1992, in press
3. Ekelund L, Haskell WL, Johnson JL, Shaley FS, Criqui MH, Sheps DS: Physical fitness as a predictor of cardiovascular mortality in asymptomatic north american men. *N Engl J Med* 1988;319:1379–1384
4. Ehsani AA, Heath GW, Hagberg JM, Sobel BS, Holloszy JO: Effects of 12 months of intense exercise training on ischemic ST-segment depression in patients with coronary artery disease. *Circulation* 1981;64:1116–1124
5. Laughlin MH, McAllister RM: Exercise training-induced coronary vascular adaptation. *J Appl Physiol* 1992;73:2209–2225
6. Scheuer J: Effects of physical training on myocardial vascularity and perfusion. *Circulation* 1982;66:491–495
7. Laughlin MH: Effects of exercise training on coronary transport capacity. *J Appl Physiol* 1985;58:468–476
8. Laughlin MH, Overholser KA, Bhatte M: Exercise training increases coronary transport reserve in miniature swine. *J Appl Physiol* 1989;67:1140–1149
9. DiCarlo SE, Blair RW, Bishop VS, Stone HL: Daily exercise enhances coronary resistance vessel sensitivity to pharmacological activation. *J Appl Physiol* 1989;66:421–428

10. Scheuer J, Tipton CM: Cardiovascular adaptations to physical training. *Annu Rev Physiol* 1077;39:221–251
11. Leon AS, Bloor CM: Effects of exercise and its cessation on the heart and its blood supply. *J Appl Physiol* 1968;24:485–490
12. Wyatt HL, Mitchell J: Influences of physical conditioning and deconditioning on coronary vasculature of dogs. *J Appl Physiol* 1978;45:619–625
13. Anversa P, Ricci R, Olivetti G: Effects of exercise on the capillary vasculature of the rat heart. *Circulation* 1987;75(suppl I):I-12–I-18
14. Bloor CM, Leon AS: Interaction of age and exercise on the heart and its blood supply. *Lab Invest* 1970;22:160–165
15. Breisch EA, White FC, Nimmo LE, McKirnan MD, Bloor CM: Exercise-induced cardiac hypertrophy: a correlation of blood flow and microvasculature. *J Appl Physiol* 1986;60:1259–1267
16. Laughlin MH, Tomanek RJ: Myocardial capillarity and maximal capillary diffusion capacity in exercise-trained dogs. *J Appl Physiol* 1987;63:1481–1486
17. Hudlicka O: What makes blood vessels grow? *J Physiol* 1991;444:1–24
18. White FC, McKirnan MD, Breisch EA, Guth BD, Liu Y, Bloor CM: Adaptation of the left ventricle to exercise-induced hypertrophy. *J Appl Physiol* 1987;62:1097–1110
19. Rowell LB: *Human Circulation*. New York: Oxford University Press, 1986
20. Gwirtz PA, Stone HL: Coronary vascular response to adrenergic stimulation in exercise-conditioned dogs. *J Appl Physiol* 1984;243:315–320
21. Oltman CL, Parker JL, Adams HR, Laughlin MH: Effects of exercise training on vasomotor reactivity of porcine coronary arteries. *Am J Physiol* 1992, in press
22. Bove AA, Dewey JD: Proximal coronary vasomotor reactivity after exercise training in dogs. *Circulation* 1985;71:620–625
23. Rogers PJ, Miller TD, Bauer BA, Brum MM, Bove AA, Vanhoutte PM: Exercise training and responsiveness of isolated coronary arteries. *J Appl Physiol* 1991;71:2346–2351
24. Steno-Bittel L, Laughlin MH, Sturek M: Exercise training alters Ca release from coronary smooth muscle sarcoplasmic reticulum. *Am J Physiol* 1990;259:H643–H647
25. Steno-Bittel L, Laughlin MH, Sturek M: Exercise training depletes sarcoplasmic reticulum Ca in coronary smooth muscle. *J Appl Physiol* 1991;71:1764–1773
26. Muller JM, Myers PR, Tanner MA, Laughlin MH: The effect of exercise training on sensitivity of porcine coronary resistance arterioles to bradykinin. *FASEB J* 1991;5:A658
27. Muller JM, Myers PR, Tanner MA, Laughlin MH: Adenosine-induced vasodilator responses of coronary resistance arterioles from exercise trained pigs. *Med Sci Sport Exerc* 1992;24:S116
28. Muller JM, Myers PR, Tanner MA, Laughlin MH: Myogenic responses of coronary arterioles from exercise trained pigs. *FASEB J* 1992;6:A2080
29. Parker JL, Mattox ML, Laughlin MH: Relaxation responses of near

resistance arteries from exercise trained yucatan pigs. *FASEB J* 1992;6: A2081

30. Tipton CM, Carey RA, Eastin WC, Erickson HH: A submaximal test for dogs: evaluation of effects of training, detraining and cage confinement. *J Appl Physiol* 1974;37:271–275

31. Sere PA: Citrate synthase. *Meth Enzymol* 1969;13:3–5

32. Kuo L, Davis MJ, Chilian WM: Endothelium-dependent, flow-induced dilation of isolated coronary arterioles. *Am J Physiol* 1990;259:H1063–H1070

33. Liang IYS, Stone HL: Effect of exercise conditioning on coronary resistance. *J Appl Physiol* 1982;53:631–636

34. Daniel TO, Ives HE: Endothelial control of vascular function. *NIPS* 1989;4:139–142

35. Dzau VJ, Gibbons GH: The role of the endothelium in vascular remodeling, in Rubanyi GM (ed): *Cardiovascular Significance of Endothelium-derived Vasoactive Factors*. Mount Kisco, NY: Futura Publishing Co, Inc, 1991, pp 281–291

36. Kuo L, Chilian WM, Davis MJ: Coronary arteriolar myogenic response is independent of endothelium. *Circ Res* 1990;66:860–866

37. Kuo L, Davis MJ, Chilian WM: Myogenic activity in isolated subepicardial and subendocardial coronary arterioles. *Am J Physiol* 1989;255:H1558–H1562

38. Tschudi M, Richard V, Buhler FR, Luscher TF: Importance of endothelium-derived nitric oxide in porcine coronary resistance arteries. *Am J Physiol* 1991;260:H13–H20

39. Holtz J, Giesler M, Bassenge E: Two dilatory mechanisms of anti-anginal drugs on epicardial coronary arteries in vivo:indirect, flow-dependent, endothelium-mediated dilation and direct smooth muscle relaxation. *Z Kardiol* 1983;72(suppl 3):98–106

40. Lamping KG, Dole WP: Flow-mediated dilation attenuates constriction of large coronary arteries to serotonin. *Am J Physiol* 1988;255:H1317–H1324

41. Hull SS, Kaiser L, Jaffe MD, Sparks HV: Endothelium-dependent flow induced dilation of canine femoral and saphenous arteries. *Blood Vessels* 1986;23:183–198

42. Pohl U, Holtz J, Busse R, Bassenge E: Crucial role of endothelium in the vasodilation response to increased flow in vivo. *Hypertension Dallas* 1986;8:37–44

43. Rubanyi GM, Romero JC, Vanhoutte PM: Flow-induced release of endothelium-derived relaxing factor. *Am J Physiol* 1986;250:H1145–H1149

44. Feigl EO: Coronary physiology. *Physiol Rev* 1983;63:1–205

45. Kuo L, Davis MJ, Chilian WM: Endothelial modulation of arteriolar tone. *NIPS* 1992;7:5–9

46. Heistad DD, Armstrong ML, Marcus ML, Piegors DJ, Mark AL: Augmented responses to vasoconstrictor stimuli in hypercholesterolemic and atherosclerotic monkeys. *Circ Res* 1984;54:711–718

47. Shimokawa H, Tomoike H, Nabeyama S, Yamamoto H, Araki H, Nakamura M: Coronary artery spasm induced in atherosclerotic miniature swine. *Science* 1983;221:560–562

48. Selke FW, Armstrong ML, Harrison DG: Endothelium-dependent vascular relaxation is abnormal in the coronary microcirculation of atherosclerotic primates. *Circulation* 1990;81:1586–1593

49. Chilian WM, Dellsperger KC, Layne SM, Eastham CL, Armstrong MA, Marcus ML, Heistad DD: Effects of atherosclerosis on the coronary microcirculation. *Am J Physiol* 1990;258:H529–H539

50. Cohen RA, Zitnay KM, Haudenschild CC, Cunningham LD: Loss of selective endothelial cell vasoactive functions caused by hypercholesterolemia in pig coronary arteries. *Circ Res* 1988;63:903–910

51. Creager MA, Cook JP, Mendelsohn ME, Gallagher SJ, Coleman SM, Loscalzo J, Dzau VJ: Hypercholesterolemia attenuates endothelium mediated vasodilation in man. *J Clin Invest* 1990;86:228–234

52. Cox DA, VIta JA, Treasure CB, Fish RD, Alexander RW, Ganz P, Selwyn AP: Atherosclerosis impairs flow-mediated dilation of coronary arteries in humans. *Circulation* 1989;80:458–465

53. Kuo L, Davis MJ, Cannon MS, Chilian WM: Pathophysiological consequences of atherosclerosis extend into the coronary microcirculation. Restoration of endothelium-dependent responses by L-Arginine. *Circ Res* 1992;70:465–476

Chapter 11

Blood Volume Response to Training

Victor A. Convertino, PhD

Numerous investigations have established that individuals who are trained for endurance athletic events exhibit dramatically greater total circulating blood volumes than untrained, more sedentary persons. The magnitude of average blood volumes in men trained for highly competitive sports can be as high as 104 ml/kg of body weight compared with 75 to 85 ml/kg in nonathletes.[1,2] More commonly, average blood volumes of 90 to 93 ml/kg have been reported in endurance-trained men compared with 75 ml/kg in their nontrained counterparts.[2,3] Female endurance athletes also demonstrate this hypervolemic relationship with average blood volumes as high as 89 ml/kg compared with only 62 ml/kg in nontrained women.[2] Furthermore, aerobic capacity (maximal oxygen uptake) correlates with blood volume (Figure 1). There are no significant differences in the hematocrit and hemoglobin concentration between trained and untrained persons, suggesting that both plasma and red cell components of blood can contribute to the expanded blood volume (hypervolemia) and total circulating hemoglobin observed in endurance-trained athletes compared with their untrained counterparts. Clearly, these cross-sectional observations support the notion that endurance-trained athletes exhibit 20–25% larger blood volume than untrained persons.

Although cross-sectional differences in blood volumes between trained and untrained individuals argue for a cause–effect relationship with exercise, they fail to separate the exercise effect from possible contributions from genetic and environmental factors. An

Claimer: Portions of this chapter and its illustrations have been previously published as a peer-reviewed article (Reference 6) and are presented here with permission from the editor of *Medicine and Science in Sports and Exercise*.

From Fletcher GF, (ed): *Cardiovascular Response to Exercise*. Mount Kisco, NY, Futura Publishing Company, Inc., © 1994.

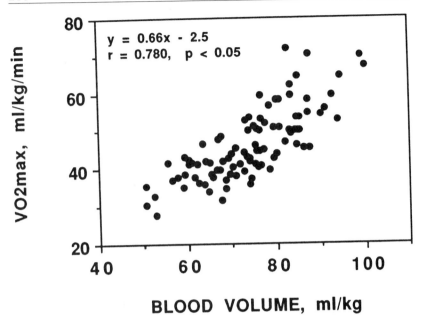

FIGURE 1. *Cross-sectional relationship between total blood volume and maximal oxygen uptake (VO_2max) in 97 men. First order correlation coefficient is 0.780 and linear regression of best fit is VO_2max = 0.66 (blood volume) − 2.51. Reproduced from Reference 6 with permission.*

understanding of hypervolemic adaptation during exercise training requires the use of longitudinal studies to measure blood volume changes in the same individuals before and after training in order to define the exercise stimulus and time course dynamics, and identify mechanisms and physiological advantages.

Dynamics of Hypervolemia During Exercise Training

The average blood volume expansion in humans reported from most longitudinal training studies lasting 3 to 120 days ranges from 5–10%,[4–13] with the largest expansion measured at 16% after 8 months of exercise training.[14] These results are much less than the 20–25% difference observed in cross-sectional comparisons between highly trained competitive athletes and nonathletes. However, intensive exercise training for 2 months failed to induce hypervolemia in young athletes whose initial blood volume was above 80 ml/kg.[15,16] Taken together, these data suggest that a hypervolemia induced by endurance exercise training is limited by such factors as initial fitness levels, duration of previous exposure to exercise training, or genetic components.

Despite the natural interest in athletic populations, the assessment of a hypervolemic response to exercise training in women and elderly people from average fitness populations is a clinically relevant issue. Although data have been reported from both cross-sectional[2] and longitudinal[7,9] investigations on women, suggesting that their hypervolemic response to training is similar to that of men, one study was specifically designed to assess this comparison. Akgun and coworkers[4] demonstrated that 2 months of endurance training for 30 minutes daily, 6 days a week on a cycle ergometer induced expansion of blood, plasma, and red cell mass by 7, 8, and 7%, respectively, in six women compared with 10, 11, and 9% in nine age-matched men. Similarly for aging, we have recently reported that 24 60- to 80-year-old men and women who increased their maximal aerobic capacity by 12% with 6 months of exercise training expanded their blood, plasma, and red cell volumes by 12, 11, and 14%, respectively.[17] It is therefore clear that female and elderly populations have equal capacity compared with young men and athletes to expand their blood volume during exercise training.

Figure 2 presents a hypothesized time course relationship (drawn lines) for changes in blood, plasma, and red cell volumes during exercise training based on a compilation of longitudinal studies from the literature.[4-8,9-11,13,18] The striking rate at which exercise-induced hypervolemia occurs is demonstrated by the observation that only one exposure to exercise can increase blood volume within 24 hours.[18,19] Training-induced hypervolemia appears to reach a plateau around 10 to 14 days of training. Up to this time, virtually all of the blood volume expansion can be explained by increased plasma volume with virtually no change in red cell mass.[6,8,10,11,18,20,21] As the duration of training continues beyond 2 to 4 weeks, the increase in blood volume is distributed more equally between increases in the plasma volume and the red cell mass.[4,6,7,12,13,22] However, little is known regarding the mechanisms of red blood cell adaptation to endurance exercise training and more long duration exercise training studies designed to address this issue

Changes in Vascular Volumes

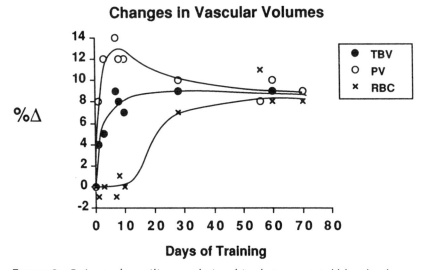

FIGURE 2. *Estimated curvilinear relationships between total blood volume (TBV, closed circles), plasma volume (PV, open circles), red blood cell mass (RBC, x's), and the duration of exercise training. Data points represent a compilation of results from eight independent longitudinal studies.[4–8,10,11,13]*

are required. Consequently, the remainder of this chapter emphasizes the characteristics and mechanisms of plasma volume expansion during endurance exercise training and how it affects performance. It also must be appreciated that interpretation of the time course for hypervolemia based on the results of different studies may be influenced by different stimuli such as varying intensity, frequency, duration, and mode of exercise. Despite this limitation, description of the time course of changes in blood volume with varying durations of training using cross-study comparisons provides useful information about the hypervolemic adaptation to exercise training.

Numerous investigators have taken advantage of the rapid expansion of plasma volume within the first 24 hours after exercise to examine mechanisms of hypervolemia using training durations of less than 10 days. Figure 3 presents the average responses of blood volume and its components in eight persons who underwent exercise training at an intensity of 65% of their maximal oxygen uptake (VO_2max) for 2 continuous hours daily for 8 consecutive days. Blood

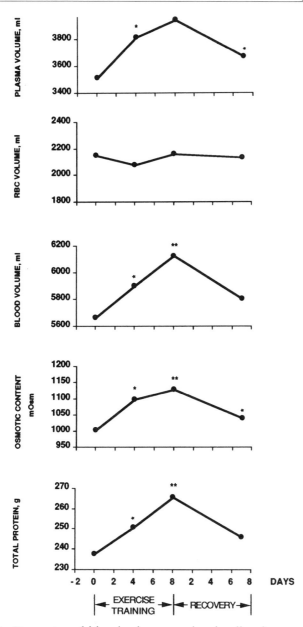

FIGURE 3. *Dynamics of blood, plasma and red cell volumes, and total circulating plasma proteins and osmotic contents during 8 days of exercise training and after 7 days of cessation of training. Values represent the average of eight persons. * indicates* $p<0.05$ *from day 0; ** indicates* $p<0.05$ *from days 0 and 4. Data modified from Reference 21.*

volume increased in a linear fashion to 8% by the end of training. The hypervolemia resulted from a 12% increase in plasma volume with no change in red cell mass. Plasma osmolality and protein concentration remained constant, suggesting the presence of an effective homeostatic mechanism designed to defend the constancy of osmotic and electrochemical properties of fluids within the vascular space to assure normal physiological function. A constancy of plasma solute concentrations in the face of increasing plasma volume during exercise training requires proportionate increases in both the total circulating protein and osmotically active electrolytes (Figure 3). Plasma and blood volume, as well as circulating solutes, returned toward the pretraining level when the persons discontinued exercise for 7 days. The rapid return of blood volume to pretraining levels demonstrates that the termination of physical activity represents the removal of a primary stimulus for maintaining chronic hypervolemia.[21,23]

Characteristics of the Exercise Stimulus

Since characteristics of heat acclimation can be induced partially by endurance training,[24] it is reasonable that elevation in body temperature during exercise might be considered a primary stimulus for training-induced hypervolemia. To test this hypothesis, blood volume was measured in four persons before and after they underwent 8 consecutive days of exposure to exercise for 2 continuous hours at 65% VO_2max, and compared with the blood volume responses in four persons who underwent a similar body temperature stimulus when their rectal temperature profiles were equal by sitting in a heat chamber for 2 hours with ambient temperature at 42°C and 93% relative humidity.[20] With this design, effects of elevated body temperature could be isolated from other exercise factors contributing to the total stimulus of the hypervolemia. The average sweat rates were 800 to 900 ml/hr and the plasma volume reduction was 9–12% during heat and exercise exposures for both groups, corroborating similar thermal challenges. After the 8 days of exercise training or passive heat exposure, the increase in plasma volume in the resting group was 5% compared with 12% in the exercise group. The increases in total circulating osmotic solutes and total protein were proportionately less in the group that rested in the heat but did not have the exercise stimulus. The original hypothesis was not supported by these data; the stimulus for plasma and blood volume expansion during endurance exercise training is a combination of a thermal factor and some other exercise factor(s) that may be related to increased metabolism and blood flow demands during exercise but not during the resting state. When exercise and heat exposure were combined[25] using the same frequency (8 days) and duration (2 hr/day) to induce the same elevation in body temperature as that induced in the persons who underwent exercise training and passive heat exposure alone,[20] a plasma volume expansion (17%) equal to the sum of that reported by exercise alone (12%) and heat alone (5%) was observed. Thus, the thermal and exercise factors that stimulate hypervolemia appear to be additive.

Mechanisms of Training-induced Hypervolemia

Hypervolemia induced by exercise training must depend on mechanisms that can increase total circulating plasma proteins and electrolytes (Figure 3) in order to maintain osmotic constancy across capillary and tissue membranes. Indeed, exercise-induced plasma expansion is accompanied by proportionate increases in the total circulating protein without a change in plasma protein concentration.[20,21,26,27] Since capillary membranes are relatively permeable to plasma electrolytes, increased total circulating protein represents a primary mechanism for expansion of plasma volume during exercise training by increasing oncotic pressure across capillary membranes and subsequently promoting osmotic compartmentalization of water in the vascular space. There appear to be two phases of circulating plasma protein expansion. The initial phase occurs early after exercise. Since the increase in total circulating protein and plasma within hours of exercise is so rapid, the mechanism may involve a rapid shift of protein and fluid from the cutaneous interstitial spaces to intravascular spaces from lymphatic flushing.[27] This mechanism serves to replace plasma rapidly, immediately after exercise. However, to avoid a chronic deficit in interstitial protein and fluid volume, a second slower phase probably includes de novo synthesis of protein with a subsequent expansion of total body water.[6,28–30]

There must be mechanisms activated by exercise that enhance water replacement (intake) and/or reduce excretion (output) to support an expansion of plasma volume and total body water. Exercise training increases 24-hour loss of body water primarily because of the additional sweating during the acute exercise period. Sweat loss is completely compensated for by an increase in 24-hour water intake,[6] suggesting that thirst mechanisms contribute significantly to the replacement and expansion of body water during recovery from exercise. In addition, the 24 hours of recovery after exercise is accompanied by an average 20% reduction in the total urine output.[6] There is no change in glomerular filtration rate,[6] suggesting that the mechanism of reduced urine excretion during exercise training must be postglomerular. Free water clearance actually is more positive during exercise training, supporting the notion that antidiuretic hormone action on renal tubular water reabsorption probably is an unlikely explanation for decreased urine output during exercise training.[31] Exercise training reduces osmotic clearance mainly resulting from a 50% reduction in the clearance of sodium,[6] suggesting that a primary renal mechanism for increasing water retention and expanding body water involves an enhanced capacity for renal tubular reabsorption of sodium. When persons are given an aldosterone antagonist (spironolactone) during exercise training, normal plasma volume expansion is attenuated compared with that of a control group that had no drug.[11] By the end of training, plasma volumes and circulating plasma proteins of the drug and control groups were similar, reinforcing the important role of increased total circulating proteins in training-induced hypervolemia. However, the attenuated hypervolemia during the early phase of training was associated with greater renal sodium and water excretion. These data suggest that an aldosterone-sodium retention mechanism is an important factor in the exercise training–induced hypervolemia, particularly during the early phase. Since there is no change in 24-hour resting plasma aldosterone levels,[10,22] increased renal tubular sodium reabsorption may represent an increase in the sensitivity of receptors to aldosterone as an adaptation to exercise training. Thus, the balance between the increased water loss through sweating and the water gain through drinking and renal retention translates to a net gain of body water that is reflected in the chronic expansion of blood volume with training.

The expansion of blood volume with exercise training raises a relevant clinical issue regarding the distribution of the fluid and the subsequent effects on the mechanisms associated with maintenance of vascular pressures. Clearly, the fluid volume within a given vascular space could not increase without an increase in total effective vascular capacitance or a rise in vascular pressure, both of which have clinical implications. In a recent study,[22] 10 weeks of endurance exercise training did not alter total vascular capacitance in the face of a 9% increased blood volume. Arterial pressure was not altered, but central venous pressure was elevated by 16%. This observation has been corroborated more recently in a cross-sectional comparison demonstrating that average resting central venous pressure was 7.6 mm Hg in seven endurance-trained persons compared with 4.8 mm Hg in moderately fit persons.[32] An increase in venous pressure usually provides a stimulus to receptors on the low pressure side of the circulation to promote diuresis and prevent volume expansion. A chronically expanded blood volume and central venous pressure without altered plasma levels of vasopressin, atrial naturetic peptide (ANP), and aldosterone supports the notion that the sensitivity of volume reflex control may become attenuated with exercise training.[22,33] Thus, the hypervolemia associated with exercise training is associated with elevated venous pressure and perhaps a resetting of volume/pressure control mechanisms.

Physiological Advantages of Training-induced Hypervolemia

The expansion of blood volume during exercise training provides the functional advantages of increased thermoregulatory and cardiovascular stability during exercise.[27,34,35] Figure 4 presents data that demonstrate this point by illustrating that increased plasma volume during training is associated with greater sweat rates (evaporative cooling) and lower heart rates during exercise of equal relative intensity (65% VO_2max). Because training increases maximal aerobic capacity, these results demonstrate the important benefit that trained persons can exercise at higher absolute work rates while maintaining the same body temperature with less cardiovascular challenge.[34]

Several longitudinal exercise-training studies have demonstrated that the magnitude of the hypervolemia induced by exercise training is associated with increased sweat rate and evaporative

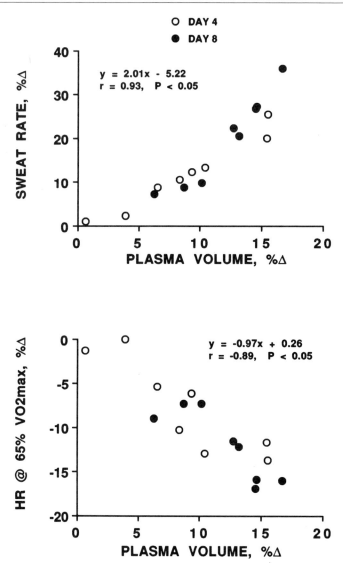

FIGURE 4. *Relationships between the percent increase in plasma volume and the percent increase in sweat rate (top panel) and percent reduction in heart rate during exercise at 65% VO$_2$max (bottom panel) at 4 days (open circles) and 8 days (closed circles) of exercise training. Modified from Reference 34.*

cooling during exercise.[6,10,20,21,28,29,34] Various methods including hypohydration,[36] hyperhydration,[36,37] saline infusion,[38,39] and albumin infusion[40,41] have been used to compare temperature regulation at different blood volumes during exercise to determine if this relationship was causal. In all cases, a reduction in blood volume or restriction of fluid intake resulted in higher core temperature during exercise. Exercise training can induce adaptation of heat-dissipating mechanisms that are independent of hypervolemia. However, increased heat dissipation during exercise with acute hypervolemia clearly demonstrates the contribution of volume alone to both increased sweating[36,37,40] and greater skin blood flow.[37,39] Since the chronic hypervolemia of exercise training reflects increased total body water,[6,28,30] it seems reasonable that more interstitial fluid will be available to the sweat glands to provide water to the skin surface for evaporative cooling as well as greater vascular volume to provide optimal skin blood flow to enhance conductive heat exchange. The hypervolemia induced by endurance exercise training is therefore associated with greater thermoregulatory stability (*ie*, lower body core temperature) during exercise at the same intensity.

Hypervolemia induced by endurance exercise training is associated with a reduction in heart rate[20,21,28–30,34,35] and elevated stroke volume[42] during exercise at the same intensity. Furthermore, the training-induced hypervolemia and exercise bradycardia are closely related such that a 1% increase in plasma volume has been associated with a 1% reduction in exercise heart rate (Figure 4). The most likely explanation for the effects of hypervolemia on increased stroke volume and reduced heart rate during exercise is a Frank-Starling effect. Acute expansion of blood volume by intravenous infusion of dextran,[43] albumin,[44] or whole blood[45] produces increased cardiac stroke volume during exercise but maintains cardiac output with a lower heart rate. The importance of a Frank-Starling effect caused by training-induced hypervolemia was eloquently demonstrated by the experiments of Coyle and associates,[23] who reduced blood volume in previously trained persons by terminating their training (detraining). They observed that the relative hypovolemia after detraining caused a reduction in stroke volume and increased heart rate to maintain the same cardiac output at the same intensity of exercise compared with before the detraining period. The elevated stroke volume during exercise after endurance training may result from greater venous return and right atrial filling pressure associated with a greater pressure gradient from the central venous reservoir to the right atrium as a consequence of the chronically induced training hypervolemia.[22,32] The interaction between hypervolemia and altered sympathetic control of the cardiac response during exercise after training is not clear, but probably represents some optimal coupling between the volume available and the time allowed for cardiac filling. It is clear that hypervolemia contributes significantly to improve cardiovascular reserve and stability during exercise by increasing stroke volume.

Summary

Expansion of blood volume is a well-documented phenomenon of exercise training, independent of age and gender. Plasma volume expansion can account for nearly all of the exercise-induced hypervolemia up to 2 weeks; after this time expansion of both plasma and red cell volumes occur. The stimulus for the expansion of blood volume by exercise training includes the additive effect of a thermal factor and exercise factors. Exercise training induces the increase in total circulating proteins, which elevates the oncotic pressure across capillary membranes to compartmentalize fluid selectively within the vascular space. The mechanism of increased circulating proteins is not clear, but may include a rapid phase provided by lymphatic flow followed by a slower phase of de novo synthesis. Exercise training also provides a stimulus to increase thirst and to activate various renal mechanisms, probably through neurohormonal control. The increase in thirst aids in the oral replacement of fluids during recovery from exercise. The primary renal mechanism is lower urine volume associated with increased tubular sodium reabsorption, perhaps mediated by increased receptor sensitivity to aldosterone. The combination of increased water intake and reduced urine volume output during the 24 hours of recovery from each exercise training session results in a net increase in the total body fluid retention. With the added effect of increased vascular oncotic force due to circulating proteins, a greater proportion of the total body water expansion is distributed in the vascular space, thus increasing plasma and blood volume. The stimulus for increased red cell mass is unclear. Expanded total blood volume increases the ability to maintain a high stroke volume and a lower heart rate for cardiovascular stability and to enhance heat dissipation (thermal stability) by increasing the amount of water available for sweating and the amount of blood flow to the skin.

References

1. Dill DB, Braithwaite K, Adams WC, Bernauer EM: Blood volume of middle-distance runners: effect of 2,300-m altitude and comparison with non-athletes. *Med Sci Sports* 1974;6:1–7
2. Kjellberg SR, Rudhe U, Sjostrand T: Increase of the amount of hemoglobin and blood volume in connection with physical training. *Acta Physiol Scand* 1949;19:146–151
3. Brotherhood J, Brozovic B, Pugh LGCE: Hematological status of middle- and long-distance runners. *Clin Sci Mol Med* 1975;48:139–145
4. Akgun N, Tartaroglu N, Durusoy F, Kocaturk E: The relationship between the changes in physical fitness and in total blood volume in subjects having regular and measured training. *J Sports Med* 1974;14:73–77
5. Convertino VA, Keil LC, Greenleaf JE: Plasma volume, renin, and vasopressin responses to graded exercise after training. *J Appl Physiol* 1983;54:508–514
6. Convertino VA: Blood volume: its adaptation to endurance training. *Med Sci Sports Exerc* 1991;23:1338–1348
7. Fortney S, Senay LC: The effects of a modest training program on the responses of females to work in a hot environment. *J Appl Physiol* 1979;47:978–984
8. Green HJ, Thomson JA, Ball ME, Hughson RL, Houston ME, Sharratt MT: Alterations in blood volume following short-term supramaximal exercise. *J Appl Physiol* 1984;56:145–149
9. Holmgren A, Mossfeldt F, Sjostrand T, Strom G: Effect of training on work capacity, total hemoglobin, blood volume, heart volume and pulse rate in recumbent and upright position. *Acta Physiol Scand* 1960;50:72–83
10. Kirby CR, Convertino VA: Plasma aldosterone and sweat sodium concentrations after exercise and heat acclimation. *J Appl Physiol* 1986;61:967–970
11. Luetkemeier MJ: The mechanism of exercise-induced plasma volume expansion. *Doctoral Dissertation.* The Ohio State University, 1988, pp 1–127
12. Oscai LB, Williams BT, Hertig BA: Effect of exercise on blood volume. *J Appl Physiol* 1968;24:622–624
13. Ray CA, Cureton KJ, Ouzts HG: Postural specificity of cardiovascular adaptations to exercise training. *J Appl Physiol* 1990;69:2202–2208
14. Stevens GHJ, Foresman BH, Shi X, Stern SA, Raven PB: Reduction in LBNP tolerance following prolonged endurance exercise training. *Med Sci Sports Exerc* 1992;24:1235–1244
15. Frick MH, Sjogren AL, Perasalo J, Pajunen S: Cardiovascular dimen-

sions and moderate physical training in young men. *J Appl Physiol* 1970;29:452–455

16. Glass HI, Edwards RHT, de Garreta AC, Clark JC: [11]CO red cell labeling for blood volume and total hemoglobin in athletes: effect of training. *J Appl Physiol* 1969;26:131–134

17. Carroll JF, Convertino VA, Wood CE, Graves JE, Pollock ML: The influence of six months of exercise training on resting plasma volume and hormone levels in older men and women. *Med Sci Sports Exerc* 1992;24:S158

18. Pugh LGCE: Blood volume changes in outdoor exercises of 8-10 hour duration. *J Physiol (Lond)* 1969;200:345–351

19. Gillen CM, Lee R, Mack GW, Tomaselli CM, Nishiyasu T, Nadel ER: Plasma volume expansion in humans after a single intense exercise protocol. *J Appl Physiol* 1991;71:1914–1920

20. Convertino VA, Greenleaf JE, Bernauer EM: Role of thermal and exercise factors in the mechanism of hypervolemia. *J Appl Physiol* 1980;48:657–664

21. Convertino VA, Brock PJ, Keil LC, Bernauer EM, Greenleaf JE: Exercise training-induced hypervolemia: role of plasma albumin, renin, and vasopressin. *J Appl Physiol* 1980;48:665–669

22. Convertino VA, Mack GW, Nadel ER: Elevated central venous pressure: a consequence of exercise training-induced hypervolemia? *Am J Physiol* 1991;29:R273–R277

23. Coyle EF, Hemmert MK, Coggan AR: Effects of detraining on cardiovascular responses to exercise: role of blood volume. *J Appl Physiol* 1986;60:95–99

24. Piwonka RW, Robinson S, Gay VL, Manlis RS: Preacclimatization of man to heat by training. *J Appl Physiol* 1965;20:379–384

25. Shvartz E, Convertino VA, Keil LC, Haines RF: Orthostatic fluid-electrolyte and endocrine responses in fainters and nonfainters. *J Appl Physiol* 1981;51:1404–1410

26. Koch G, Rocker L: Plasma volume and intravascular protein masses in trained boys and fit young men. *J Appl Physiol* 1977;43:1085–1088

27. Senay LC, Mitchell D, Wyndham CH: Acclimatization in a hot humid environment: body fluid adjustments. *J Appl Physiol* 1976;40:786–796

28. Bass DE, Kleeman CR, Quinn M, Henschel A, Hegnauer AH: Mechanisms of acclimatization to heat in man. *Medicine* 1955;34:323–380

29. Bass DE, Buskirk ER, Iampietro PF, Mager M: Comparison of blood volume during physical conditioning, heat acclimatization, and sedentary living. *J Appl Physiol* 1958;12:186–188

30. Wyndham CH, Benade AJA, Williams CG, Strydom NB, Goldin A, Heyns AJA: Changes in central circulation and body fluid spaces during acclimatization to heat. *J Appl Physiol* 1968;25:586–593

31. Wade CE: Response, regulation, and action of vasopressin during exercise: a review. *Med Sci Sports Exerc* 1981;16:506–511

32. Shi X, Andresen JM, Potts JT, Foresman BH, Stern SA, Raven PB: Aortic baroreflex control of heart rate during hypertensive stimuli: effect of fitness. *J Appl Physiol* 1993;74:1555–1562

33. Mack GW, Shi X, Nose H, Tripathi A, Nadel ER: Diminished baroreflex

control of forearm vascular resistance in physically fit humans. *J Appl Physiol* 1987;63:105–110

34. Convertino VA: Heart rate and sweat rate responses associated with exercise-induced hypervolemia. *Med Sci Sports Exerc* 1983;15:77–82
35. Wyndham CH, Rogers GG, Senay LC, Mitchell D: Acclimatization in a hot humid environment: cardiovascular adjustments. *J Appl Physiol* 1976;40:779–785
36. Greenleaf JE, Castle BL: Exercise temperature regulation in man during hypohydration and hyperhydration. *J Appl Physiol* 1971;30:847–853
37. Nadel ER, Fortney SM, Wenger CB: Effect of hydration state on circulatory and thermal regulations. *J Appl Physiol* 1980;49:715–721
38. Deschamps A, Levy RD, Cosio MG, Marliss EB, Magder S: Effect of saline infusion on body temperature and endurance during heavy exercise. *J Appl Physiol* 1989;66:2799–2804
39. Fortney SM, Vroman NB, Beckett WS, Permutt S, LaFrance ND: Effect of exercise hemoconcentration and hyperosmolality on exercise responses. *J Appl Physiol* 1988;65:519–524
40. Fortney SM, Nadel ER, Wenger CB, Bove VR: Effects of blood volume on sweating rate and body fluids in exercising humans. *J Appl Physiol* 1981;51:1594–1600
41. Sawka MN, Hubbard RW, Francesconi RP, Hortsman DH: Effect of acute plasma volume expansion on altering exercise-heat performance. *Eur J Appl Physiol* 1983;51:303–312
42. Green HJ, Jones LL, Painter DC: Effects of short-term training on cardiac function during prolonged exercise. *Med Sci Sports Exerc* 1990;22:488–493
43. Hopper MK, Coggan AR, Coyle EF: Exercise stroke volume relative to plasma-volume expansion. *J Appl Physiol* 1988;64:404–408
44. Fortney SM, Wenger CB, Bove JR, Nadel ER: Effect of blood volume on forearm venous and cardiac stroke volume during exercise. *J Appl Physiol* 1983;55:884–890
45. Fortney SM, Nadel ER, Wenger CB, Bove JR: Effect of acute alterations of blood volume on circulatory performance in humans. *J Appl Physiol* 1981;50:292–298

Chapter 12

Effects of High Altitude and Training on Oxygen Transport and Exercise Performance

Robert L. Johnson, Jr., MD, Robert F. Grover, MD, PhD, and Arthur C. DeGraff, Jr., MD

Human performance pushed to its limits by stress has evoked interest throughout history. Periodically, events requiring the achievement of some practical goal heighten this interest. For example, during World War II, the development of aircraft capable of flying at extreme altitudes stimulated intense research in respiratory physiology related to acute responses to high altitude and mechanisms of acclimatization. The Summer Olympics of 1968 in Mexico City at 2,250 m altitude further stimulated interest in exertion at moderate altitude and how best to train athletes for endurance events at such altitudes. It was found that high-altitude acclimatization induced major changes in the oxygen transport system, including raising the oxygen-carrying capacity of blood, altering blood volume, stimulating ventilation, and enhancing the release of oxygen from red cells to tissues. Naturally, questions then arose whether such changes induced by high-altitude acclimatization might enhance physical performance at sea level.

It is well established that the performance of endurance events is impaired at high altitude. Mean running speeds achieved in the longer events at the 1968 Summer Olympic Games in Mexico City were slower with respect to previous records set at low altitude (Figure 1). No world records were matched or broken in Mexico City at distance events greater than 800 m.[1] However, the reduced air density at high altitude appears to provide an advantage during

From Fletcher GF, (ed): *Cardiovascular Response to Exercise*. Mount Kisco, NY, Futura Publishing Company, Inc., © 1994.

223

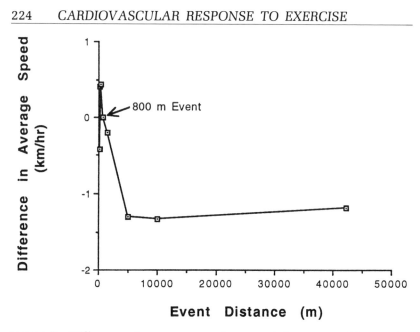

Event   Distance   (m)

FIGURE 1. *Differences in average running speeds for events of increasing distance, comparing winning runners in Mexico City with previous record holders for those events.[1] No records were broken for events greater than an 800-m distance.*

shorter events. Records were set at 100-m and 400-m distances, where wind resistance is more important than endurance in determining running times and average speeds achieved. Total duration of these events did not exceed 2 minutes. Eight hundred meters appeared to be an exercise break point, beyond which more than 50% of the energy must be derived from aerobic sources. At events of 5,000 m or greater, average speed achieved during the event fell by about 1.3 km/hr.

Determinants of Maximal Oxygen Uptake at Sea Level

Before examining the effects of high altitude on exercise performance, it would be useful to review some of the physiological determinants of aerobic exercise at sea level (Table 1). Each component in this scheme can be quantified and the approximate

TABLE 1.   Determinants of Aerobic Exercise Capacity

O_2 tension in ambient air
Ventilatory capacity
Rate limits of alveolar-capillary gas exchange
O_2 affinity of hemoglobin
O_2 carrying capacity of blood
Maximal cardiac output
Distribution of the cardiac output
Rate limits of O_2 exchange between muscle capillaries and mitochondria
Mitochondrial volume and oxidative enzyme levels in muscle

limitation imposed by each on oxygen uptake can be estimated.[2,3] We made the measurements required for such estimates in 1966 in five college students before and after 3 weeks of bed rest and after 8 weeks of endurance training.[4] Similar measurements were made in six Olympic bicyclists from Sweden who were studied in 1967 in Dallas after the "Little Olympics" in Mexico City[5] (Table 2).

With endurance training, the primary improvements that occur in these different steps of oxygen transport are in the maximal cardiac output and stroke volume and in the blood oxygen extraction by muscle as indicated by an increase in the arteriovenous oxygen difference. Thus, training primarily affects the cardiovascular system, not the lungs. The higher diffusing capacity observed in the Olympic athletes is not a consequence of training, but reflects the normal relationship between diffusing capacity and cardiac output resulting from functional recruitment of the pulmonary capillary bed.

From the measurements listed in Table 2, we can estimate the oxygen transport capacity that can be maintained by each step. For example, we can estimate the oxygen transport capacity that can be sustained by a given level of ventilation without allowing alveolar oxygen tension to fall below 110 mm Hg. We can estimate the oxygen transport capacity that can be maintained by a given oxygen-diffusing capacity without the oxygen saturation of blood leaving the lung falling below 95%. Table 3 has been constructed from these kinds of calculations.[2,3]

Note that in sedentary college students the combined oxygen transport system is unbalanced, and exercise is primarily limited by the deconditioned cardiovascular component. Deconditioning by bed rest exaggerates this imbalance. Conversely, with increasing fitness, oxygen transport capacity becomes more uniformly distributed among the different steps. Ultimately, as in top Olympic

TABLE 2. Average Functional Capacities of the Heart and Lungs at Peak Exercise in Five College Students and Six Olympic Athletes

		College Students		Olympic Athletes
	Control	After Bed Rest	After Training	
Maximum O_2 uptake (1/min)	3.30	2.43*	3.91*	5.38†
Maximum voluntary ventilation (1/min)	191	201	197	219
CO_2 diffusing capacity [(ml/min)/mm Hg]	49.3	42.6	49.5	66.1†
O_2 diffusing capacity [(ml/min)/mm Hg]	72.0	62.2	72.3	96.5†
Maximal cardiac output (1/min)	20.0	14.8*	22.8*	30.4†
Maximal heart rate (beats per minute)	193	197	191	182
Maximal stroke volume (ml)	104	74*	120*	167†
Blood O_2 capacity (ml/l)	219	205	208	224
Arteriovenous O_2 difference (ml/l)	129	99*	156*	193†

*Significantly different from control.
†Significantly different from college students after training.

TABLE 3. Oxygen Transport Capacity of Each Step at Sea Level

	Five College Students			Six Olympic Bicyclists
	Control	After Bed Rest	Training	
Ventilation	4.6	4.9	5.8	6.5
Lung diffusion	5.0	4.4	5.1	6.8
Cardiac output	3.6	2.7	4.3	6.3
Tissue diffusion	3.5	2.6	4.2	—
Measured	3.3	2.4	3.9	5.4

endurance athletes, components of the oxygen transport system become almost equally matched so that there is no clear site of limitation (*ie,* no bottleneck in the system). These data fit well with the concept of symmorphosis proposed by Weibel, Taylor, and Hoppeler,[6] which postulates that in an optimally designed system, there should be a quantitative match among the different functional components of the defined system. Such optimal design appears to exist in the oxygen transport system of the top endurance athlete. Again, the data indicate that the principal effects of training are on the cardiovascular system, through an increase in stroke volume and cardiac output, and an increase in blood oxygen extraction in tissues.

Oxygen Affinity of Hemoglobin

As indicated in Table 1, the affinity of hemoglobin for oxygen is one of the determinants of aerobic exercise capacity. Alterations in the position of the oxyhemoglobin dissociation curve can provide optimization of matching between the rate of loading of oxygen onto hemoglobin in the lung and unloading from hemoglobin in muscle. Changes in blood pH, P_{CO_2}, temperature, and red cell 2,3 diphosphoglycerate (2,3 DPG) can shift the position of the curve to optimize matching (Figure 2).

The position of the oxyhemoglobin dissociation curve can be described quantitatively with one convenient number, the oxygen tension at 50% oxyhemoglobin saturation, referred to as the P_{50}. An increased P_{50} indicates a "shift to the right" and reduced oxygen affinity; a decreased P_{50} indicates a "shift to the left" and increased oxygen affinity. The difference between the alveolar oxygen tension and P_{50} is an index of the pressure gradient driving oxygen into blood in the lung. Likewise, the difference between the P_{50} and the mitochondrial oxygen tension in the tissues is an index of the pressure gradient driving oxygen from blood into mitochondria in muscle. Hence, a reduced P_{50} enhances oxygen loading in the lung whereas an increased P_{50} enhances unloading in muscle. An optimal P_{50} will then partition the total oxygen tension difference between alveoli and mitochondria into a gradient available for loading oxygen in the lung and a gradient available for unloading in tissues,

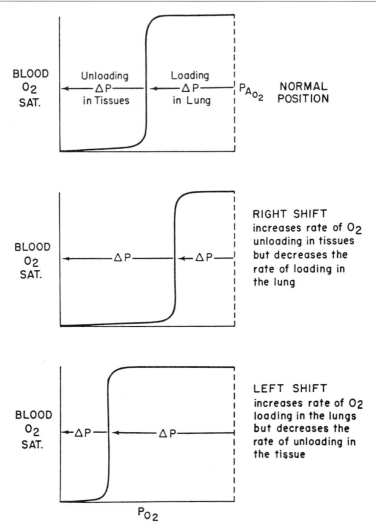

FIGURE 2. *Exaggeration of the S-shaped oxyhemoglobin dissociation curve illustrating the importance of the position of this curve in optimizing oxygen transport. Reproduced from Reference 29 with permission.*

such that the relative magnitude of each gradient matches the relative resistance offered by the corresponding step.

Hemoglobin can act the way a controlling enzyme acts in a metabolic pathway. Thus, P_{50} can be shifted to optimize the rate of oxygen transport analogous to the K_m of a controlling enzyme. For example, at heavy exercise, when a cardiovascular limit is approached causing tissue oxygen tension to fall, generation of lactic acid can increase P_{50} in the muscle capillaries and enhance unloading of oxygen in tissues; increasing temperature will augment this. At the same time, acidosis stimulates ventilation and raises the alveolar oxygen tension. Impaired oxygenation of blood leaving the lung (hypoxemia) will stimulate the carotid body to increase ventilation further, raise alveolar oxygen tension, cause respiratory alkalosis, lower the P_{50} in lung capillaries, and increase the oxygen tension gradient loading oxygen into blood passing through the lung. P_{50} also is altered metabolically by the level of 2,3 DPG in red cells, which tends to stabilize the deoxygenated configuration of the hemoglobin molecule, thereby reducing oxygen affinity. These regulatory mechanisms controlling P_{50} are not only important during exercise at sea level, but also can be important at high altitude.

Determinants of Maximal Oxygen Uptake at High Altitude

The primary physiological effects of high altitude results from the lowered oxygen tension of inspired air. With ascent from sea level to high altitude, total atmospheric pressure decreases progressively, causing a parallel fall in the oxygen tension of inspired air after humidification in the trachea (Table 4).

Based on average measurements in the trained college students, we can predict maximal oxygen consumption at different altitudes[7]

TABLE 4. Barometric Pressures and Oxygen Pressures
in the Lung at Various Altitudes

Location	Altitude Meters	Feet	Barometric Pressure (mm Hg)	Inspired O_2 Tension (mm Hg)
Dallas, Tex	120	400	755	150
Mexico City	2,250	7,500	580	110
Leadville, Colo.	3,100	10,200	535	100
Mt. Evans, Colo.	4,300	14,200	465	87

(Figure 3). Oxygen saturation of blood leaving the lung is plotted on the vertical axis versus oxygen consumption on the horizontal axis. As oxygen consumption increases with increasing work, a point will be reached beyond which blood remains in lung capillaries for too short a time to equilibrate with alveolar oxygen tension. Consequently, oxygen saturation of blood leaving the lung begins to fall sharply as oxygen consumption increases further. These curves represent limits imposed by a normal diffusing capacity on oxygen saturation of blood leaving the lung at increasing levels of oxygen consumption at different altitudes before acclimatization. The diagonal straight line indicates the limit imposed on oxygen consumption by a normal maximal cardiac output of 23 l/min at different arterial oxygen saturations, assuming a tissue oxygen extraction of 80%. The intersection of the cardiac output limit and the limit

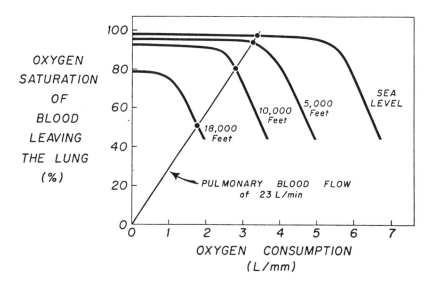

FIGURE 3. *Theoretical upper limits to oxygen uptake imposed by the alveolar capillary membrane and cardiac output at sea level and during acute exposure to altitudes of 5,000, 10,000, and 18,000 ft. The diagonal line indicates the limit imposed at different arterial oxygen saturations at a maximal cardiac output of 23 l/min. The curved lines indicate the limit imposed on arterial blood oxygen saturation by a normal membrane-diffusing capacity and capillary blood volume. Reproduced from Reference 7 with permission.*

imposed by diffusion at different altitudes predicts the maximal oxygen uptake during acute exposure at that altitude. One can see that above an altitude of about 5,000 feet or 1,500 m, the lungs begin to impose a significant limit on maximal rate of oxygen uptake. This prediction agrees with direct observations that $\dot{V}O_2$max is reduced about 8% for each 1,000-m increase in altitude above 700 m.[8] Hence, above 10,000 feet (*ie*, 3,000 m), the lungs now become the primary site of limitation, rather than the cardiovascular system.

Mechanisms of Acclimatization

What then are the mechanisms of acclimatization to high altitude that modify these responses and how does acclimatization affect physical performance at high altitude and at sea level?

As stated, the immediate consequence of ascent to high altitude is a fall in alveolar oxygen tension. The first and most important component of acclimatization is then an increase in ventilation, which lessens the fall in alveolar oxygen tension. This is enhanced over the first several days to a week by renal compensation for the associated hypocapnia and respiratory alkalosis, and finally results in a resetting of the respiratory center to a lower P_{CO_2} and higher alveolar oxygen tension than on arrival, both at rest and exercise.

There is an increase in red cell 2,3 DPG that by itself tends to raise P_{50} of hemoglobin over the first 48 hours. Hemoglobin concentration and hematocrit progressively rise and increase the oxygen-carrying capacity of blood. There is a decrease in cross-

TABLE 5.   Mechanisms of Acclimatization

Ventilation
    Carotid body stimulation
    Renal compensation
    Resetting the respiratory center
Alveolar-capillary gas exchange
Oxyhemoglobin dissociation curve
    Increased 2, 3 DPG in red cells
    Decreased P_{50}
Increased hematocrit and O_2 capacity of blood
Reduction in muscle fiber size reduces diffusion distance
Mitochondrial volume and enzyme content

sectional area of skeletal muscle fibers[9,10] that reduces diffusion distance and increases the diffusing capacity of muscle.

In addition, there are important secondary effects of the chronic reduction in alveolar oxygen tension. During the first 10 days plasma volume decreases (hemoconcentration), pulmonary vascular resistance increases, pulmonary artery pressure rises, and maximal cardiac output falls. These secondary effects may have an important bearing on the effects of training at high altitude, on exercise performance at altitude, and on subsequent performance at sea level.

Rates and Magnitudes of Change During Acclimatization

Ventilation

Over the first week at high altitude, ventilation increases progressively, both at rest and particularly during exercise. At a given work load performed above 1,500 m, this progressive increase in exercise ventilation raises alveolar oxygen tension about 10 mm Hg (Figure 4).

Hemoglobin Concentration and Blood Volume

Hemoglobin concentration rises within hours of arriving at high altitude by between 1 and 2 g/dl because of a contraction in plasma volume (hemoconcentration) (Figure 5). Although this increases the oxygen-carrying capacity of the blood, it also initially results in a decrease in blood volume. The hypoxemia of altitude stimulates red cell production, but the response varies among individuals. After approximately 3 weeks, total red cell volume was found to be measurably increased in about half of a group of 11 individuals studied during acclimatization to 4,300 m on Pikes Peak in 1991. In them, the increase in red cell volume restored blood volume, whereas in those individuals not increasing their red cell volume, blood volume remained reduced.

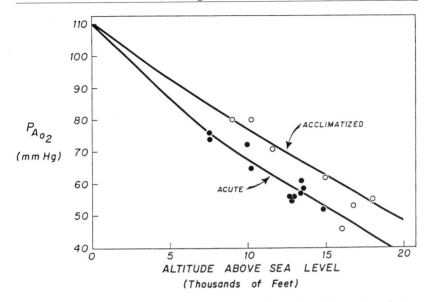

Figure 4. *Alveolar oxygen tensions at peak levels of exercise during either simulated or actual exposure to different altitudes. The closed circles represent the relationship during acute simulated exposure and the open circles represent the relationship during chronic exposure to high altitude. Reproduced from Reference 7 with permission.*

Oxygen Affinity of Hemoglobin

In addition to the initial increase in blood hemoglobin concentration, the 2,3 DPG concentration in red cells also rises in the first 48 hours at altitude[11] (Figure 6). A corresponding increase occurs in the P_{50} measured at standard pH and P_{co_2} as the hemoglobin molecule is stabilized in the desaturated configuration by the 2,3 DPG. Although respiratory alkalosis at high altitude tends to counterbalance the effect of 2,3 DPG, nevertheless, the in vivo position of the oxyhemoglobin dissociation curve was still right-shifted after 10 days at 3,100 m.[12] While this increase in P_{50} at 3,100 m favors the unloading of oxygen to the tissues at submaximal exercise, it will tend to impair oxygen loading in the lung at maximal exercise, where alveolar capillary diffusion is more important. At higher altitudes impairment of oxygen loading by an increased P_{50} could

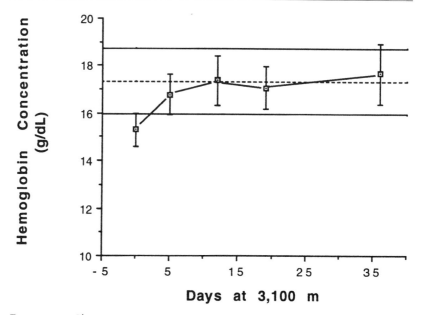

FIGURE 5. *Changes in average blood hemoglobin concentrations in residents from Dallas during a 7-week stay in Leadville, Colorado, at a 3,100-m altitude.*

negate any potential advantage at the tissue level even at low levels of exercise (Figure 2). In fact, based on these qualitative considerations, we would predict that a reduction rather than an increase in P_{50} might be more likely to enhance oxygen transport at higher altitude (Figure 7). A more quantitative analysis confirms this impression[2,11] (Figure 8).

Animals native to high altitude, such as llamas, alpacas, vicunas, and vizcachas of the Andes, have a low P_{50}, favoring the loading of oxygen in the lungs in their hypoxic environment. Interestingly, even though the low P_{50} persists after these animals are transported to sea level, this does not appear to pose a handicap. Paradoxically, sheep with a relatively high P_{50} also do well at high altitudes,[13] although they are at a distinct disadvantage during acute hypoxia.[14]

Significantly enhanced survival under hypoxic conditions can be conferred on animals by artificially lowering the P_{50}.[15] Likewise,

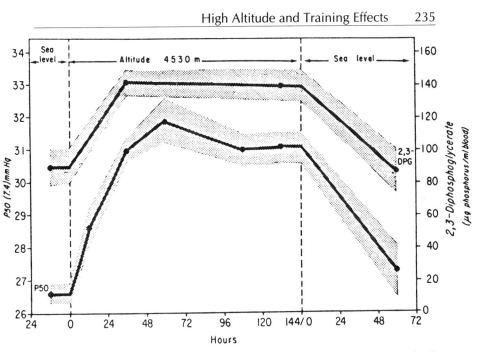

FIGURE 6. *Changes in 2,3 DPG and P₅₀ during short-term exposure to high altitude and after return to sea level. Increased concentrations of 2,3 DPG in the red cells increases the oxygen tension of oxyhemoglobin at 50% saturation with oxygen (P₅₀). Reproduced from Reference 11 with permission.*

humans with a chronically reduced P_{50} due to a genetic variant hemoglobin (chronically left-shifted dissociation curve) show no reduction in $\dot{V}O_2$max on going to 3,100 m altitude,[16] whereas individuals with a normal hemoglobin show a 25–30% reduction.[17] Conversely, an increase in P_{50} can enhance tissue release of oxygen, and so an increased P_{50} conferred by an elevated 2,3 DPG might improve oxygen transport on return to sea level.

Other secondary effects of atmospheric hypoxia occur at high altitude. For example, pulmonary vascular resistance increases because of hypoxic pulmonary vasoconstriction, resulting in modest pulmonary hypertension[18] (Figure 9), but the effect of this increased right ventricular afterload on oxygen transport and exercise performance is uncertain.

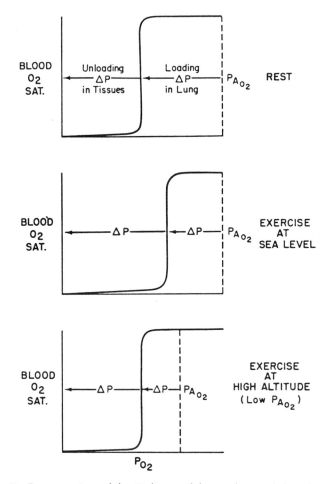

FIGURE 7. *Exaggeration of the S-shape of the oxyhemoglobin dissociation curve to illustrate how changes in the position of the curve can change the partition of the total oxygen pressure gradient between alveolar air and mitochondria during exercise at sea level and high altitude. Reproduced from Reference 3 with permission.*

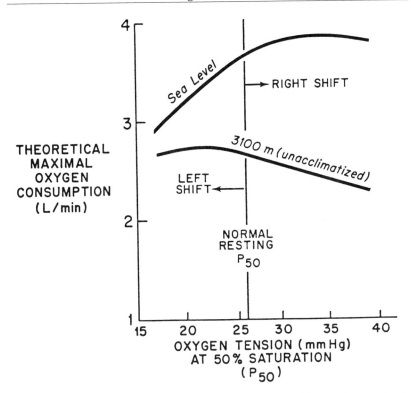

FIGURE 8. *Theoretical effect of shifting the position of the oxyhemoglobin dissociation curve on maximal oxygen uptake at sea level and at high altitude.[2]*

Cardiac Output

During acute exposure to hypoxia, submaximal cardiac output is higher at any given oxygen uptake, and maximal cardiac output is well maintained even though maximal oxygen consumption is significantly reduced by hypoxemia. With acclimatization, however, maximal cardiac output falls and may remain reduced indefinitely[3] (Figure 10). In part this may be because of the initial fall in blood volume, which may persist for several weeks. Possibly the modestly increased afterload on the right ventricle (pulmonary hypertension) has an added depressant effect on stroke volume and cardiac output. As the maximal cardiac output declines during acclimatization, the relationship between cardiac output and oxygen uptake returns to normal.

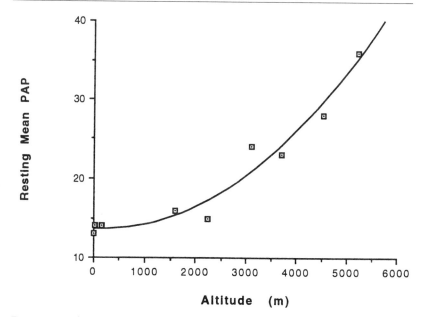

FIGURE 9. *The increase in resting pulmonary artery pressure that occurs with chronic exposure to high altitude.*[18]

Some Predicted Effects of Acclimatization

Given the measured effects of high-altitude acclimatization on different components of the oxygen transport system, how might we expect the observed changes to affect maximal oxygen uptake at high altitude and at sea level? The increase in ventilation and alveolar oxygen tension should enhance oxygen uptake in the lungs at high altitude by increasing the driving pressure for loading oxygen into blood passing through the lungs. The combined effects of raising alveolar oxygen tension and increasing the hemoglobin concentration on maximal oxygen uptake at 18,000 feet (5,500 m) are illustrated in Figure 11.[7] As in Figure 3, the curved lines indicate the limits imposed by diffusing capacity of the lung on oxygen saturation of blood leaving the lung capillaries at different levels of oxygen consumption. When a critical level of oxygen consumption is exceeded, oxygen saturation begins to fall sharply as oxygen consumption rises further. Note, however, that as alveolar oxygen tension increases from 44 mm Hg to 54 mm Hg during acclimatiza-

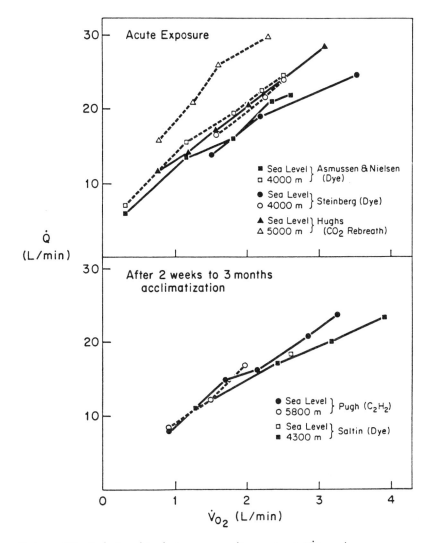

FIGURE 10. *Relationship between cardiac output (Q̇) and oxygen consumption (V̇O₂) during increasing work loads at sea level and during acute and chronic exposure to high altitude. Reproduced from Reference 3 with permission.*

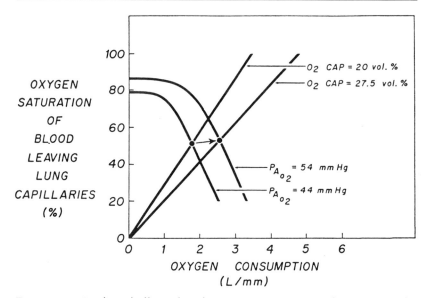

FIGURE 11. *Predicted effect of acclimatization on maximal oxygen uptake as a result of the increased alveolar ventilation and increased oxygen-carrying capacity of blood that occur during chronic exposure to 18,000 feet. Reproduced from Reference 7 with permission.*

tion, the curve shifts to the right. The straight diagonal lines indicate the limits imposed by a maximal cardiac output of 23 l/min at different arterial oxygen saturations. One line represents the relationship with a normal sea level hemoglobin concentration (O_2 capacity of 200 ml per liter of blood) and the other the relationship for polycythemic blood after acclimatization to 18,000 feet. Intersections of these diagonal straight lines with the corresponding limits imposed by diffusion (curved lines) indicate the expected rise in maximal oxygen consumption. In this instance the predicted increase (arrow) would be from 1.8 l/min before acclimatization to 2.5 l/min after acclimatization.

The increase in red cell 2,3 DPG may reduce the oxygen tension gradient for loading oxygen onto hemoglobin in the lung by increasing the P_{50}, but this potentially detrimental effect may be offset by the respiratory alkalosis. At the same time, the increase in 2,3 DPG may increase the oxygen tension gradient between capillary blood in tissues and the mitochondria; this effect may be enhanced further by an increase in capillary density,[9,10] which results in a decreased diffusion distance. These latter two effects would tend to enhance oxygen delivery and extraction in muscle. Whereas the increase in hemoglobin concentration in the blood should enhance oxygen transport by the cardiac output, this effect may be nullified at peak exercise by the decrease in maximal cardiac output and/or the decrease in arterial saturation.

Return to Sea Level

On return to sea level, the persistent increased ventilation during exercise may be detrimental because it diverts oxygen delivery from muscles of locomotion to muscles of breathing without significantly enhancing oxygen uptake by the lungs. Respiratory alkalosis may impair oxygen extraction in the tissues. The low maximal stroke volume and cardiac output at high altitudes plus hypoxia will have reduced the level of training that could be sustained at high altitude. Although functional response of the right ventricle may have improved by working against a higher afterload during exercise, the functional response of the left ventricle may have deteriorated because of the reduction in training level and reduction in left ventricle output. The early increase in hemoglobin concentration and hematocrit at altitude increase the oxygen-carrying capacity of the blood, but for the most part these are a consequence of a reduction in plasma volume. Hence, this potential advantage is lost when plasma volume re-expands after return to sea level. On the other hand, if red cell volume has increased by high altitude acclimatization, this would persist and could enhance oxygen transport at sea level.

At altitude, blood volume often is reduced but may return to sea level values in some individuals during the first few weeks at high altitude. When this does occur, then with descent to sea level, plasma volume expansion may increase blood volume above pre-ascent values, which would be an advantage. This increase in 2,3 DPG induced by high altitude may enhance oxygen extraction in the tissues if not counterbalanced by the continued respiratory alkalosis.[12] 2,3 DPG levels generally fall to normal within 48 hours after descent so the duration of this potentially useful effect is brief.[11] An increase in tissue capillary density, induced by high altitude, may enhance tissue oxygen extraction both at high altitude and at sea level, but the time course of such changes is unknown. Thus, the net effect of acclimatization to high altitude on maximal exercise capacity at sea level is difficult to predict.

It becomes apparent from this discussion that rates of development of changes in different components of the oxygen transport system that occur during high altitude acclimatization, the duration of stay at high altitude, and the different rates of regression of high altitude changes after return to sea level will be crucial in determining effects on maximal exercise capacity both at high altitude and after return to sea level. Insufficient experimental data are available to make accurate predictions; however, we can examine some actual data measuring exercise performance before and after high-altitude acclimatization and immediately upon return to sea level.

Measured Responses to Brief Acclimatization to Altitudes Between 2,250 Meters and 4,300 Meters

Figure 12 compares predicted and measured values of maximal oxygen consumption at various altitudes. Predicted values before and after acclimatization (solid and dashed lines, respectively) are based on the alveolar oxygen tension and hemoglobin concentration, assuming an unchanged maximal cardiac output. The data points represent measured values from the literature[7] before and after acclimatization (filled and open circles, respectively). Measured data seem to fall randomly around the predicted unacclimatized (solid) line, and although there appears to be no clear effect of acclimatization, paired data (joined by vertical lines) before and after acclimatization at 10,000 ft and at 7,500 ft do show improvement in maximal oxygen uptake. However, other studies[17,19] have failed to show any such improvement with acclimatization. Furthermore, maximal oxygen consumption after acclimatization (open circles) never achieves the levels predicted (dashed line) based on the increases in ventilation and oxygen-carrying capacity of the blood that occurs with prolonged exposure. Let us examine a number of these studies in more detail.

In 1967, just before the 1968 Olympic Games in Mexico City, the Swedish Olympic bicycling team was tested first in Sweden, then in

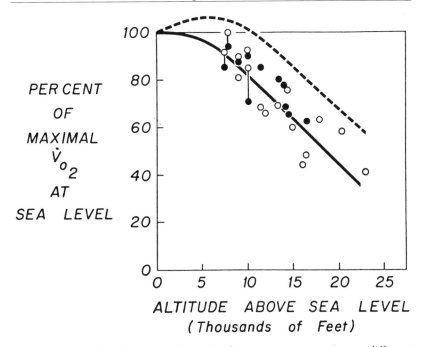

PER CENT
OF
MAXIMAL
$\dot{V}_{O_2}$
AT
SEA LEVEL

ALTITUDE ABOVE SEA LEVEL
(Thousands of Feet)

FIGURE 12. *Predicted values of maximal oxygen consumption at different altitudes above sea level before (solid line) and after (dashed line) acclimatization. Closed symbols are measurements made during acute or simulated exposure and the open symbols are measurements made after acclimatization. Lines connecting open and closed symbols indicate paired measurements on the same subjects. Above 14,000 feet there is little data to suggest improvement in $\dot{V}_{O_2}$max by acclimatization for short intervals of several weeks. Reproduced from Reference 7 with permission.*

Mexico City after 3 weeks of acclimatization at 2,250 m, and finally in Dallas several days after leaving Mexico City[5] (Figure 13). After 3 weeks in Mexico City, maximal oxygen uptake was 82.5% of control levels measured in Sweden, whereas hemoglobin concentration had risen 14% and ventilation at peak exercise had risen 15%. Two days after descent to Dallas, maximal oxygen uptake was still depressed to 96.1% of control levels in Sweden, even though hemoglobin remained increased and ventilation at peak exercise was still elevated. Hence, acclimatization to 2,250 m for 3 weeks did not augment exercise performance upon return to low altitude. Although measurements during acute exposure to the altitude of

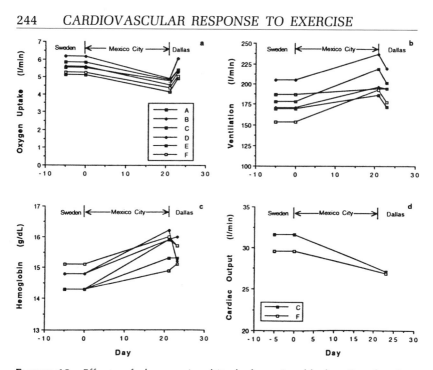

FIGURE 13. Effects of changes in altitude from Stockholm, Sweden (sea level) to Mexico City (2,250 m) and then to Dallas (120 m) on maximal oxygen uptake (a), ventilation (b), blood hemoglobin concentration (c), and maximal cardiac output (d).[5]

Mexico City were not obtained in these Olympic athletes, other studies indicate significant improvement in maximal oxygen uptake during 10 days to 3 weeks of continuous exposure to an altitude of 2,250 m.[20,21]

The effects of acclimatization were examined in two high school endurance track runners from Dallas who spent 36 days in Leadville, Colorado, at an altitude of 3,100 m.[22] Maximal oxygen uptake, breathing an inspired oxygen tension in Dallas equivalent to 3,100 m, fell to 71% of that measured in Dallas breathing air, and ventilation was 90% of that breathing air (Figure 14). After 32 days in Leadville, maximal oxygen consumption had increased to 83% of control, breathing air in Dallas. Ventilation had increased to 48% above that at peak exercise in Dallas and hemoglobin concentration in blood had increased to 20% above that measured in Dallas. In only one of the two runners were blood gas measurements during

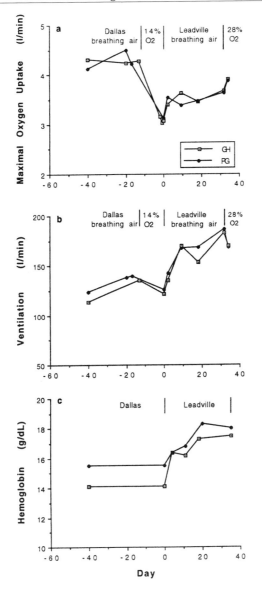

FIGURE 14. *Effects of acclimatization to 3,100-m altitude in Leadville, Colorado, for 36 days and a simulated return to sea level on maximal oxygen uptake (**a**), ventilation (**b**), and blood hemoglobin concentration (**c**) in two endurance runners from Dallas, Texas.*

rest and exercise measured both at simulated high altitude in Dallas and after 5 weeks of acclimatization in Leadville. After 5 weeks of acclimatization arterial oxygen saturation during exercise was higher at a given oxygen consumption in Leadville than during high altitude simulation in Dallas owing to the compensatory increase in ventilation and alveolar oxygen tension during acclimatization (Figure 15) as predicted from earlier data (Figures 4 and 11). On the other hand, when exposed to an inspired oxygen tension in Leadville equivalent to that in Dallas, maximal oxygen consumption was still only 88% of control levels in Dallas whereas ventilation was still 35% above that at peak exercise in Dallas. Hence, acclimatization to 3,100 m altitude for more than 4 weeks did not enhance exercise capacity after a simulated return to sea level.

In 1964, Reeves and Grover[17] tested five members of the

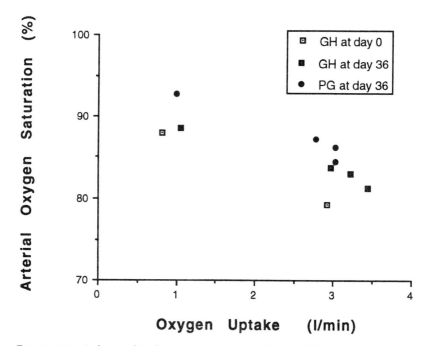

Oxygen Uptake (l/min)

FIGURE 15. *Relationship between arterial oxyhemoglobin saturation and oxygen uptake in endurance runners from Dallas during increasing exercise work loads during simulated acute exposure to an altitude of 3,100 m and after 7 weeks of acclimatization to 3,100 m in Leadville, Colorado.*

Kentucky state champion track team, first at low altitude (1,000 ft or 300 m), then during a 3-week sojourn in Leadville at 10,200 ft (3,100 m), and finally within 7 days after returning to low altitude. On arrival at high altitude, $\dot{V}O_2$max was reduced to 73% of that at low altitude. Statistically significant improvement in $\dot{V}O_2$max was not observed during acclimatization between days 1 and 3 and days 16 and 18, although three of the four runners did improve. Upon return to low altitude, $\dot{V}O_2$max returned to pre-ascent values but did not exceed them. Combining the two studies of young athletes acclimatizing for 2 to 7 weeks in Leadville, a modest but statistically significant improvement in $\dot{V}O_2$max does occur with acclimatization at 3,100 m but $\dot{V}O_2$max was not enhanced at low altitude.

In another study of acclimatization, maximal oxygen uptake was measured first at low altitude and during acute exposure to an oxygen tension equivalent to an altitude of 4,300 m, and repeated after 2 weeks of acclimatization on the summit of Mt. Evans, Colorado (4,300 m), followed by re-exposure to a sea level inspired oxygen tension. These studies were carried out on four of the five college students who had participated in the bed rest–training study mentioned earlier.[23] Breathing an inspired oxygen tension in Dallas similar to that at an altitude of 4,300 m caused maximal oxygen uptake to fall to 68% of that measured breathing air (Figure 16). During acclimatization on Mt. Evans, students maintained training by exercising at 60% of their maximal work load for 15 minutes, followed by 3 minutes at 70% of maximal, and then to maximal for 3 to 5 minutes every second or third day breathing either air or 30% oxygen for serial measurements during acclimatization. On the third day on Mt. Evans, $\dot{V}O_2$max was 70% of that measured in Dallas, with virtually no improvement over the next 10 days despite a 10.5% increase in hemoglobin concentration. At the end of 2 weeks, when inspired oxygen tension was raised to the value in Dallas, $\dot{V}O_2$max increased but was still only 92% of the pre-ascent value. Hence, 2 weeks of acclimatization to 4,300 m did not improve $\dot{V}O_2$max at either high or low altitude.

Buskirk et al.[19] tested six members of the Pennsylvania State University varsity track team, first at low altitude (1,000 ft or 300 m) followed by 7 weeks at 4,000 m in the Andes, and finally on return to low altitude. $\dot{V}O_2$max was reduced by 29% on day 3 at 4,000 m, and was still reduced by 26% after 48 days of acclimatization; the postaltitude values were similar to the prealtitude ones. Here again, altitude acclimatization resulted in little or no improvement in

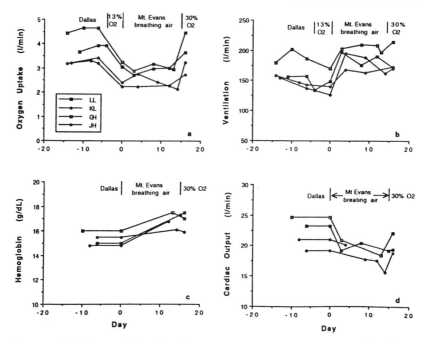

FIGURE 16. *Effects of simulated acute exposure to a 4,300-m altitude in Dallas, 2 weeks of acclimatization to 4,300 m (Mt. Evans, Colorado), and simulated rapid return to Dallas in four college students who had, before ascent, undergone 8 weeks of endurance training in Dallas (Tables 2 and 3).*

exercise capacity either at high altitude or after return to low altitude.

Collectively, these studies provide evidence that the reduction in $\dot{V}O_2$max on arrival at high altitudes between 2,200 and 4,000 m show modest improvement over 2 to 7 weeks at altitude. Acclimatization is associated with a progressive increase in ventilatory response to exercise, an increase in hemoglobin concentration (which may be associated in the early stages with a decrease in blood volume due to a decrease in plasma volume), followed by a slow and variable increase in red cell mass, sometimes restoring blood volume. Red cell concentrations of 2,3-DPG increase and the P_{50} of blood measured under standard conditions increases, although this may be partially or completely reversed in vivo by the Bohr shift induced by respiratory alkalosis. Alveolar hypoxia induces an increase in pulmonary vascular resistance and modest pulmonary hyperten-

TABLE 6.   Living at High Altitude and Training at Low Altitude
vs. Living and Training at Low Altitude

Training group living at:	Maximum O_2 Uptake [ml/min]/kg]		Blood Volume (ml)	
	Pre	Post	Pre	Post
High alt 2,800 m	64.9	67.7*	4387	4882*
Low alt 1,200 m	65.1	65.9	4678	4532

*$p<.05$ compared with control measurements.

sion. Maximal cardiac output and stroke volume become depressed during acclimatization. Acutely upon return to sea level or to sea level inspired oxygen tensions, maximal oxygen uptake during incremental exercise usually is still less than pre-ascent rather than being augmented despite the increased oxygen-carrying capacity of blood and persistence of an increased exercise ventilation.

The most likely explanation for the reduction in maximal oxygen uptake in physically-trained athletes after return from training at high altitude is the restriction imposed by high altitude on the level of training that can be sustained during chronic hypoxia. Stroke volume[20] and maximal cardiac output fall,[23–27] probably in part because of a fall in circulating blood volume and reduction in preload on both ventricular chambers; thus, sustained training of the left ventricle is restricted.

More recently, Levine and colleagues[28] at the University of Texas used a different strategy in using high-altitude acclimatization as a potential means for improving exercise performance in athletes. They divided a group of young athletes into two groups. For 3 weeks, both groups trained each day in Salt Lake City at an altitude of 1,200 m. Ten athletes lived in Salt Lake City whereas 9 athletes lived at a higher altitude of 2,800 m (Table 6).

In the group living at high altitude and training at a lower altitude, performance was significantly enhanced compared with the group living and training at lower altitude. Contrary to previous data obtained by other investigators showing that early acclimatization to high altitude decreases plasma volume, Levine et al. found a significant increase in plasma volume (when measured at 1,200 m) during 3 weeks of living at 2,800 m without a significant associated increase in hemoglobin concentration. These findings by Levine and his associates suggest that it may be possible to obtain the potential advantages of living at high altitude without the disadvantages of restricted training, and hence may have a place in training athletes for endurance events at sea level.

Summary: Sites of Exercise Limitation

1. In average humans at sea level, determinants of $\dot{V}o_2$max are not well matched. Primary limitation is imposed by the cardiovascular system.
2. In top athletes at sea level, determinants of $\dot{V}o_2$max are well matched. There is no clear site of primary limitation.
3. In both average men and top athletes at high altitude, $\dot{V}o_2$max becomes limited primarily by the diffusing capacity of the lungs.
4. $\dot{V}o_2$max falls acutely at high altitude but may recover partially during acclimatization at altitudes less than 4,300 m despite a fall in maximal cardiac output.
5. Acclimatization is associated with increased exercise ventilation, polycythemia, increased P_{50} of blood, reduced diffusion distances in skeletal muscle, modest pulmonary hypertension, and a reduced submaximal and maximal cardiac output.
6. Training at high altitude does not enhance $\dot{V}o_2$max at sea level.
7. Living at high altitude while training at low altitude may enhance $\dot{V}o_2$max at low altitude but mechanisms are not clear.

References

1. Stiles M: Athletic performance at Mexico City, in Vogel JHK (ed): *Advances in Cardiology.* Basel, Switzerland, S. Karger, 1970, pp 17–23
2. Johnson RL Jr.: Heart lung interactions in the transport of oxygen, in Scharf S, Cassidy SS, (eds): *Heart-Lung Interaction in Health and Disease.* New York, Marcel Dekker, 1989, pp 5–41
3. Johnson RLJ: Oxygen transport, in Willerson JT, Sanders CA (eds): *Clinical Cardiology.* New York, San Francisco, London, Grune & Sratton, 1977, pp 74–84
4. Saltin B, Blomqvist G, Mitchell JH, Johnson RL Jr, Wildenthal K, Chapman CB: Response to exercise after bed rest and after training. *Circ* 1968;38(suppl VII):VII-1–VII-78

5. Blomqvist G, Johnson RL Jr, Saltin B: Pulmonary diffusing capacity limiting human performance at altitude. *Acta Physiol Scand* 1969;76(3):284–287

6. Weibel ER, Taylor CR, Hoppeler H: The concept of symmorphosis: A testable hypothesis of structure-function relationship. *Proc Nat Acad Sci USA* 1991;88(22):10357–10361

7. Johnson RL Jr: Pulmonary diffusion as a limiting factor in exercise stress. *Circ Res* 1967;20(suppl I):I-154–I-160

8. Grover RF, Weil JV, Reeves JT: Cardiovascular adaptation to exercise at high altitude, in Pandolf KB (ed): *Exercise and Sports Sciences Reviews*. New York, Macmillan, 1986, pp 269–302

9. Hoppeler HE, Kleinert E, Schlegel C, Claassen H, Howald H, Kagar SR, Cerretelli P: Morphological adaptations of human skeletal muscle to chronic hypoxia. *Int J Sports Med* 1990;11(suppl 1):S3–S9

10. Kayser B, Hoppeler H, Claassen H, Cerretelli P: Muscle structure and performance capacity of Himalayan Sherpas. *J Appl Physiol* 1991;70(5):1938–1942

11. Lenfant C, Torrance J, English E, Finch C, Reynafarje C, Ramos J, Faura J: Effect of altitude on oxygen binding by hemoglobin and on organic phosphate levels. *J Clin Invest* 1968;47:2652–2656

12. Grover RF, Lufschanowski R, Alexander JK: Alterations in the coronary circulation of man following ascent to 3100 m altitude. *J Appl Physiol* 1976;41(6):832–838

13. Reeves JT, Grover EB, Grover RF: Pulmonary circulation and oxygen transport in lambs at high altitude. *J Appl Physiol* 1963;18(3):560–566

14. Banchero N, Grover RF: Effect of different levels of simulated altitude on oxygen transport in the llama and sheep. *Am J Physiol* 1972;222:1239–1245

15. Eaton JW, Skelton TD, Berger E: Survival at extreme altitude, protective effect of increased hemoglobin-oxygen affinity. *Science* 1974;183(743)

16. Hebbel RP, Eaton JW, Kronenberg RS, Zanjani ED, Moore LG, Berger EM: Human llamas: Adaptations to altitude in subjects with high hemoglobin oxygen affinity. *J Clin Invest* 1978;62:593–600

17. Reeves JT, Grover RF, Cohn JE: Regulation of ventilation during exercise at 10,200 ft in athletes born at low altitude. *J Appl Physiol* 1967;22(3):546–554

18. Grover RF: Chronic hypoxic pulmonary hypertension, in Fishman AP (ed): *The Pulmonary Circulation. Normal and Abnormal*. Philadelphia, University of Pennsylvania Press, 1990, pp 283–299

19. Buskirk ER, Kollias J, Akers RF, Prokop EK, Reategui EP: Maximal performance at altitude and on return from altitude in conditioned runners. *J Appl Physiol* 1967;23(2):259–256

20. Balke B, Nagel FJ, Daniels J: Altitude and maximum performance in work and sports activity. *JAMA* 1965;194:646

21. Saltin B: Aerobic and anaerobic work capacity at 2300 m. *Med Thorac* 1967;24:205–210

22. DeGraff AC Jr, Grover RF, Johnson RL Jr, Hammond JW Jr, Miller JM: Diffusing capacity of the lung in Caucasians native to 3,100 m. *J Appl Physiol* 1970;29(1):71–76

23. Saltin B, Grover RF, Blomqvist CG, Hartley H, Johnson RL Jr: Maximal oxygen uptake and cardiac output after 2 weeks at 4,300 m. *J Appl Physiol* 1968;25(3):400–409
24. Alexander JK, Grover RF: Mechanism of reduced cardiac stroke volume at high altitude. *Clin Cardiol* 1983;6:301–303
25. Alexander JK, Hartley LH, Modelski M, Grover RF: Reduction of stroke volume during exercise in man following ascent to 3,100 m altitude. *J Appl Physiol* 1967;23(6):849–858
26. Hartley LH, Alexander JK, Modelski M, Grover RF: Subnormal cardiac output at rest and during exercise in residents at 3,100 m altitude. *J Appl Physiol* 1967;23(6):839–848
27. Klausen K: Cardiac output in man in rest and work during and after acclimatization to 3,800 m. *J Appl Physiol* 1966;21(2):609–616
28. Levine BD, Stray-Gunderseon J, Duhaime Snell P, Friedman DB: Living high—training low: The effect of altitude acclimatization/normoxic training in trained runners. *Med Sci Sports Exerc* 1991;23:S25
29. Mitchell JH, Wildenthal K, Johnson RL Jr: The effects of acid-base disturbances on cardiovascular and pulmonary function. *Kidney Int* 1972;1(5):375–389

Part 4

Exercise as a Trigger of Onset of Acute Cardiovascular Disease

Chapter 13

Exercise as a Trigger of Onset of Myocardial Infarction and Sudden Cardiac Death

James E. Muller, MD, Murray Mittleman, MD, and Geoffrey Tofler, MBBS

Exercise appears to be capable of both preventing and causing acute myocardial infarction and sudden cardiac death. This paradox leaves a residua of uncertainty in clinical recommendations and a need for research on the mechanisms of these opposing effects.

Although it has been difficult to obtain conclusive evidence in a single study that exercise prevents acute cardiovascular disease, there is general agreement that the circumstantial evidence of a beneficial effect is substantial. Numerous prospective studies have shown an association between increasing levels of regular physical exertion and decreasing numbers of cardiovascular events. Small-scale interventional studies have shown that individuals performing regular exercise develop favorable changes in traditional cardiovascular risk factors and in other variables that might prevent cardiovascular disease. A large-scale randomized evaluation of the effect of exercise training on myocardial infarction and cardiac death (The National Exercise and Heart Disease Project) showed a trend toward a beneficial effect, but a more extensive test of the exercise hypothesis through a larger randomized trial was not deemed feasible.[1] This level of understanding leads to recommendations to the public and to patients that exercise, particularly in moderation, is a useful means to reduce the risk of cardiovascular disease. The American

From Fletcher GF, (ed): *Cardiovascular Response to Exercise.* Mount Kisco, NY, Futura Publishing Company, Inc., © 1994.

255

Heart Association has recently identified a sedentary lifestyle as a risk factor comparable in magnitude to hypertension, hypercholesterolemia, and cigarette smoking.[2]

The recommendation for an exercise program is made with caution because it is universally accepted that in rare circumstances, exercise actually may trigger the condition it is supposed to prevent. This risk is accepted because the frequency of triggering is quite low. The number of arrests during rehabilitation training was only 0.66 per 10,000 patient-hours and during exercise testing the number rose to only 4 per 10,000 tests.[3] However, when viewed from the perspective of relative risk, comparing periods of nonexertion with periods of exertion, the likelihood of a cardiac arrest was sixfold higher during the exertion of the rehabilitation program and 164-fold higher during exercise tests. These large increases in relative risk, which appear to increase with increased levels of exertion, highlight the difficulty in determining the proper level of exertion to recommend.

Although these issues are unlikely to be resolved by a randomized trial of varying levels of exertion, answers may be provided through advances in the understanding of the mechanism of onset of acute cardiovascular disease. Over the past 10 years, studies of circadian variation and triggering have produced new insights into disease onset. Understanding triggering is particularly important for the question of exertion, because studies indicate that the protective effect of regular exertion persists only during the period of months or years that the individual engages in regular exertion. This finding, that the protective effect of exercise requires continued exertion, is compatible with the hypothesis that regular exertion produces its beneficial effect by preventing triggering of disease onset, and not by producing a permanent change in the degree of atherosclerosis.

The final and most compelling reason to understand the role of exertion in triggering of infarction and sudden death is that such knowledge may be beneficial in the prevention of cardiac events not clearly related to exertion but possibly triggered by similar stressors. Although it is likely that less than 10% of nonfatal myocardial infarctions may be attributable to heavy physical exertion, these are the cases in which the mechanisms causing this catastrophic event are the most clearly revealed and amenable to study.

Epidemiologic Evidence of Triggering

Triggering of myocardial infarction (MI) onset was described in the original 1910 description of infarction by Obraztsov and Strazhesko.[4] The hypothesis that activities frequently trigger MI was challenged in the 1930s when studies of many patients revealed that in many instances, it occurred without an obvious precipitating event. A controversy developed with investigators for[5,6] and against[7,8] the view that triggers were frequent. The debate was suspended, however, with widespread acceptance of the conclusion of Master, based on an uncontrolled study using retrospective questionnaires, that activities are of little importance in triggering onset.[9]

Interest in the triggering hypothesis was renewed by findings that MI, sudden cardiac death, stroke, and transient myocardial ischemia show a prominent circadian variation with a morning increase in frequency.[10] Early studies had been ambiguous, because objective data on onset times were lacking. Doubts were dispelled in 1985 by the demonstration of the circadian pattern of MI onset using sequential creatinine kinase levels and back-extrapolation to define onset time objectively.[11] This study, based on data from the Multicenter Investigation of Limitation of Infarct Size (MILIS) Study, led us to examine the frequency of possible triggers reported by the MILIS patients.[12] Almost half (48.5%) of 849 patients indicated exposure to one or more possible triggers, including emotional upset (18.8%), moderate physical activity (14.4%), and heavy physical activity (8.7%). Similar frequencies were reported by Sumiyoshi.[13]

Tofler et al. analyzed the frequency and predictors of infarction occurring soon after heavy physical exertion among the 3,339 patients entered into the Thrombolysis in Myocardial Infarction (TIMI) II Study.[14] Myocardial infarction occurred during moderate or marked exertion in 18.7% of the patients. The most powerful multivariate predictors of exertion-associated infarction were absence of other chest pain in the 48 hours before infarction, male gender, exertional pain in the prior 3 weeks, and absence of any rest pain in the prior 3 weeks. The increasing likelihood of exertion-associated infarction with increased presence of these four variables is shown in Figure 1.

All of these studies, however, suffered from a lack of appropri-

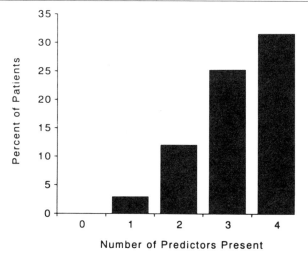

FIGURE 1. *The relation between the likelihood of infarction beginning during exertion and the number of predictors present with odds ratio >2.0 (ie, when the variable was present, onset was more than twice as likely to occur during exertion as during rest); 0% (0/64) (no predictors); 25.3% (444/1755) (three predictors); and 31.6% (44/139) (when all four of the predictors were present). The predictors were male gender, absence of other chest pain in the prior 48 hours, absence of any rest pain in the prior 3 weeks, and exertional angina in the prior 3 weeks. Adapted from Reference 14 with permission.*

ate control data. To compute the relative risk of MI during physical exertion, it is necessary to adjust for usual frequency of exertion. This need shaped the design of the Onset Study, described below.

The role of psychosocial factors in causation of MI and sudden cardiac death has been difficult to determine. Type A personality has been advanced as a risk factor for infarction, but the findings have been mixed and controversial. It has been proposed that hostility is the virulent core of the Type A personality.[15] Other epidemiologic evidence of psychosocial triggering is found in the increased cardiovascular mortality following an earthquake in Greece[16] and during the first week of SCUD missile attacks on Israel during the recent Gulf War.[17]

Indirect evidence of triggering comes from the circannual pattern of MI incidence, which falls to its nadir during the summer months in North America, but reaches its peak during the same months in

Australia where it is winter.[18] This phenomenon is likely to be caused by circannual variation in exposure to, or susceptibility to, triggers.

The Acute Risk Factor Concept

The findings of circadian variation and triggering have led to a new concept of an acute risk factor that supplements the traditional concept of a chronic risk factor. The acute risk factor results from a combination of an external stress (physical or mental) and the individual's reactivity to that stress resulting in increased hemodynamic, vasoconstrictive, or prothrombotic forces, as shown in Figure 2. It is possible that regular exertion achieves its protective effect by modifying an individual's reactivity to a physical, and possibly even to a mental, stress.

The extent of atherosclerosis changes slowly with time (chronic risk factors); however, hemodynamic, vasoconstrictive, and prothrombotic forces (acute risk factors) may be generated rapidly by external stresses. The proposed combined contribution of chronic and acute factors required to exceed the threshold to initiate MI is represented schematically in Figure 3. In this figure, the spikes indicate transient increases in risk resulting from a stress such as anger or physical exertion. These spikes rise from a baseline of chronic risk.

A rabbit model of atherosclerotic plaque rupture and thrombosis[19] has been developed to explore triggering hypotheses. New Zealand white rabbits are maintained on a cholesterol-rich diet for more than 4 months. They are then injected with Russell viper venom (a procoagulant and endothelial toxin) and histamine (a pressor in rabbits). Eight of 10 rabbits developed atherosclerotic plaque rupture and thrombus after this pharmacological triggering.[20] This model can now be used to identify mechanisms of triggering and to test preventive measures.

Little et al.[21] have shown that minimal coronary stenoses often are the cause of plaque rupture and have compared the incidence of MI and death in morning versus afternoon cardiac rehabilitation classes. Although there was no significant increase in cardiac events among patients exercising in the morning versus those exercising in

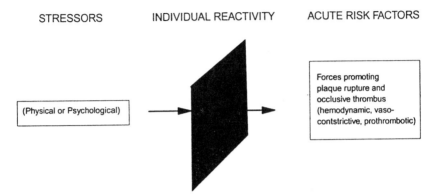

FIGURE 2. *Physical or psychological stressors as modified by individual reactivity produce acute risk factors.*

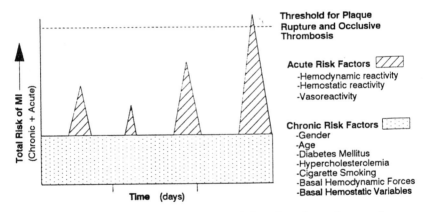

FIGURE 3. *A schematic representation of the chronic and acute factors required to exceed the threshold to initiate an acute cardiovascular event. The spikes indicate transient increases in risk resulting from a stress such as anger or physical exertion. Increases in hemodynamic, vasoconstrictive, and prothrombotic forces are acute risk factors for disease onset. They are superimposed on a background of traditional chronic risk factors.*

the afternoon, many patients presumably were taking β-blockers, and since the number of events was small, the power to detect an increase in risk was low.

Although our understanding of triggering mechanisms of infarction remains limited, our knowledge of triggering of transient myocardial ischemia is extensive. Willich et al. have shown that episodes of transient ischemia can be prevented by β-blockade without elimination of the morning increase of platelet aggregability.[22] Panza et al.[23] have shown that peripheral vascular resistance is increased in the morning and Parker et al.[24] have demonstrated that the morning increase in transient ischemia is dependent on initiation of activity.

The Myocardial Infarction Onset Study

For the past 4 years, investigators in 53 hospitals have worked together to identify and characterize triggering of onset of acute MI. More than 1,250 patients have now been interviewed concerning the activities during the hours before their infarction. A new epidemiologic technique, termed the *case-crossover design*, has been used to obtain appropriate control data to identify triggering.[25] The interview covers a 26-hour period before the infarction to include a 2-hour "hazard period" immediately before MI onset, and the comparable 2-hour "control period" at the same time on the preceding day.

Figure 4 illustrates the method by showing hazard and control periods. Each patient contributes information about both periods, and therefore serves as both a case and a self-matched control. Relative risks are computed using standard methods for matched-pair case-control studies. Instead of concordant and discordant pairs of subjects, however, there are individual patients whose two exposure periods were either concordant or discordant.

All the information comes from two types of discordant patients: patients exposed in the hazard period but not the control period, and patients exposed in the control period but not the hazard period. The number exposed in the hazard period only divided by the number exposed in the control period only is the estimate of the relative risk.

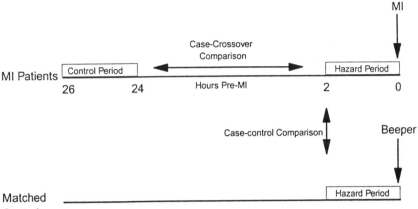

FIGURE 4. *A diagram indicating the case-crossover method. The frequency of a potential trigger in the "hazard" period, the 2 hours before MI onset, is compared with its frequency in the same 2-hour "control" period on the prior day.*

A traditional case-control comparison is also made. Age- and gender-matched neighborhood controls are given a beeper that is set off at the same time of day as the patient experienced the MI. The controls are then questioned about events in the "hazard period" prior to beeper activation.

The interviews obtained from the 1,250 postinfarction patients in the Onset Study have provided the following quantitative information about triggering of MI.

Waking/Activity and Effect of β-Blockade

Wake-time adjustment was found to sharpen the morning peak of MI onset.[26] The risk of onset in the 2 hours following awakening is 2.3 (95% CI: 1.9, 2.7) times higher than during other times of the day. The timing of onset was no different in men versus women, smokers versus nonsmokers, old versus young, diabetics versus nondiabetics, or hypertensives versus nonhypertensives.

We assessed the effect of aspirin and β-blockers on the circadian pattern of onset.[27] β-blocker usage was associated with a statistically significant decrease in the morning peak in infarctions observed in nonusers. The implication of this finding is that triggering by waking and commencement of activity can be prevented by the use of β-blockers. Regular users of aspirin had a similar pattern of wake-time–adjusted onset as those not using aspirin.

Physical Exertion

The relative risk of MI onset in the 2-hour period after strenuous exertion (≥6 metabolic equivalents [mets]) was found to be 4.6 (95% CI:2.3, 9.1).

It was noted that β-blockers lowered the point estimate of the relative risk of triggering by an episode of heavy physical exertion. The relative risk for MI triggering by heavy exertion was 5.4 (95% CI: 2.42, 12.2) among non–β-blocker users. The point estimate for the relative risk among β-blocker users was 2.0. This result was not statistically significant but the study does not yet have sufficient power to test this hypothesis adequately.

Anger

A seven-level self-report scale was developed for the Onset Study. The risk of MI onset was elevated three-fold (95% CI: 1.4, 6.4) in the 2 hours following an outburst of anger above level 3 on our scale.

Caffeine

Reported intake of caffeinated beverages in the 2 hours before MI onset was almost identical to reported intake in the same 2-hour period the day before. The relative risk was 0.94 (95% CI: 0.64, 1.4).[30] These findings are consistent with a meta-analysis of the relation between chronic coffee consumption and risk of heart disease, which concluded that there was no association.[31]

A large epidemiologic study similar to the Onset Study has been conducted in Germany. This study, entitled TRIMM, has produced results on triggering similar to those of the Onset Study.[32]

Modifiers of Susceptibility to Triggering of Myocardial Infarction

It appears likely that a number of factors may alter the risk of MI, given exposure to a potential trigger. β-Blockers, aspirin, captopril, and estrogen use have, with varying levels of proof, been shown to prevent MI.[33-36] Although knowledge of mechanisms of their preventive effects remains incomplete, it is possible that they act by reducing susceptibility to triggering. In the MILIS Study[11] and the TIMI Study,[14] it was found that prior β-blocker usage was associated with an apparent elimination of the morning peak of infarction, but the power to detect a peak was limited. The BHAT study demonstrated selective prevention of sudden death in the morning of β-blockade.[37]

The Onset Study has demonstrated conclusively that β-blockers decrease the peak in infarct onset after awakening and commencement of activity. The finding that β-blockers can prevent MIs, triggered in the hours after awakening raises the possibility that they also may reduce susceptibility to other triggers such as physical exertion and anger. A possible mechanism through which β-blockers may reduce susceptibility to triggers is via the reduction of peak systolic arterial pressures associated with potential triggering activities. Such a decrease might lower the probability of rupture of a vulnerable plaque.

Aspirin is well documented to provide both secondary and primary prevention of MI,[33,38] presumably by reduction of platelet aggregability. It has been reported to exert a selective beneficial effect in the morning,[39] when platelet aggregability is known to surge. However, its effect on the morning peak of MI is not yet clarified. Preliminary findings from the Onset Study indicate that a substantial increase in MI after awakening persists despite aspirin therapy, but the Onset Study is not randomized and lacks the power of the Physicians Health Study.

General Theory of Triggering of Coronary Thrombosis

A general hypothesis of the manner in which daily activities might trigger coronary thrombosis has been proposed.[10] The hypothesis presented in Figure 5 adds the concept of triggering activities to the general scheme of the role of thrombosis in the acute coronary syndromes advanced by Falk,[40] Davies and Thomas,[41] Fuster et al.,[42] Willerson et al.,[43] and others. It is further hypothesized that plaque rupture with occlusive thrombosis occurs at a critical moment, when a threshold combination of hemodynamic, prothrombotic, and vasoconstrictive forces are rapidly generated by external stresses.

The initial step in the process leading to coronary thrombosis is the development, with advancing age, of a vulnerable atherosclerotic plaque. Plaque vulnerability is defined functionally as the susceptibility of a plaque to rupture. Development of such vulnerability is a poorly understood process, but is presumably a dynamic, potentially reversible disorder caused by changes in the constituents of the plaque, its blood supply via the vasa vasorum, and/or the functional integrity of the overlying endothelium.

The theory that onset of thrombosis is unrelated to daily activities presumably would attribute disease onset solely to evolution of the plaque, and the diagram (Figure 5) therefore would lead directly from the plaque to occlusive coronary thrombosis. In the present formulation, however, it is proposed that onset frequently might begin when a physical or mental stress triggers a hemodynamic change sufficient to rupture a vulnerable plaque. However, if such a trigger does not occur during vulnerability, the plaque may change and become nonvulnerable.

The rupture in the plaque may be major or minor, depending on factors such as the amount and type of collagen exposed.[44] A major plaque rupture produces a thrombogenic focus sufficiently intense to cause occlusive coronary thrombosis leading directly to MI or sudden cardiac death. A minor rupture leads only to a mural thrombus that fails to produce symptoms, or leads to unstable angina or non–Q-wave MI. At this point, mental stress or physical activity may trigger increases in coagulability or vasoconstriction. Such a coagulability increase may trigger growth of the thrombus, or vasoconstriction may lead to complete occlusion of an already compromised lumen, leading to infarction or sudden death. Since normal individuals and even patients with coronary artery disease are exposed constantly to potentially triggering activities that do not produce coronary thrombosis, it seems likely that development of plaque vulnerability is the rarest event in the chain of causation described above.

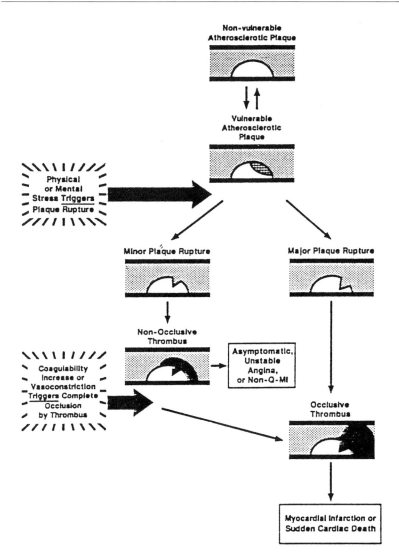

FIGURE 5. *Illustration of a hypothetical method by which daily activities may trigger coronary thrombosis. Three triggering mechanisms, 1) physical or mental stress producing hemodynamic changes leading to plaque rupture, 2) activities causing a coagulability increase, and 3) stimuli leading to vasoconstriction, have been added to the well known sheme depicting the role of coronary thrombosis in unstable angina, MI and sudden cardiac death. See text for detailed discussion. Adapted from Reference 10 with permission.*

A synergistic combination of triggering activities may account for thrombosis. For example, the combination of physical exertion (producing a minor plaque rupture) followed by cigarette smoking (producing an increase in coronary artery vasoconstriction and a relatively hypercoagulable state) may be needed to cause disease onset. Thus, the onset of infarction, in some cases, may be the result of the unfortunate simultaneous occurrence of several events each by itself of little consequence, but catastrophic when occurring together.

Significance

The primary immediate value of recognizing the circadian variation of acute onset of MI is the emphasis that can be placed on pharmacological protection during the morning hours for patients already receiving anti-ischemic therapy. Although no scientific studies have been performed to test the hypothesis, it seems reasonable that long-acting anti-ischemic agents would have an advantage over short-acting agents in providing protection against MI in the morning when the effects of short-acting agents taken the night before may begin to attenuate.

As noted above, the finding that more infarcts occur in the morning raises questions about the desirability of exercise in the morning. At present, the evidence that exercise is beneficial in reducing the risk of infarction[2] is substantial and, although theoretical concerns can be raised, there is no evidence that exercise in the morning is more hazardous than exercise at other times of the day, and even a sizeable increase in relative risk of morning versus evening exercise would produce only a very low absolute risk.

Research Implications

The hypothetical mechanism of triggering of coronary thrombosis described can serve as a means to evaluate the probable preventive effects of regular moderate exercise. Table 1 indicates six

TABLE 1. Mechanisms Through Which Fitness Could Prevent MI

Proinfarction process	Beneficial effect of exercise
Plaque formation	Reduction of LDL, elevation of HDL
Plaque vulnerability	Reduction of LDL, elevation of HDL
Plaque rupture	Less systolic hypertension
Hypercoagulability	Increased fibrinolysis, PGI_2, decreased platelet Aggregability
Vasoconstriction	PGI_2 increased
Occlusion	Artery size increased

LDL, low density lipoproteins; HDL, high density lipoproteins; PGI_2, prostaglandin I_2.

ways in which a known effect of chronic exercise could interrupt the causative chain leading to MI and sudden cardiac death. As this process is better understood it may be possible to identify more precisely the needed changes and thereby formulate a more appropriate exercise prescription. Knowledge of the manner in which strenuous exertion triggers onset also might lead to methods to block the linkage between the exercise and disease onset.

Resolution of the paradox that exercise can both protect against and cause MI and sudden death would be of great benefit in determining the proper form of safe and beneficial exercise. However, its greatest benefit is likely to be improved understanding and better methods of prevention of most infarcts and sudden deaths, which are not associated with heavy physical exertion but are likely to be caused by more subtle variants of the processes causing exertion-related events.

Acknowledgement

We are grateful for the assistance of Ms. Kathleen Carney in the preparation of the chapter.

References

1. Stern MJ, Cleary P: National Exercise and Heart Disease Project: long-term psychosocial outcome. *Arch Intern Med* 1982;142(6): 1093–1097
2. American Heart Association Committee on Exercise. *Circulation* 1992;86:340–344

3. Cobb LA, Weaver D: Exercise: a risk for sudden death in patients with coronary heart disease. *J Am Coll Cardiol* 1986;7:215–219

4. Obraztsov VP, Strazhesko ND: The symptomatology and diagnosis of coronary thrombosis. Works of the First Congress of Russian Therapists. Vorobeva VA, Konchalovski MP (eds): Comradeship Typography of A.E. Mamontov, 1910;26–43

5. Fitzhugh G, Hamilton BE: Coronary occlusion and fatal angina pectoris. Study of the immediate causes and their prevention. *JAMA* 1933;100:475–480

6. Sproul J: A general practitioner's views on the treatment of angina pectoris. *N Engl J Med* 1936;215:443–452

7. Parkinson J, Bedford DE: Cardiac infarction and coronary thrombosis. *Lancet* 1928;1:4–11

8. Phipps C: Contributory causes of coronary thrombosis. *JAMA* 1936;106:761–762

9. Master AM: The role of effort and occupation (including physicians) in coronary occlusion. *JAMA* 1960;174:942–948

10. Muller JE, Tofler GH, Stone PH: Circadian variation and triggers of onset of acute cardiovascular disease. *Circulation* 1989;79:733–743

11. Muller JE, Stone PH, Turi ZG, Rutherford JD, Czeisler CA, Parker C, Poole WK, Passamani E, Roberts R. Robertson T, Sobel BE, Willerson JT, Braunwald E, The MILIS Study Group: Circadian variation in the frequency of onset of acute myocardial infarction. *N Engl J Med* 1985;313:1315–1322

12. Tofler GH, Stone PH, Maclure M, Edelman E, Davis VG, Robertson T, Antman EM, Muller JE, The MILIS Study Group: Analysis of possible triggers of acute myocardial infarction (The MILIS Study). *Am J Cardiol* 1990;66:22–27

13. Sumiyoshi T: Evaluation of clinical factors involved in onset of myocardial infarction. *Jpn Circ J* 1986;50:164–173

14. Tofler GH, Muller JE, Stone PH, Forman S, Solomon RE, Knatterud GL, Braunwald E, the TIMI Research Group: Modifiers of timing and possible triggers of acute myocardial infarction in the TIMI II population. *J Am Coll Cardiol* 1992;20:1045–1055

15. Suarez EC, Williams RB Jr: The relationships between dimensions of hostility and cardiovascular reactivity as a function of task characteristics. *Psychosom Med* 1990;52:558–570

16. Trichopoulos D, Katsouyanni K, Zavitsanos X, Tzonou A, Dalla-Vorgia P: Psychological stress and fatal heart attack: the Athens (1981) earthquake natural experiment. *Lancet* 1983;1:441–444

17. Meisel SR: Effect of Iraqi missile war on incidence of acute myocardial infarction and sudden death in Israeli civilians. *Lancet* 1991;338:660–661

18. Ornato JP, Siegel L, Craren EJ, Nelson N: Increased incidence of cardiac death attributed to acute myocardial infarction during winter. *Coron Art Dis* 1990;1:199–203

19. Constantinides P: Plaque fissures in human coronary thrombosis. *J Atheroscler Res* 1966;1:1–17

20. Picon PD, Friedl SE, Ye B, Gebara O, Johnstone E, Saxton JM,

Federman M, Aretz HT, Tofler GH, Muller JE, Abela GS: Pharmacological triggering of plaque rupture and arterial thrombosis in an atherosclerotic rabbit model (abstract). *J Am Coll Cardiol* 1993;21:435A

21. Little WC, Constantinescu, M, Applegate RJ, Kutcher MA, Burrows MT, Kahl FR, Santamore WP: Can coronary angiography predict the site of a subsequent myocardial infarction in patients with mild to moderate coronary artery disease? *Circulation* 1988;78:1157–1166

22. Willich SN, Phojola-Sintonen S, Bhatia S, Snook TL, Muller JE, Curtis DG, Williams GH, Stone PH: Suppression of silent ischemia by metoprolol without altering the morning increase of platelet aggregability in patients with stable coronary artery disease. *Circulation* 1989;79:557–565

23. Panza JA, Epstein SE, Quyyumi AA: Circadian variation in vascular tone and its relation to sympathetic vasoconstrictor activity. *N Engl J Med* 1991;325:986–990

24. Parker JD, Jimenez AH, Farrell B, et al: The morning increase in myocardial ischemia is dependent on the time of onset of physical activity (abstract). *Circulation* 1990;(suppl III):391

25. Maclure M: The case-crossover design: A method for studying transient effects on the risk of acute events. *Am J Epidemiol* 1991;133:144–153

26. Maclure M, Sherwood J, Andrade S, Goldberg RJ, Toffler GH, Muller JE: Increased risk of myocardial infarction onset within the two hours after awakening (abstract). *Circulation* 1990:82(4)supplement

27. Mittleman M, Maclure M, Sherwood J, Toffler GH, Muller JE, for the Onset Study Investigators: Beta blocker usage is associated with a reduction in the post-awakening peak of myocardial infarction onset (abstract). *J Am Coll Cardiol* 1993;21:436A

28. Mittleman MA, Maclure M, Sherwood JB, et al: Three-fold increase in risk of myocardial infarction onset following episodes of anger. Abstract submitted to the Epidemiology Council Meeting AHA March 1994.

29. Speilberger CD, Jacobs G, Russel S, et al: Assessment of anger: The state-trait anger scale, in Butcher JN, Speilberger CD (eds): *Advances in Personality Assessment*, vol 2. Hillsdale, NJ, Lawrence Erlbaum Associates, 159–187

30. Mittleman M, Maclure M, Sherwood J, Goldberg R, Tofler GH, Muller JE: Caffeinated beverage consumption is not responsible for triggering of myocardial infarction (abstract). *Int Heart Health Con* May 1992

31. Greenland S: Coffee, myocardial infarction, and coronary death: An update of the 1987 meta-analysis. *Epidemiol Rev* 1992, in press

32. Willich SN, Lowel H, Lewis M, Arntz R, Bauer R, Winther K, Keil U, Schroder R, et al: Association of wake-time and the onset of myocardial infarction. Triggers and mechanisms of myocardial infarction (TRIMM) pilot study. TRIMM Study Group. *Circulation* 1991;84(suppl VI):62–67

33. Lewis HD Jr, Davis JW, Archibald DG, Steinke WE, Smitherman TC, Doherty JE III, Schnaper HW, LeWinter MM, Linaries E, Pouget JM, Sabharwal SC, Chesler E, DeMots H: Protective effects of aspirin

against acute myocardial infarction and death in men with unstable angina: results of a Veterans Administration Cooperative Study. *N Engl J Med* 1983;309:396–403

34. Beta-blocker Heart Attack Trial Research Group. A randomized trial of propranolol in patients with acute myocardial infarction. Mortality results. *JAMA* 1982;247:1707–1714

35. Moye LA, Pfeffer MA, Braunwald E: Rationale, design, and baseline characteristics of the survival and ventricular enlargement trial. SAVE Investigators. *Am J Cardiol* 1991;68(14):70D–79D

36. Stampfer MJ, Colditz GA: Estrogen replacement therapy and coronary heart disease: a quantitative assessment of the epidemiologic evidence. *Prev Med* 1991;20:47–63

37. Peters RW, Muller JE, Goldstein S, Byington R, Friedman LM: Propranolol and the circadian variation in the frequency of sudden cardiac death: the BHAT experience (abstract). *Circulation* 1988;76(suppl IV):IV–364

38. Steering Committee of the Physicians' Health Study Research Group. Final report of the ongoing Physicians' Health Study. *N Engl J Med* 1989;321:129–135

39. Ridker PM, Manson JE, Buring JE, Muller JE, Hennekens CH: Circadian variation of acute myocardial infarction and the effect of low-dose aspirin in a randomized trial of physicians. *Circulation* 1990;82:897–902

40. Falk E: Plaque rupture with severe pre-existing stenosis precipitating coronary thrombosis. *Br Heart J* 1983;50:127–134

41. Davies MJ, Thomas AC: Plaque fissuring—the cause of acute myocardial infarction, sudden ischemic death, and crescendo angina. *Br Heart J* 1985;53:363–373

42. Fuster V, Steele PM, Chesebro JH: Role of platelets and thrombosis in coronary atherosclerotic disease and sudden death. *J Am Coll Cardiol* 1985;5(suppl):175B–184B

43. Willerson JT, Campbell WB, Winniford MD, Schmitz J, Apprill P, Firth BG, Ashton J, Smitherman T, Bush L, Buja LM: Conversion from chronic to acute coronary artery disease: speculation regarding mechanisms (editorial). *Am J Cardiol* 1984;54:1349–1354

44. Badimon L, Badimon JJ, Turitto VT, et al: Platelet thrombus formation on collagen type I. A model of deep vessel injury. Influence of blood rheology, von Willebrand factor, and blood coagulation. *Circulation* 1988;78:1431–1432

45. Myers MG, Basinsk A: Coffee and coronary heart disease. *Arch Intern Med* 1992;152:1767–1772

Chapter 14

Sudden Cardiac Death During Exercise

David S. Siscovick, MD, MPH

Sudden death during exercise raises the concern that bouts of exercise might trigger the onset of catastrophic acute cardiac events.[1] Plausible pathophysiological mechanisms for a potentially adverse acute cardiovascular response to exercise include the occurrence of exercise-induced myocardial ischemia and cardiac arrhythmias.[2,3] Recent epidemiologic studies demonstrate that the occurrence of sudden cardiac death during exercise is not a coincidence or chance occurrence; acute bouts of exercise occasionally trigger cardiac arrest.[4,5]

In this chapter we briefly review the findings of population-based studies that examine the risk of sudden cardiac death during exercise among apparently healthy adults in the community. Based on these data, we estimate the incidence of sudden cardiac death during exercise, identify several factors that might alter the risk, and put into perspective the risks and benefits of exercise that relate to sudden cardiac death. Finally, we suggest that although exercise occasionally triggers sudden cardiac death, the overall effect of exercise reflects the net balance of the transient risk associated with the acute cardiovascular response to bouts of exercise and cardiac benefits related to habitual exercise.

Magnitude of the Problem

Among community-dwelling adults, sudden cardiac death occurs most commonly in the setting of atherosclerotic coronary heart

From Fletcher GF, (ed): *Cardiovascular Response to Exercise.* Mount Kisco, NY, Futura Publishing Company, Inc., © 1994.

disease (CHD).[6] CHD remains the leading cause of death in the United States, accounting for approximately 35% of all deaths.[7] Approximately half of all deaths attributed to CHD among middle-aged men in the Framingham Heart Disease Study occurred suddenly (within 1 hour of symptom onset), and half of the sudden cardiac deaths occurred among men without a prior history of clinical coronary heart disease.[8]

Population-based studies from Seattle and King County (Washington) suggest that approximately 6% of incident sudden cardiac death cases occur during exercise, such as racket sports and jogging.[4] An additional 9% of cases occur during less intense physical activity, such as walking and lawn and garden activities. Overall, 15% of sudden cardiac deaths occur during leisure-time physical activity. Although these data indicate the magnitude of the problem of sudden cardiac death during acute bouts of exercise, rates of sudden death during exercise in defined populations are needed to determine the risk of sudden cardiac death during exercise.

Risk of Sudden Cardiac Death During Exercise

Several studies have estimated the risk of sudden cardiac death during exercise among adults in the community. Vouri[9] reported the incidence of sudden cardiac death during jogging/running and cross-country skiing among men, aged 20 to 69 years, in Finland. During a 9-year period (1970 through 1978), there were 235 cardiac deaths during exercise. Population surveys were used to estimate the number of Finnish men who engaged in specific sports. Incidence rates for sudden death during exercise were lowest for younger men, with similar rates for middle-aged and older men. For men aged 50 to 69 years, there was one sudden death during cross-country skiing annually per 31,000 men who engaged in the sport.

Thompson et al.[5] identified all sudden cardiac deaths during jogging in Rhode Island from 1975 through 1981 and estimated the number of persons engaged in jogging from population surveys. The incidence of death during jogging among apparently healthy joggers was one death per 15,240 joggers per year. In a community-based study of physical activity and primary cardiac arrest in Seattle and King County (Washington), we observed a similar rate of sudden cardiac death during vigorous exercise, one cardiac arrest per 20,000 exercisers per year.[4]

The rates reported from studies of somewhat more selected groups are higher than rates reported from community-based studies. For example, among joggers at the aerobics center in Dallas, Texas and marathon runners in South Africa, rates of three to four deaths during exercise per 20,000 joggers or runners per year have been reported.[10,11] Several factors may account for the higher rates observed in these groups, including characteristics of the study population, the nature of the exercise, and the time spent in exercise. For example, joggers at the aerobics center in Dallas may be at higher risk of CHD or spend more time in exercise than persons in the community and, the intensity and time spent in exercise among marathon runners far exceeds that expected in the community.

Although these data reflect the low absolute risk of sudden death during exercise among apparently healthy men, the occurrence of sudden death during exercise may not be a random event. To determine whether exercise transiently increases the risk of sudden cardiac death, it is necessary to determine if the risk is increased during exercise, compared with the risk at other times. Each of the three community-based studies noted previously examined this question. Vouri[9] reported that the risk of sudden cardiac death during cross-country skiing in Finland was increased 4.5-fold, compared with that during more sedentary activities. Thompson et al.[5] found that the risk of sudden death during jogging in Rhode Island was increased sevenfold. In our community-based study in Seattle, we observed a similar increase in risk during vigorous exercise compared with the risk at other times.[4] These observations suggest that the occurrence of sudden death during exercise is not a coincidence or random event; exercise occasionally precipitates sudden cardiac death.

Influence of Other Factors

Despite broad participation in exercise in the community, sudden death during exercise is a rare event. It is likely that the transient risk associated with bouts of exercise is modified by the presence of other factors. Several studies have examined whether other factors, including the intensity of exercise, habitual activity level, gender, prior morbidity, and age, influence the cardiac risks of exercise. Vouri[9] demonstrated that the increase in risk during exercise was greater for strenuous than nonstrenuous exercise. There was a ninefold increase in risk during strenuous exercise, but only a threefold increase during nonstrenuous exercise.

Because regular participation in exercise influences the acute cardiovascular response to bouts of exercise through biochemical and physiological responses to exercise training,[12,13] we determined whether the amount of regular exercise influenced the magnitude of the transient increase in risk of primary cardiac arrest during exercise.[4] With increasing amounts of time spent in exercise on a regular basis, there was a reduction in the transient increase in risk during exercise. Among apparently healthy men who spent less than 20 minutes a week engaged in vigorous exercise, the risk was increased 56-fold. However, among habitually active men who spent more than 20 minutes per day engaged in vigorous exercise, the risk was increased only fivefold. In short, regular exercise reduced the transient increase in risk associated with acute bouts of exercise; men who were physically inactive were at the greatest risk of sudden cardiac death during exercise. However, even among regular exercisers, the risk of sudden death during exercise was increased compared with the risk at other times.

Few published studies examine the influence of gender on the risk of sudden death during exercise, in part because among middle-aged persons both CHD and sudden cardiac death occur most commonly among men. Nevertheless, both Finnish and U.S. community-based studies of sudden cardiac death during exercise suggest that the risk is lower among women compared with men. Vouri[9] noted that sudden cardiac death during exercise was 14 times less frequent among women than men, despite the fact that the proportion of women and the frequency of participation in recreational activity in Finland was similar to that of men. In our studies of exercise and primary cardiac arrest in Seattle, sudden death during exercise was nine times less frequent among women than men (unpublished data). The extent to which gender differences in risk reflect differences among men and women in the prevalence of CHD, the biochemical or physiological response to exercise, or characteristics of exercise remains unknown.

Because case series demonstrate a high prevalence of structural cardiac abnormalities among persons who experience sudden cardiac death during exercise,[14] some suggest that persons occasionally experience sudden death during exercise, but not from exercise. Alternatively, structural cardiac abnormalities might provide a substrate for exercise-induced sudden cardiac death. Among adults, the presence of clinical CHD increases the absolute risk of sudden cardiac death during exercise.[15,16] However, the magnitude of the transient increase in risk during exercise compared with other times is similar to that observed among apparently healthy persons.[5] For men with prior clinical CHD, the risk during strenuous exercise also is increased sixfold. These findings result from the fact that men with prior clinical coronary disease are at greater risk of sudden cardiac death both during and not during exercise.

Since coronary disease increases the absolute risk of sudden death during exercise, it has seemed reasonable to speculate that coronary risk factors such as hypercholesterolemia, hypertension, cigarette smoking, obesity, diabetes, and family history of premature CHD might increase the risk of exercise-related acute cardiac events. Data from the Lipid Research Clinics Program Coronary Primary Prevention Trial suggest that the risk of sudden death during exercise may be increased among apparently healthy, middle-aged, hypercholesterolemic men.[17] Whether other CHD risk factors alter the risk of sudden cardiac death during exercise has not been investigated. In addition, prior research has not examined whether factors that can trigger cardiac arrhythmias, such as alcohol and caffeine consumption, influence the risk of sudden death during exercise.

Environmental factors also may influence risk. Vouri observed that the risk of sudden cardiac death during exercise was increased at low ambient temperatures (personal communication). High ambient temperatures also may increase risk, but available data do not specifically address this question. The potential role of high altitude on risk also has not been examined. In short, although it is plausible that environmental factors that influence the acute cardiac response to bouts of exercise also may influence the risk of sudden cardiac death during exercise, few studies of exercise-related sudden cardiac death examine these potential effect modifiers.

Net Balance of Risks and Benefits

To put the cardiac risks and benefits of exercise into perspective, we examined both the risk of primary cardiac arrest during exercise and the potential benefit of habitual exercise in the same population.[4] We not only identified the circumstances surrounding the occurrence of primary cardiac arrest among apparently healthy men in Seattle and King County (Washington) during a 14-month period, but we also estimated the time spent in and out of exercise in the community. We used these data to demonstrate that the overall incidence of primary cardiac arrest in the population reflects the weighted average of the risk during and not during exercise, where the weights are the amount of time spent in and out of exercise. In short, we demonstrated the extent to which the transient increase in risk of primary cardiac arrest during exercise detracts from the cardiac benefits associated with exercise.

Among men who engaged in vigorous exercise, such as jogging and racket sports, the transient increase in risk during exercise was outweighed by a decrease in risk at other times, so that the overall risk was lower among active men than sedentary men. As expected, men who did not engage in exercise were not at risk for events during exercise. However, these sedentary men had the highest overall rates of primary cardiac arrest. The overall incidence of primary cardiac arrest among men who engaged in vigorous exercise for more than 20 minutes per week was only 40% that of sedentary men.[4,18] These findings suggest that although the risk of primary cardiac arrest was transiently increased during exercise, habitual exercise was associated with a reduced risk of primary cardiac arrest.

Conclusions

The occurrence of sudden cardiac death during exercise is not a coincidence or random event. Although case series demonstrate that these events occur in the setting of structural cardiac abnormalities, acute bouts of exercise occasionally precipitate sudden cardiac death. When viewed in terms of the population at risk, however, the occurrence of sudden cardiac death during exercise among apparently healthy persons in the community is a rare event.

Other factors may need to be present for exercise to trigger the occurrence of sudden cardiac death. Host factors, such as the presence of clinical or subclinical coronary disease, characteristics of the "exposure," such as the intensity of exercise and whether the exercise is usual or unusual for the person, and environmental factors, such as ambient temperature, may influence the risk of sudden cardiac death during exercise. However, additional research is needed to examine the role of other factors in exercise-related sudden cardiac death.

The extent to which the transient risk of sudden cardiac death during exercise detracts from the cardiac benefits of habitual exercise in the community has been clearly demonstrated.[4] Given these data, clinical observations of sudden death during acute bouts of exercise and epidemiologic studies that suggest that habitual exercise is associated with an overall reduced risk of CHD and sudden cardiac death are not contradictory. In short, exercise has cardiac risks and benefits; overall, the cardiac benefit of regular exercise outweighs the transient cardiac risk during exercise.

Biochemical and physiological responses during acute bouts of exercise and the adaptation to exercise training suggest that epidemiologic observations of exercise-related cardiac risks and benefits are biologically plausible.[19,20] Neurohumoral or other mechanisms may be involved in transiently increasing risk during exercise and/or decreasing overall risk as a consequence of exercise training.[19] Animal studies suggest that both acute and habitual exercise alter the balance of sympathetic and vagal activity and, thus, at least in part explain the cardiac risks and benefits of exercise.[13,20]

To identify optimal levels of exercise that minimize the cardiac risks and maximize the benefits of exercise, there is a need for "physiology and epidemiology to get together," as suggested by British epidemiologist Jeremy Morris.[21] In addition, since factors other than the intensity, frequency, duration, and type of exercise may influence both the risks and benefits of exercise, research related to the cardiovascular response to exercise also should consider the potential influence of the circumstances surrounding exercise and other factors on the cardiac risks and benefits of exercise.[22]

References

1. Rennie D, Hollenberg NK: Cardiomythology and marathons. *N Engl J Med* 1979;301:103–104

2. Durstine JL, Pate RR: Cardiorespiratory responses to acute exercise, in Blair SN, Painter P, Pate RR, Smith LK, Taylor CB, (eds): *Resource Manual for Guidelines for Exercise Testing and Prescription.* Philadelphia: Lea and Febiger, 1988, pp 48–54

3. American College of Sports Medicine. *Guidelines for Exercise Testing and Prescription.* 4th ed. Philadelphia: Lea and Febiger, 1991

4. Siscovick DS, Weiss NS, Fletcher RH, Lasky T: The incidence of primary cardiac arrest during vigorous exercise. *N Engl J Med* 1984;311:874–877

5. Thompson PD, Funk EJ, Carleton RA, Sturner MD: Incidence of death during jogging in Rhode Island from 1975-1980. *JAMA* 1982;247:2535–2538

6. Myerburg RJ, Castellanos A: Cardiac arrest and sudden cardiac death, in Braunwald E, (ed): *Heart Disease.* Philadelphia: WB Saunders Co, 1988, pp 742–777

7. NCHS Advance Report of Final Mortality Statistics, 1989. Hyattsville, MD: US Department of Health and Human Services; Public Health Service, CDC, 1992, Monthly vital statistics report; 40:8, suppl 2.

8. Schatzkin A, Cupples LA, Heeren T, Morelock S, Kannel WB: Sudden death in the Framingham Heart Study. *Am J Epidemiol* 1984;120:888–899

9. Vouri I: The cardiovascular risks of physical activity. *Acta Med Scand* 1984;Suppl 711:205–214

10. Gibbons LW, Cooper KH, Meyer BM, Ellison RC: The acute cardiac risk of strenuous exercise. *JAMA* 1980;244:1799–1801

11. Noakes TD, Opie LH, Rose AG: Marathon running and immunity to coronary heart disease: fact versus fiction. *Clin Sports Med* 1984;3:527–543

12. Saltin B: Cardiovascular and pulmonary adaptation to physical activity, in Bouchard C, Shephard RJ, Stephens T, Sutton JR, McPherson BD (eds): *Exercise, Fitness, and Health.* Champaign, IL: Human Kinetics Books, 1990, pp 187–203

13. Billman GE, Schwartz PG, Stone HL: The effects of daily exercise on susceptibility to sudden cardiac death. *Circulation* 1984;69:1182–1189

14. Waller BF, Roberts WC: Sudden death while running in conditioned runners aged 40 years or over. *Am J Cardiol* 1980;45:1292–1300

15. Haskell WL: Cardiovascular complications during exercise training of cardiac patients. *Circulation* 1978;57:920–924

16. Van Camp SP, Peterson R: Cardiovascular complications of outpatient cardiac rehabilitation programs. *JAMA* 1986;256:1160–1163

17. Siscovick DS, Ekelund LG, Johnson JL, Truong Y, Adler A: Sensitivity of exercise electrocardiography for acute cardiac events during moderate and strenuous physical activity. *Arch Intern Med* 1991;151:325–330

18. Siscovick DS, Weiss NS, Hallstrom AP, Inui TS, Peterson DR: Physical activity and primary cardiac arrest. *JAMA* 1982;248:3113–3117

19. Duncan JJ, Farr JE, Upton SJ, Hagan RD, Oglesby ME, Blair SN: The effects of aerobic exercise on plasma catecholamines and blood pressure in patients with essential hypertension. *JAMA* 1985;254:2609–2613

20. Billman GE, Schwartz PG, Gagnol GP, Stone HL: Cardiac response to

submaximal exercise in dogs susceptible to sudden cardiac death. *J Appl Physiol* 1985;59:890–897
21. Morris JN, Clayton DG, Everitt MG, Semmence AM, Burgess EH: Exercise in leisure time: coronary attack and death rates. *Br Heart J* 1990;63:325–334
22. Siscovick DS, Weiss NS, Fletcher RH, Schoebach VJ, Wagner EH: Habitual vigorous exercise and primary cardiac arrest: effect of other risk factors on the relationship. *J Chron Dis* 1984;37:625–631

Chapter 15

Relative Risk of Morning Versus Evening Exercise

William Little, MD, David M.
Herrington, MD, John Zornosa, MD,
and Paul Murray, MD

There is a circadian variation in the onset of myocardial infarction (MI) and other ischemic cardiac events with the peak incidence occurring between 6:00 AM and noon. Muller[1] has proposed that this increased frequency of MI in the morning is caused by the circadian variation of potential triggers of plaque rupture and development of occlusive thrombosis. These potential triggers of MI include morning surges of cortisol and catecholamines,[1,2] increases in blood pressure and heart rate,[3] and increases in platelet aggregability,[2,4] blood viscosity,[5] and vasomotor tone in conjunction with diminished fibrinolytic activity.[6]

Exercise produces a tremendous increase in serum catecholamines[7] and also may be associated with alterations in platelet effects and fibrinolytic activity.[8] Furthermore, exercise is associated with a marked increased incidence of cardiac events.[9] Thus, we speculated that the joint effects of circadian variation and exercise on potential triggers of myocardial ischemia might be synergistic, making it more dangerous to exercise in the morning than the afternoon. We examined this hypothesis by conducting a series of clinical studies designed to determine the association between morning exercise and the risk of cardiac events.

To examine if it is safer to exercise in the evening than in the mornings, we first evaluated the incidence of cardiac events in two groups of patients with known cardiac disease who underwent supervised exercise in cardiac rehabilitation programs conducted in

From Fletcher GF, (ed): *Cardiovascular Response to Exercise*. Mount Kisco, NY, Futura Publishing Company, Inc., © 1994.

either the morning or the afternoon.[10] The study subjects were participants in the Cardiac Rehabilitation Program at Wake Forest University referred to as the morning, or AM, exercise group, and the Rehabilitation Program at Georgia Baptist Medical Center referred to as the afternoon, or PM, exercise group. Admission criteria for patients entering the two programs were the same and included recent myocardial infarction, cardiovascular surgery, or percutaneous transluminal coronary angioplasty, new-onset angina pectoris, or other cardiac conditions such as cardiomyopathies, valvular heart disease, and arrhythmias.

The exercise program for each individual was designed to achieve 50–85% of their symptom-limited functional capacity as demonstrated on a graded exercise treadmill test. This aerobic exercise included walking, jogging, swimming, or bicycling for a 40-minute stimulus phase, after a 10-minute warmup, and followed by a 10-minute cool-down phase. The frequency of exercise was 3 days per week; Monday, Wednesday, and Friday. The AM exercise was performed from 7:30 to 8:30 AM and the PM exercise was performed for 1 hour between the hours of 3:00 and 5:00 PM (starting on the hour of their choice). We analyzed the records of all patients enrolled in the two programs from January 1980 to December 1989.

We defined cardiac events as syncope, documented sustained arrhythmias, myocardial infarction, or sudden death. Angina was not included as a defined cardiac event because this may not have been completely reported by the patient or was not always noted on the record. Each program used a standardized report form to document serious events that occurred on the facility grounds. These forms were filed separately and a copy also was placed in the patient's record. All patient charts were reviewed to record hours of exercise and collect records of the cardiac events.

Participants in the AM rehabilitation program contributed 168,111 patient-hours of observed exercise compared with 84,491 patient-hours from the PM rehabilitation program. The average monthly enrollment in the two programs was 183 ($\pm$8) and 98 ($\pm$11). Despite the larger number of patients in the AM program compared with the PM program, individuals in the two programs contributed a similar number of hours of observation per month (7.8 $\pm$ 1.4 vs. 7.1 $\pm$ 0.8 hours in AM vs. PM, $p = 0.31$). The number of patient-hours of observation was evenly distributed over the 10 years of follow-up in the AM group. In the PM group there were fewer participants and patient-hours of observation in 1982–1983 as compared with the other years.

There were five cardiac events in the AM group, for an incidence of 3.0 ± 1.3 (rate $\pm$ S.E.)/100,000 patient-hours of exercise (Figure 1). The PM group had two cardiac events for an incidence rate of 2.4 ± 1.6/100,000 patient-hours of exercise. The risk ratio of cardiac events occurring in the AM group compared with the PM group was 1.27 (95% confidence intervals 0.25–6.55). There was no statistically significant difference between the risk of exercising in the morning versus the evening. Thus, we found that the incidence of severe cardiac events in patients with known ischemic cardiac disease undergoing regular supervised submaximal exercise was very low, whether the patients exercised in the morning or the evening.

It is important to recognize that our patients underwent regular submaximal exercise. Our results may not be directly applicable to patients with intermittent maximal exercise. Such exercise may have a much higher risk of cardiac events than habitual exercise.[9] The implications of these observations for exercising persons without established heart disease also is unknown, although the risk of cardiac events during exercise in such patients should be even lower than we observed in patients with documented coronary artery disease.

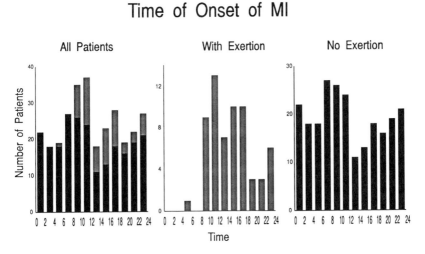

FIGURE 1. *Risk of cardiac events during regular supervised submaximal exercise performed between 7:30 and 8:30 (AM) and 3 and 5 (PM).*

Even though we studied a large exercise experience (>200,000 hours) in high-risk patients, there were so few events that it is impossible to exclude with certainty an increased risk of exercising in the AM versus PM. To do so would require an extremely large number of patients and years of observation. For example, based on observed event rates in the PM exercise groups, more than 1,000,000 patient-hours of exercise would be required to have the power to exclude a twofold increase in AM exercise risk. However, the absolute risk is so low that even if the relative risk of exercise was twofold greater in the AM group, the absolute increase in risk for AM exercise would be of no clinical significance (approximately 0.4%/year of patient exercise). Although the scientific question of a possible synergism between the increased risks of MI in the morning and exercise remains unanswered, these data suggest that the answer to the clinical question of when patients should perform regular, submaximal exercise is clear—both AM and PM are safe.

When studying rare outcomes such as exertionally related cardiac events, a case-control study is a more efficient method for determining the risk associated with a certain exposure or behavior such as AM exertion. Therefore, we also conducted a case-control study among 295 consecutive patients admitted to North Carolina Baptist Hospital Cardiac Care Unit with MI who were interviewed within 48 hours of admission.[11] Patients were questioned regarding the exact time of onset of chest pain and their activity during the 30 minutes before pain onset. Activity was graded in metabolic equivalents (mets) as rest (<3 mets) or during exertion (>3 mets).

Most (79%) of the MIs occurred in the absence of exertion (<3 mets). The peak incidence of these nonexertionally related MIs was between 6:00 and 8:00 AM (Figure 2). This is coincident with the peak activity of many potential triggers of MI that include surges in heart rate, blood pressure, catecholamines, cortisol, platelet aggregability, coronary vascular tone, plasma viscosity, and fibrinolytic activity associated with awakening and assumption of the upright posture.[1]

A smaller proportion (21%) of the MIs were temporarily associated with exertion. These occurred throughout the day with a peak occurrence near midday (Figure 2). Because of customary sleeping patterns, few patients are active between midnight and 6:00 AM, thus, few exertionally-related MIs occurred during this time period.

For the purposes of the case-control analysis, time of onset of chest pain was divided into AM (6:00–noon) or PM (anytime other than 6:00–noon). Table 1 shows the distribution of MIs with and

Risk of Cardiac Events
During Exercise

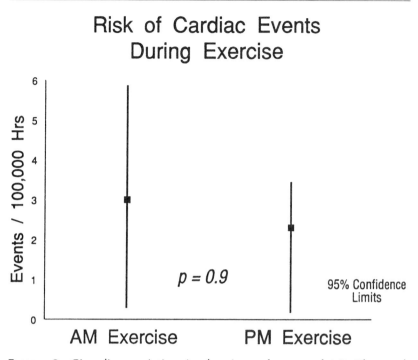

FIGURE 2. *Circadian variation in the time of onset of MI. The peak incidence in all patients was between 10:00 AM and noon. The peak incidence of MI associated with exertion was in the midday. Considering only patients with MI unassociated with exertion (no exertion), the peak incidence is in the early morning between 6:00 and 8:00 AM.*

without exertion according to time of onset of chest pain. The odds ratio for the association between exertion and AM MIs was not significantly different from unity whether or not events that occurred between midnight and 6 AM were excluded [1.28 (0.71, 2.30), midnight–6 AM events excluded: 0.84 (0.53, 3.12)]. After adjustment for age and gender using a logistic regression model, there remained no significant association between exertion and AM onset of chest pain ($p > 0.47$).

These data also may help to explain the lag observed in several studies between time of peak activity for circadian varying triggers (6:00–8:00 AM) and time of peak incidence of MIs (10:00 AM–noon).[1] Without separating out the exertionally-related events that occur uniformly throughout the day, the early morning (6:00–8:00 AM)

TABLE 1. Distribution of Myocardial Infarctions With and Without Exertion* According to Time of Onset** of Chest Pain

Time of onset	Exertion	No exertion	p value
Midnight–6:00 AM events included:			
AM	22	70	
PM	40	163	0.41
Midnight–6:00 AM events excluded:			
AM	22	70	
PM	39	105	0.59

*≤, or 0.3 metabolic equivalent.
**AM = 6:00 AM–noon, PM = noon–6:00 AM.

peak incidence of the nonexertional MIs is partially obscured and the apparent peak incidence in the combined group is slightly later in the day (10:00 AM–noon) (Figure 2).

In conclusion, there does not appear to be an important synergism between circadian varying triggers of MI and exertion. Although circadian influences on incidence of MI are clearly evident in nonexertional persons, we found no such relationship present in MI occurring in association with exertion. In fact, even among persons with documented coronary artery disease, the risk of untoward cardiac events during regular, submaximal exercise is very low regardless of whether the exercise is performed during the morning or afternoon.

Acknowledgments

The authors gratefully acknowledge the assistance of Judy Fleurant in preparing this chapter.

References

1. Muller JE, Tofler GH, Stone PH: Circadian variation and triggers of onset of acute cardiovascular disease. *Circulation* 1989;79:733–743

2. Brezinski DA, Tofler GH, Muller JE, Pohjola-Sintonen S, Willich SN, Schafer AI, Czeisler CA, Williams GH: Morning increase in platelet aggregability. *Circulation* 1988;78:35–40

3. Panza JA, Epstein SE, Quyyumi AA: Circadian variation in vascular tone and its relation to α-sympathetic vasoconstrictor activity. *N Engl J Med* 1991;325:986–990

4. Tofler GH, Brezinski D, Schafer AI, Czeisler CA, Rutherford JD, Willich SN, Gleason RE, Williams GH, Muller JE: Concurrent morning increase in platelet aggregability and the risk of myocardial infarction and sudden cardiac death. *N Engl J Med* 1987;316:1514–1518

5. Ehrly AM, Jung J: Circadian rhythm of human blood viscosity. *Biorheology* 1973;10:577–583

6. Andreotti F, Davies GJ, Hackett DR, Khan MI, De Bart ACW, Aber VR, Maseri A, Kluft C: Major circadian fluctuations in fibrinolytic factors and possible relevance to time of onset of myocardial infarction, sudden cardiac death and stroke. *Am J Cardiol* 1988;62:635–639

7. Dimsdale JE, Hartley H, Guiney T, Ruskin JN, Greenblatt D: Postexercise peril: plasma catecholamines and exercise. *JAMA* 1984;251:630–632

8. Small M, Simpson I, McGhie I, Douglas JT, Lowe GDO, Forbes CD: The effect of exercise on thrombin and plasmin generation in middle-aged men. *Haemostasis* 1987;17:371–376

9. Siscovick DS, Weiss NS, Fletcher RH, Lasky T: The incidence of primary cardiac arrest during vigorous exercise. *N Engl J Med* 1984;311:874–877

10. Murray PM, Pettus CW, Miller HS, Cantwell JD, Bergey DB, Thiel JE, Little WC: Should patients with coronary artery disease exercise in the morning or afternoon? *Arch Intern Med* 1993;153:833–836

11. Zornosa J, Smith M, Little WC: Effect of activity on circadian variation in time on onset of acute myocardial infarction. *Am J Cardiol* 1992;69:1089–1090

Chapter 16

The Relative Risk of Myocardial Infarction During Exercise

Paul D. Thompson, MD

Anecdotal reports have linked vigorous physical exertion with the onset of acute myocardial infarction (MI).[1–7] Despite such reports, there are inadequate data from the general population to compare the risk of MI during exercise with that during sedentary activities. Several factors have limited collection of adequate data. The stuttering onset of many acute coronary syndromes obscures their relation to exertion and interferes with defining an accepted time interval for classifying exercise-related events. Furthermore, and compared with exercise-related sudden cardiac death (SCD), ascertainment of exercise-related MIs is difficult. SCDs in metropolitan areas are generally evaluated by one medical examiner's office, whereas acute MIs often are distributed among several hospitals. This renders complete case collection more difficult. Consequently, this chapter is necessarily speculative. Nevertheless, we review studies that determined the percentage of MIs related to exercise and discuss the limitations of this approach. We also estimate the incidence of exercise-related MIs from figures on the incidence of exercise-related SCD and suggest mechanisms by which vigorous exercise might initiate an acute coronary event.

Percentage of MI's Related to Vigorous Exertion

Approximately 10% of acute MIs in the general population occur during or immediately after unusual physical exertion. Master

From Fletcher GF, (ed): *Cardiovascular Response to Exercise.* Mount Kisco, NY, Futura Publishing Company, Inc., © 1994.

et al.[8] in 1939 reported that 8.5% of 1,440 "acute coronary occlusions" occurred during moderately heavy physical work. An additional 2% occurred during unusually severe physical effort. Cases involving workmen's compensation were excluded because of concerns about the patient's veracity in such instances. Romo[9] estimated that 6.3–6.9% of Finnish men and 1.9–2.7% of Finnish women suffered cardiac events (excluding SCD) during strenuous activity. Matsuda et al.[10] reported that 11% of MI patients were engaged in heavy exertion at the onset of their acute MI. Patients enrolled in the Multicenter Investigation of Limitation of Infarct Size study (MILIS) identified moderate or heavy physical exercise as a possible trigger of their MI in 14.1% and 8.7%, respectively.[11]

Such results suggest that exercise initiates acute cardiac events. Nevertheless, these studies cannot provide definitive information on the relative risks of exercise because they rarely determine the relative amount of time spent in various activities. For example, the MILIS results indicate that heavy physical activity was associated more frequently with the onset of MI in men and in patients without prior symptoms of cardiac disease.[11] Similarly, 9 of 26 consecutive MI patients (35%) under age 35 years had the onset of symptoms during or immediately after vigorous exercise.[2] Such observations may reflect either an increase in the risk of activity for these persons or an increase in the amount of time spent in physically active pursuits. Experience with the incidence of SCD during exercise suggests that the latter is operative. The relative risk of SCD during exertion is higher in young persons[12,13] in part because the risk of nonexertion-related SCD is so low. Furthermore, younger men spend more time in vigorous activity,[13] and the absolute death rate per hour of exercise is actually lower in younger age groups.[12]

Few studies have compared the frequency of acute MIs during exercise with the expected rate to determine if such events were randomly distributed. Twelve percent of Toronto men enrolled in a cardiac rehabilitation program were engaged in sporting or other vigorous activity at the onset of their MI.[14] This frequency is six times the expected rate based on the activities of other men from the same city. These results suggest that exercise increases the risk of an acute MI, but must be cautiously accepted because patients electing to participate in cardiac rehabilitation may have been habitually more active than otherwise comparable men.

Estimated Incidence of MIs During Exercise

If we assume that similar processes initiate both acute MI and SCD in the asymptomatic population, we can estimate the incidence of exercise-related MIs from the incidence of exercise-related SCD. Acute MI and SCD appear to result from similar pathological events. Acute coronary thrombosis is found in more than 90% of MI patients studied acutely during the event.[15] Similarly, atherosclerotic plaque rupture and coronary thrombosis are found at necropsy in 73% or more of SCD cases.[16,17] SCD victims not demonstrating acute coronary lesions often demonstrate chronic high-grade stenoses with myocardial scarring.[16] Consequently, it is likely that similar pathological processes produce both exercise-related MI and SCD in previously asymptomatic persons.[18]

Indeed, coronary arteriography performed acutely in 13 patients presenting with either exercise-related acute MI ($n = 7$) or SCD ($n = 6$) demonstrated similar coronary artery pathology in both groups.[5] Coronary occlusion was present in three of the MI patients (an additional patient had received thrombolytic therapy) and in all of the SCD victims. Associated spasm was observed in one MI and two SCD patients, and eccentric lesions suggestive of plaque rupture were noted in three of the MI and five SCD patients.

The number of exercise-related MIs and SCDs in 3,617 hyperlipidemic men participating in the Lipid Research Clinics (LRC) Primary Prevention Trial was determined over a mean period of 7.4 years.[19] There were 54 MIs and 8 SCDs yielding a cumulative incidence of exercise-related events of 2% and a yearly incidence of 1 MI and 1 SCD per 500 and 3,300 men, respectively. This frequency of SCD is considerably higher than that for the general population[12,13] and probably reflects the increased prevalence of occult coronary disease among hyperlipidemic men. The incidence of SCD during exercise in asymptomatic middle-aged men in the general population is estimated at 1 death per 15,000[12] to 1 death per 18,000 men[13] per year. Despite this low absolute incidence, the hourly death rate during exertion is at least five times higher than during more sedentary activities.[12,13] If the ratio of nonfatal to fatal events is similar for the LRC and the general population (an assumption that can be challenged given the yearly exercise tests and frequent medical contact among the LRC men), the incidence of MI during physical activity is 1 in 2,000 to 2,500 men per year and probably increased compared with more sedentary pursuits.

These estimates are for asymptomatic men without prior history of coronary disease. Experience from cardiac rehabilitation programs demonstrates that, in contrast to the asymptomatic population, exercise-related cardiac arrests are 2.6[20] to 7[21] times more frequent than MI. This probably represents the increased risk of ventricular fibrillation in patients with myocardial scarring and left ventricular dysfunction.[22]

How Might Exercise Initiate a Myocardial Infarction?

Children and Young Adults

Different pathological conditions are associated with exercise-related SCD in children and adults. SCD in adults is almost invariably associated with atherosclerotic coronary artery disease, whereas a variety of congenital cardiac abnormalities such as hypertrophic cardiomyopathy and anomolous coronary arteries are found in young individuals dying during exertion.[23] Coronary artery abnormalities including anomolous origin and course[24] as well as abnormal coronary drainage[3] also are reported in young patients who suffer MI during exercise. Consequently, coronary arteriography is indicated in all children and young adults with exercise-related cardiac events.

The mechanism by which anomolous coronary arteries produce cardiac ischemia and acute MI is not defined. Origin of the left main coronary artery from the anterior sinus of Valsalva with its subsequent course between the aorta and pulmonary artery is the most frequent coronary anomaly associated with exercise-related events[25] (Figure 1). The increased stroke volume during exercise may distend the major vessels and compress the coronary between the pulmonary artery and aorta.[25] This mechanism seems unlikely, however, in the absence of pulmonary hypertension.[24] In addition, SCD has been reported in patients whose anomolous artery did not pass between the great vessels.[26]

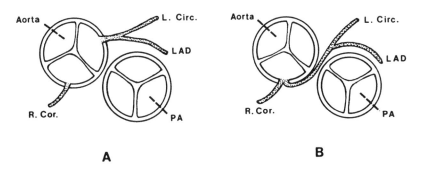

FIGURE 1. A: *Normal origin of the right coronary artery (R. COR.) and left main from the anterior and left sinuses of Valsalva, respectively.* **B:** *Anomolous origin of the left main from the anterior sinus with an abnormal course between the aorta and pulmonary artery (PA).*

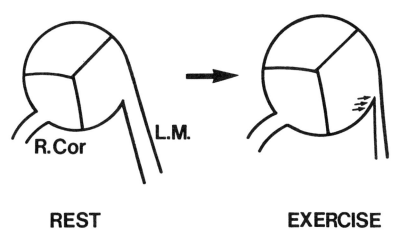

FIGURE 2. *Acute take-off angle of the left main coronary artery L.M. from the aorta. Aortic dilatation during exercise could compress the vessel. Right coronary take-off is normal.*

An alternative explanation is that anomolous coronaries exit at an abnormally acute angle from the aorta[25] (Figure 2). An increase in stroke volume could compress the coronary lumen. Indeed, acute coronary take-offs have been identified in SCD victims who had no other pathological findings.[27]

Adults

Coronary artery plaque rupture with thrombosis is present in most acute MIs in adults. The following discusses mechanisms by which exercise could initiate these events (Table 1).

Master et al.[8] suggested that exertion had no provocative role in the acute coronary event and that exercise increased myocardial oxygen demand and thereby amplified the symptoms of an established infarct. This suggestion ignores the observation that many exercise-related MIs occur after exercise.

Exercise can induce inappropriate vasoconstriction[28] in coronary segments whose vasodilatory capacity has been altered by atherosclerosis.[29] Alternatively, spasm-induced arterial constriction may lead to arterial injury and thrombus formation.[30] Coronary spasm has been documented in 3 of 13 victims of exercise-related MI or SCD studied soon after the event, but it is unclear if spasm was the primary event or the result of endothelial damage.[5]

Exercise also could initiate plaque disruption. Mechanical and physical forces contribute to plaque disruption.[31] Increases in blood pressure during exercise could produce plaque fissuring. Left ventricular end-diastolic volume increases and end-systolic volume decreases in normal persons during upright exercise.[32] These volumetric changes could alter the configuration of the epicardial arteries and coronary wall stress. Also, exercise-induced coronary spasm distorts the vessel wall and could initiate plaque disruption.[5]

Exercise also can enlarge an existing plaque rupture or render a

Table 1. Mechanisms for Exercise-related MI in Adults

Exercise amplifies symptoms of existing infarct
Exercise induces coronary spasm producing:
  An infarct
  Arterial injury → thrombosis → infarct
Exercise induces plaque rupture via:
  Increased blood pressure and shear forces
  Altered coronary artery shape
  Exercise-induced spasm
Exercise renders a fissured plaque more thrombogenic by:
  Deepening the fissure
  Increasing thrombogenicity
Exercise directly induces thrombogenesis

---

fissured plaque more thrombogenic. Davies et al.[17] examined the coronary arteries of patients with atherosclerosis who died from noncardiac events. Nine percent of patients had minor plaque fissures, suggesting that most minor plaque disruptions are repaired without sequelae. Deep plaque rupture, however, with exposure of collagen type I is more likely to initiate thrombosis.[33] By increasing blood pressure, altering coronary geometry, or inducing spasm vigorous exercise could deepen an existing plaque fissure and render the injury more thrombogenic. In addition, platelet aggregation at sites of endothelial injury could be exacerbated by the exercise-induced increase in catecholamines.[29] Angioplasty produces a localized coronary plaque disruption to reduce coronary stenosis. Reports of coronary occlusion during stress testing after a recent angioplasty[33,34] suggest that exercise may increase an existing coronary lesion's thrombogenicity by any of the above mechanisms.

Finally, exercise may directly induce thrombosis in normal coronary arteries. Chan et al.[4] reported a 34-year-old man who developed an anterior wall MI 30 minutes after completing a 42-km footrace. Coronary angiography 5 hours later documented occlusion of the left anterior descending coronary artery as well as a nonocclusive clot in the right coronary. The patient was treated with thrombolytic therapy and had angiographically normal coronary arteries 10 days later. The presence of probable thrombi in two coronary arteries argues against simultaneous plaque disruption in this patient and suggests a more direct thrombogenic mechanism.

Conclusion

Anecdotal reports and deductive reasoning support the hypothesis that vigorous exertion transiently increases the risk of MI for the general population. Definite conclusions on this hypothesis are not possible without epidemiologic studies documenting an increase in the incidence of MI during exercise compared with more sedentary activities.

Acknowledgments

The author thanks David S. Siscovick, MD, for reviewing and Barbara A. Potocnik for preparing the chapter.

References

1. Black A, Black MM, Gensini G: Exertion and acute coronary artery injury. *Angiology* 1975;26:759–783
2. Pic A, Broustet JP, Saliou B, Gosse P, Guern P: Coexistence of vigorous exercise and heavy smoking in triggering acute myocardial infarction in men under 35 years—fact or fiction?, in Roskamm H (ed): *Myocardial Infarction at Young Age.* Berlin, New York, Springer-Verlag, 1981, pp 108–114
3. Delaye J, Beaune J, Delahaye JP: Myocardial infarction at young age during high physical exercise, in Roskamm H (ed): *Myocardial Infarction at Young Age.* Berlin, New York, Springer-Verlag, 1981, pp 115–121
4. Chan KL, Davies RA, Chambers RJ: Coronary thrombosis and subsequent lysis after a marathon. *J Am Coll Cardiol* 1984;4:1322–1325
5. Ciampricotti R, El Gamal MIH, Bonnier JJ, Relik THFM: Myocardial infarction and sudden death after sport: acute coronary angiographic findings. *Cath Cardiovasc Diagn* 1989;17:193–197
6. Ciampricotti R, El Gamal M: Recurrent myocardial infarction and sudden death after sport. *Am Heart J* 1989;117:188–191
7. Rose E, Hughes LO, Raftery EB: Myocardial infarction associated with exercise in young men. *Int J Cardiol* 1991;31:99–101
8. Master AM, Dack S, Jaffe HL: Activities associated with the onset of acute coronary artery occlusion. *Am Heart J* 1939;18:434–443
9. Romo M: Factors related to sudden death in acute ischaemic heart disease. *Acta Med Scand* 1972;547(suppl):I–92
10. Matsuda M, Matsuda Y, Ogawa H, Moritari K, Kusukawa R: Angina pectoris before and during acute myocardial infarction: relation to degree of physical activity. *Am J Cardiol* 1985;55:1255–1258
11. Tofler GH, Stone PH, Maclure M, Edelman E, Davis VG, Robertson T, Antman EM, Muller JE: Analysis of possible triggers of acute myocardial infarction (the MILIS study). *Am J Cardiol* 1990;66:22–27
12. Thompson PD, Funk EJ, Carleton RA, Sturner WQ: Incidence of death during jogging in Rhode Island from 1975 through 1980. *JAMA* 1982;247:2535–2538
13. Siscovick DS, Weiss NS, Fletcher RH, Lasky T: The incidence of primary cardiac arrest during vigorous exercise. *N Engl J Med* 1984;311:874–877
14. Kavanagh T, Shephard RJ: The immediate antecedents of myocardial infarction in active men. *Can Med Assoc J* 1973;109:19–22
15. DeWood MA, Spores J, Notske R, Mouser LT, Burroughs R, Golden MS, Lang HT: Prevalence of total coronary occlusion during the early hours of transmural myocardial infarction. *N Engl J Med* 1980;303:897–902
16. Davies MJ: Anatomic features in victims of sudden coronary death. *Circulation* 1992;85(suppl I):I19–I24
17. Davies M, Bland J, Hangartner J, Angelini A, Thomas AC: Factors

influencing the presence or absence of acute coronary artery thrombi in sudden ischaemic death. *Eur Heart J* 1989;10:203–208

18. Davies MJ, Thomas AC: Plaque fissuring—the cause of acute myocardial infarction, sudden ischaemic death, and crescendo angina. *Br Heart J* 1985;53:363–73

19. Siscovick DS, Ekelund LG, Johnson JL, Truong Y, Adler A: Sensitivity of exercise electrocardiography for acute cardiac events during moderate and strenuous physical activity. *Arch Intern Med* 1991;151:325–330

20. Van Camp SP, Peterson RA: Cardiovascular complications of outpatient cardiac rehabilitation programs. *JAMA* 1986;256:1160–1163

21. Haskell WL: Cardiovascular complications during exercise training of cardiac patients. *Circulation* 1978;57:920–924

22. Cobb LA, Weaver WD: Exercise: a risk for sudden death in patients with coronary heart disease. *J Am Coll Cardiol* 1986;7:215–219

23. Maron BJ, Roberts WC, McAllister HA, Rosing DR, Epstein SE: Sudden death in young athletes. *Circulation* 1980;62:218–229

24. Kimbiris D, Iskandrian AS, Segal BL, Bemis CE: Anomalous aortic origin of coronary arteries. *Circulation* 1978;58:606–615

25. Cheitlin MD, De Castro CM, McAllister HA: Sudden Death as a complication of anomalous left coronary origin from the anterior sinus of valsalva: a not-so-minor congenital anomaly. *Circulation* 1974;50:780–787

26. Patterson FK: Sudden death in a young adult with anomalous origin of the posterior circumflex artery. *South Med J* 1982;75:748–749

27. Virmani R, Chun PKC, Goldstein RE, Rabinowitz M, McAllister HA: Acute takeoffs of the coronary arteries along the aortic wall and congenital coronary ostial valve-like ridges: association with sudden death. *J Am Coll Cardiol* 1984;3:766–771

28. Yasue H, Omote S, Takizawa A, et al: Circulation variation of exercise capacity in patients with Prinzmetal's variant angina: role of exercise-induced coronary arterial spasm. *Circulation* 1979;59:938–947

29. Gordon JB, Ganz P, Nabel EG, Fish D, Zebede J, Mudge GH, Alexander RW, Selwyn AP: Atherosclerosis influences the vasomotor response of epicardial coronary arteries to exercise. *J Clin Invest* 1989;83:1946–1952

30. Gertz SD, Uretsky G, Wajnberg RS, Navot N, Gotsman MS: Endothelial cell damage and thrombus formation after partial arterial constriction: relevance to the role of coronary artery spasm in the pathogenesis of myocardial infarction. *Circulation* 1981;63:476–486

31. Richardson PD, Davies MJ, Born GVR: Influence of plaque configuration and stress distribution on fissuring of coronary atherosclerotic plaques. *Lancet* 1989;2:941–944

32. Rowell LB: *Human Circulation: Regulation During Physical Stress*. New York, Oxford University Press, 1986

33. Badimon L, Badimon JJ, Turitto VT, Vallabhajosula S, Fuster V: Platelet thrombus formation on collagen type I: a model of deep vessel injury—influence of blood rheology, von Willebrand factor, and blood coagulation. *Circulation* 1988;78:1431–1442

34. Nygaard TW, Beller GA, Mentzer RM, Gibson RS, Moeller CM, Burwell LR: Acute coronary occlusion with exercise testing after initially successful coronary angioplasty for acute myocardial infarction. *Am J Cardiol* 1986;57:687–688

35. Dash H. Delayed coronary occlusion after successful percutaneous transluminal coronary angioplasty: association with exercise testing. *Am J Cardiol* 1982;52:1143–1144

Part 5

Modification of Cardiovascular Risk by Exercise

Chapter 17

Cardiovascular Fitness and Cardiovascular Disease

Steven N. Blair, PED, Harold W. Kohl, III, PhD and Carolyn E. Barlow, MS

Regular physical activity has been considered an important health habit since ancient times. Systematic study of the relation of exercise to health, however, is a relatively recent development. Some reports on the deleterious effects of sedentary habits were published early in this century,[1,2] but the careful evaluation of inactivity and cardiovascular disease was given impetus by reports in the 1950s by Professor Jeremy Morris of London.[3] Several dozen studies on physical activity and cardiovascular disease have been published over the ensuing 40 years, and recent reviews summarize these data. There is a general consensus that a sedentary lifestyle contributes to increased risk of cardiovascular disease, especially hypertension[4,5] and coronary heart disease (CHD).[6,7] Indeed, in July 1992, the American Heart Association published a revised Statement on Exercise,[8] in which physical inactivity was designated as a risk factor for CHD. This was the first official recognition by the American Heart Association of inactivity as a risk factor, and it was given status comparable to the other well-established risk factors of hypertension, hypercholesterolemia, and cigarette smoking.

Recent papers on physical inactivity and CHD, and the systematic reviews of the topic, generally show an approximate doubling of risk in sedentary compared with active study participants.[6,7] These findings are consistent across studies in men, but the results are

Supported in part by U.S. Public Health Service Research Grant AG06945 from the National Institute on Aging, Bethesda, Maryland.

From Fletcher GF, (ed): *Cardiovascular Response to Exercise.* Mount Kisco, NY, Futura Publishing Company, Inc., © 1994.

somewhat equivocal in women.[6] The prevalence of sedentary habits is substantial in the U.S. adult population, and is at least as common as the prevalence of the other risk factors.[9] This factor, and the strength of the association between inactivity and disease, combine to produce population-attributable risk estimates that are comparable to other major risk factors.[10,11] The number of deaths from CHD in the U.S. in 1986 because of sedentary habits is estimated by Hahn et al.[12] to be 205,254. If the assumptions used to derive these figures are correct, this number is second only to elevated cholesterol (253,194) in terms of population mortality burden. Obesity (190,456), hypertension (171,121), and cigarette smoking (148,879) are each responsible for fewer CHD deaths than physical inactivity.

Physical inactivity is prominent in the causal pathway to CHD, and the public health burden of sedentary living is substantial. This chapter reviews the related question of the association of physical fitness to cardiovascular disease, evaluates the data to determine if understanding of the role of inactivity in cardiovascular disease can be enhanced by the physical fitness studies, and discusses the clinical applications of physical fitness testing in adults.

Physical Fitness and Cardiovascular Disease Mortality

There are seven analyses from five recent prospective population studies on physical fitness and cardiovascular disease mortality.[11,13–18] Five of the analyses included only men, and two included both men and women.

Prospective Studies on Physical Fitness and Cardiovascular Disease

Oslo Fitness Study

Lie et al.[13] recruited a group of Norwegian male long-distance cross-country skiers aged 26 to 64 years, and 2,014 male workers aged 40 to 59 years for a study of physical fitness and cardiovascular disease. All men were free of known heart disease at baseline. Physical fitness was assessed at baseline by a near-maximal exercise test on a cycle ergometer. Smoking habits, blood pressure, and blood lipids were measured by standard methods. The participants were followed for 7 years for mortality. During this interval, 58 of the workers and 1 of the skiers died of CHD. CHD death rates were calculated for each quartile of physical fitness in the population of workers and for the cross-country skiers. The crude death rates for these groups are shown in Figure 1. The data show a strong inverse gradient across fitness quartiles in the workers. The death rates for the most physically fit workers and for the cross-country skiers are comparable, about 1%

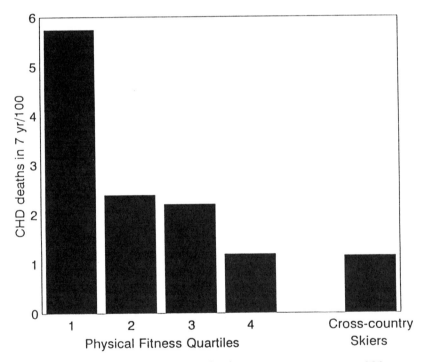

FIGURE 1. *Coronary heart disease death rates over 7 years per 100 men. The four bars on the left show the death rates by physical fitness quartiles in 2,014 who were 40 to 59 years of age at baseline and were employed in companies or government agencies in Oslo, Norway. The bar on the right shows the death rate in 87 cross-country skiers who were 43 to 64 years of age at baseline. Data for this figure were taken from Reference 13.*

over the 7-year follow-up period. This mortality rate is relatively low (based on only 59 deaths), and only crude death rates (not age-adjusted) are included in the report. Age group–specific death rates across fitness quartiles in the workers (not shown) exhibit the same strong inverse gradient, however, especially for the men in the 50- to 54- and 55- to 59-year age groups. The coronary death rate in the first fitness quartile is 4.8 times higher than the rate in the fourth fitness quartile. This high relative risk is considerably greater than the approximate doubling of risk in sedentary compared with active participants in physical activity and CHD studies.[6]

This study is relatively small, and only men were included. Study methods and statistical analyses were appropriate, although no multivariate adjusted CHD rates across fitness groups were presented.

U.S. Railroad Workers Study

Slattery and Jacobs[14] report on the association between physical fitness and mortality in a cohort of 3,043 U.S. railroad workers. The men in this study were 22 to 79 years of age at the baseline examination, which occurred from 1957 to 1960. The men were re-examined between 1962 and 1964, and were followed for mortality through 1977. Physical fitness was assessed at baseline by a submaximal exercise test on a treadmill. Fitness was determined by heart rate response after 3 minutes of walking at 3 mph up a 5% grade. There were 258 deaths caused by CHD during the 17- to 20-year follow-up in the men who were free of pre-existing cardiovascular disease at baseline.

Age-adjusted CHD death rates were 43% higher in men with an exercise heart rate of >135 beats per minute when compared with men with an exercise heart rate of <105 beats per minute. Similar results were reported for the 12 to 15 years of mortality follow-up after the second examination, and all-cause death rates followed the same pattern. The relationship between fitness and CHD mortality was attenuated (to a relative risk of 1.20) after adjustment for other risk factors, but it remained significantly elevated in the least fit workers. The relative risk for CHD death in the men with low physical fitness (1.43) compared with very physically fit men was considerably less than for the other studies on physical fitness and cardiovascular disease in healthy men reviewed here (relative risk range = 4.8–9.3).

The reasons for this lower relative risk are not clear. One possibility is that the classification scheme used to determine physical fitness may have resulted in more misclassification of exposure (and thus attenuation of effect) than in the other studies. Each railroad worker was assigned to a fitness group based on his heart rate after 3 minutes of treadmill walking, with the average heart rate for all age groups being <120 beats per minute. Other studies of fitness and CHD used maximal or near maximal (peak exercise heart rate of 90% of the predicted maximum or more) exercise test. The low level fitness assessment in the railroad study probably is not as accurate an estimate of aerobic power as the other tests, and if maximal aerobic power is actually related to risk of CHD, then the lower risk estimate may be caused by this misclassification. The long follow-up interval in the railroad study of 17 to 20 years may be another factor causing the relatively lower relative risk. The length of follow-up in the other studies ranged from 7 to 8.5 years. Longer follow-up increases the likelihood of a period effect in that individuals may be more likely to crossover into another fitness group with the longer follow-up. If this were the case, the most likely changes occurring would be a shift to the less fit categories, especially in the railroad workers where their physical activity was presumably primarily occupational. As the workers aged, they may have become less active and less fit because of job shifts and retirement. Another factor discussed by the authors is the relatively small variance in fitness in the railroad workers. Few of the railroad workers engaged in high levels of athletic training, and thus few had high levels of fitness.

Canada Health Survey

Arraiz et al.[15] report on a follow-up of The Canada Health Survey, which is a nationally representative sample of Canadian households. Physical fitness was assessed at baseline (1978–1979) by a submaximal step test. Study participants were classified into recommended and unacceptable fitness levels based on the pulse rate responses to the step test. There is no quantification of these levels given in the report. There were 93 deaths in 2,267 men and women aged 30 to 64 years during a 7-year follow-up. Thirty-seven of the deaths were caused by cardiovascular disease.

All-cause and cardiovascular disease mortality rates were higher in the unacceptable fitness category than in the recommended category. The adjusted (age, sex, body mass index, [BMI], and smoking habit) relative risk for the unacceptable group was 5.4 (95% CI = 1.9–15.9). After exclusion of participants with heart disease, stroke, or hypertension at baseline, the adjusted relative risk was 2.1 (95% CI = 0.5–8.7).

The strengths of this study are the representative population under observation, standardization of study methods, and completeness of follow-up. Weaknesses include the small number of deaths available for analysis and the submaximal fitness test.

Lipid Research Clinics Study

Ekelund et al. analyzed the mortality experience of 4,276 men aged 30 to 69 years at baseline who were enrolled in the Lipid Research Clinics Prevalence survey.[16] Physical fitness was assessed by a submaximal (to 90% of predicted maximal heart rate) exercise test on a treadmill. Men were assigned to fitness quartiles based on heart rate at stage two of the test and by total time on the treadmill. There were 45 cardiovascular disease deaths during the 8.5-year follow-up interval.

The cumulative cardiovascular disease mortality rates over 8.5 years across the fitness categories were 2.21, 1.56, 1.30, and 0.26 from low physical fitness to high physical fitness groups, respectively. These rates were not changed by age adjustment. Proportional hazards regression models were used to control for other risk factors. The relative risk for cardiovascular mortality for a difference in treadmill times of 2 SD was 3.6 after adjustment for age, smoking habits, high-density lipoprotein cholesterol, low-density lipoprotein cholesterol, and systolic blood pressure. These results are for the group of men who were free of cardiovascular disease at baseline. Similar analyses also were performed in the cohort with cardiovascular disease at baseline. The association between physical fitness and mortality was somewhat stronger in this latter group, with an adjusted relative risk for cardiovascular mortality of 4.8.

This study had excellent methods and the data were thoroughly analyzed. Excellent data on potential confounding variables were available for the analyses. There were only 45 cardiovascular disease deaths, and a submaximal exercise test was used.

Aerobics Center Longitudinal Study

We find a strong inverse association between physical fitness and mortality in prospective studies of men and women examined at the Cooper Clinic in Dallas.[11,17,18] Patients came to the clinic for preventive medical examinations and counseling. Physical fitness was determined by a maximal exercise test on a treadmill. Treadmill time distributions within age- and sex-specific groups were used to assign individuals to low (least fit quintile), moderate (second and third quintiles), and high (fourth and fifth quintiles) fitness categories. All participants were examined at least once at the Cooper Clinic sometime between 1970 and 1982. Follow-up for mortality was from the date of the baseline examination through 1985, approximately 8 years on average.

The first mortality report from this study was on 10,224 men and 3,120 women who had no history of myocardial infarction, stroke, hypertension, or diabetes at baseline.[11] Cardiovascular disease mortality for low-, moderate-, and high-fitness groups is shown in Figure 2 for both men and women. The age-adjusted relative risks for low compared with high physical fitness are approximately 9 in women and 8 in men. These values are comparable to the relative risks reported for the Lipid Research Clinics and Oslo studies.

We also have followed 1,832 male patients who were excluded from the analyses on the healthy cohort because of hypertension at baseline[17]. The fitness assessment, study design, and other methods were the same as for the healthy men and women.[11] There were 78 deaths during approximately 8 years of follow-up. Age-adjusted relative risk for men who were the least fit compared with high fitness levels was 4.5.

There were 98 men in the Aerobics Center Longitudinal Study who had a fasting blood glucose of 7.8 mM (140 mg/dl) or higher, or had physician-diagnosed noninsulin-dependent diabetes mellitus at baseline.[18] Fourteen of these men died during 8.2 years of follow-up; 10 deaths were caused by cardiovascular disease. Multivariate analyses were conducted to evaluate the relationship between

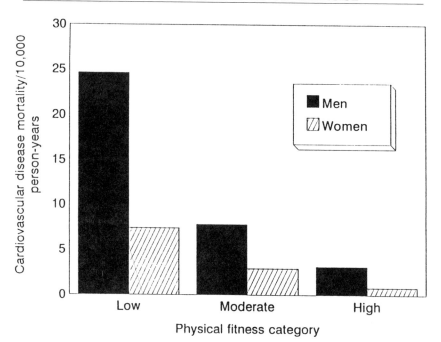

FIGURE 2. *Cardiovascular disease mortality (cause of death codes 390–448, International Classification of Diseases, 9th ed, Revised) per 10,000 person-years of follow-up (average follow-up was approximately 8 years) by physical fitness categories in 10,224 men and 3,120 women in the Aerobics Center Longitudinal Study.[11] Physical fitness was assessed at baseline by a maximal exercise test on a treadmill. The low fitness category is approximately the least fit 20%, moderate fitness is the next 40%, and high fitness is the top 40%.*

fitness and mortality after adjustment for age, resting systolic blood pressure, serum cholesterol, body mass index, family history of heart disease, smoking habit, and length of follow-up. Relative risk estimates per minute of treadmill time were 1.28 (95% CI = 0.98–1.67) for all-cause mortality and 1.25 (95% CI = 0.96–1.64) for cardiovascular mortality. These findings were comparable to the relative risks seen in this study in other glucose tolerance strata.

Strengths of these studies include a maximal exercise test for fitness assessment, the inclusion of women in the apparently healthy cohort, and extensive data on potential confounders. A major weakness is the relatively small number of cardiovascular disease deaths for some of the analyses.

Summary of Studies on Physical Fitness and Cardiovascular Mortality

The prospective studies on physical fitness and cardiovascular mortality are summarized in Table 1. Each report higher death rates in individuals in the low fitness level. In addition, other studies not reviewed in detail here on the relationship between physical fitness and fatal and nonfatal cardiovascular disease show results similar to the mortality studies.[19–21] The relationship between physical fitness and cardiovascular disease mortality holds in several studies after extensive multivariate modeling to control for potential confounding variables. The strength of the association between physical fitness and mortality is substantial in five of the six studies (ranging from about 4 to about 9 in healthy men and women), and is significantly elevated in the railroad workers study (increased risk of 45% in the low fitness level group). In general, the strength of this association is considerably greater than the relative risk for cardiovascular disease in sedentary compared with active individuals. Powell et al.[6] report a summary relative risk of about 1.9 for inactivity. The stronger inverse association in the fitness studies is perhaps because those studies have less misclassification on the exposure than is found in activity studies. Fitness measurement is relatively objective, and physical activity assessments are more crude and imprecise because of self-report bias, incomplete recall, and a large intra- and interperson variance. Thus, it may be that the studies of physical activity and CHD actually underestimate the true impact of a sedentary lifestyle on cardiovascular disease.

Clinical Applications of Exercise Testing

It is clear from the studies reviewed in this chapter that low levels of physical fitness increase the risk of death caused by cardiovascular disease. Just as for other risk factors, such as high cholesterol, the obvious clinical inference is that identification of

TABLE 1. Summary of Results from Studies on Physical Fitness and Cardiovascular Mortality

Study group	Design	Physical fitness measure	Endpoint	Main results
Company or government employees in Oslo: 2,014 men, 40–59 years at baseline[13]	Prospective, 7-yr follow-up	Submaximal exercise test, cycle ergometer	CHD death, 58 deaths	RR = 4.8, least fit quartile/most fit quartile
U.S. railroad workers: 2431 white men, 22–79 years at baseline[14]	Prospective, x̄ follow-up of approximately 20 yr	Submaximal exercise test, treadmill	CHD and CVD death, 258 CHD deaths	RR = 1.43[a] for CHD and 1.51 for CVD; adjusted RR = 1.20[b] (1.10, 1.26)[c] for CHD; low/high fitness
Canada Health Survey: 2,267 men and women, 30–64 years at baseline[15]	Prospective, 7 yr follow-up	Submaximal step test	CVD death, 37 deaths	RR = 5.4[b] (1.9,15.9)[c] unacceptable fitness/recommended level of fitness
Lipid Research Clinics study: 3,106 men, 30–69 years at baseline[16]	Prospective, 8.5-yr follow-up	Submaximal exercise test, treadmill	CHD death, CVD death, 45 deaths	RR = 6.5 (1.5,28.7)[c] for CHD death; RR = 8.5 (2.0,36.7)[c] CVD death, least fit quartile/most fit quartile. Adjusted RR = 2.8[b] (1.3,6.1)[c] for CHD; RR = 3.6[b] (1.6,5.6)[c] for CVD

Cooper Clinic patients: 3,120 women, 10,224 men[11]	Prospective, 8.2 yr of follow-up	Maximal exercise tolerance, treadmill test	CVD death, 73 deaths (7 women, 66 men)	RR = 9.25[a] (−5.1, 0.5)[d] for women; RR = 7.93[a] (−8.8, −3.3)[d] for men, low/high fitness
Cooper Clinic patients: 1,832 men who were hypertensive at baseline[17]	Prospective, x̄ follow-up of slightly more than 8 yr	Maximal exercise tolerance, treadmill test	All-cause mortality, 78 deaths	RR = 4.5[a] (2.9, 6.9)[c] first/fifth fitness quintiles
Cooper Clinic patients: 98 men with glucose intolerance[18]	Prospective, 8.2 yr of follow-up	Maximal exercise tolerance, treadmill test	CVD death, 10 deaths	RR = 1.28[b] (0.96, 1.64)[c] per each minute of lower treadmill time

[a]Relative risk adjusted for age only, although additional adjustments for other factors had a negligible effect.
[b]Relative risk adjusted for age and other major CHD risk factors.
[c]Numbers in ( ) are 95% confidence intervals.
[d]95% confidence interval for linear trend slope.
CHD, coronary heart disease; CVD, cardiovascular disease; RR, relative risk.

individuals with low fitness levels, with possible follow-up intervention, is a worthwhile procedure. There are, however, important differences between screening to detect high cholesterol or high blood pressure and screening to detect low physical fitness. A fitness evaluation requires more time, more professional staff, and greater expense, and typically has greater equipment needs. In addition, the risk of an untoward event (such as sudden death) is higher with fitness testing than for blood pressure or cholesterol screening. The use of diagnostic electrocardiogram (ECG) exercise testing has been questioned as a screening test, primarily because of high false-positive rates in asymptomatic populations.[22,23] In an apparently healthy population with a low prevalence of CHD, the number of false-positives may be greater than the number of true-positives.[22] Recent recommendations from the American College of Sports Medicine and the American Heart Association suggest that diagnostic exercise testing is not necessary, or in some cases is actually discouraged, in certain population groups.[24,25]

Exercise Testing Issues

Exercise testing in medical settings typically has focused on diagnosis and evaluation of therapeutic interventions. Several applications of exercise testing are apparent: to assist in the diagnosis of angina pectoris, for risk stratification after myocardial infarction, to evaluate the efficacy of various therapies in cardiac patients, to evaluate cardiac dysrhythmias, to evaluate pulmonary and other diseases, to screen for latent coronary artery disease, to provide a basis for a precise exercise prescription, and to assess functional capacity.[23] The first five items in this list have specific diagnostic and therapeutic applications, are generally not controversial, and are not discussed further in this chapter. Discussion of the last three applications is presented in the following paragraphs.

Exercise tests have been used to screen for latent CHD. The rationale is that if ischemia is detected, therapy, such as medical or surgical intervention, can be implemented and perhaps prevent a myocardial infarction or sudden cardiac death. Exercise testing for this purpose has been criticized because of the high rate of false-positive tests, especially in healthy populations. Redwood et al.[22] present an example that quantifies this point. If an exercise test is 95% sensitive and 95% specific (which is probably overly optimistic), the predictive accuracy of the test is 99% in a population with a disease prevalence of 90%. This example might be applicable in a population of angina patients. Instead, if the disease prevalence in the population is 2%, which is likely in an apparently healthy and asymptomatic group, the number of false-positive tests would far exceed the number of true-positive tests, and the predictive accuracy would be 28%. This latter example could lead to unnecessary concern for many individuals, increased costs of further testing, and a greater burden on the medical care systems.

Screening for latent CHD is mentioned frequently as a requirement for all adults before starting an exercise program. If a large population of incipient exercisers is screened using an exercise test with ECG monitoring, cases of undetected coronary artery disease may be discovered, and subsequently verified by additional diagnostic testing. Therapy to ameliorate, or perhaps even cure, the problem can be implemented, or the exercise can be taken under medical supervision. The issues highlighted previously argue against this approach in groups of apparently healthy individuals. Advocates of exercise test screening before initiation of an exercise program may counter that false-positives are a cost worth accepting to reduce risk and perhaps save lives of individuals with undetected disease. This concern notwithstanding, we do not believe that all adults must undergo exercise testing before starting an exercise program. This recommendation is based on two main points. First, there is no evidence that exercise-related sudden deaths are less frequent in populations that have been screened by exercise testing, compared with populations that have had less complicated and expensive or even no medical screening. Thus, there is no evidence that the benefits of mass testing outweigh the costs, and it is unwise to make broad public health recommendations without data to support efficacy. Second, the risk of cardiac arrest during exercise is a rare event, and the overall cost to benefit ratio for physical activity is favorable in population-based studies.[26] Thus, on a population basis, it is questionable if exercise testing is beneficial. Individuals at high risk for coronary artery disease or those with symptoms or a diagnosis of disease should have a medical evaluation before starting an exercise program,[24] but apparently healthy persons of any age can be encouraged to increase their physical activity, especially moderate intensity activity such as walking, without medical evaluation. Self-screening by simple scales such as the Physical Activity Readiness Questionnaire is useful in identifying individuals at high risk, who can be advised to seek medical review.[27]

Another major application of exercise testing is to provide data for a scientific exercise prescription. This purpose is certainly relevant for medically supervised rehabilitation programs, and the specifics of exercise program in those settings have been thoroughly described.[24] Many healthy individuals may benefit from an exercise test evaluation and professional counseling. It is possible that such activities may help increase a person's motivation to begin and maintain an exercise program, although data on this point are lacking. Some persons may enjoy and benefit from having the relatively rigid structure and instructions that can be provided by a formal exercise program that is based on their personal fitness level. Therefore, we do not recommend against exercise testing for apparently healthy individuals, if they choose to participate. However, we do not believe that it is sound public health policy to encourage mass exercise testing and prescription simply for the evaluation of latent CHD. This advice places additional time and expense barriers to increasing physical activity for sedentary individuals.

Exercise promotion efforts over the past 20 to 25 years emphasized the traditional exercise prescription approach. Less than 10% of adult Americans are currently exercising at that recommended level,[9] thus it seems reasonable to develop and implement other methods of encouraging the population to be physically active. The 40 to 50 million sedentary and unfit adult Americans who are at three- to fourfold higher risk of dying than their more active and fit peers, many of whom dislike rigidly prescribed, formal, and vigorous exercise programs, may be more likely to become active if a lifestyle exercise plan, rather than a rigid prescription, is recommended.[28] If this group can integrate more activity into their lives by climbing stairs instead of taking the elevator, fitting short walks into their daily routine, and generally become more active at home and at work, it seems likely that they can obtain health and functional benefits.

Physical Fitness Evaluation

Exercise testing is used to evaluate functional capacity. This is useful to determine hemodynamic impairment, to evaluate response to therapy for many patients, and to assign patients to risk strata after myocardial infarction. In addition, exercise testing can be used to assign healthy individuals to risk strata. This function is not yet widespread in medical environments, but has been used extensively in recent years in worksite health promotion programs, exercise clubs, and other related facilities. This use of exercise testing is not for diagnostic purposes, and in many situations (if testing is low level–submaximal) an exercise ECG is not obtained. The purpose is to evaluate physical fitness level. Studies on physical fitness and health support the hypothesis that low levels of fitness are associated with substantially increased risk of death during follow-up.[11,13–18] This approach to exercise testing is analogous to screening for other risk factors such as high blood pressure or high cholesterol. No one assumes that a high cholesterol level is a diagnosis of CHD—it simply indicates increased risk. The same assumption can be made for low levels of physical fitness.

Sensitivity, Specificity, and Predictive Accuracy

The applicability and appropriateness of exercise testing to evaluate fitness for the purpose of screening and risk stratification needs to be considered. This section compares fitness testing with other risk factor screening tests in terms of sensitivity, specificity, and predictive accuracy.

The Aerobics Center Longitudinal Study provides data to calculate the sensitivity, specificity, and predictive validity of several screening tests for CHD risk factors, including low physical fitness and sedentary habits. The study group consists of 25,851 men and 7,252 women ages 20 to 88 years who received a baseline preventive medical examination at the Cooper Clinic some time between 1970 and 1989. The follow-up ranged from <1 to 19 years, with an average length of 8 years. There were 284 cardiovascular disease deaths in men and 26 cardiovascular disease deaths in women during follow-up. Preliminary analyses in this database provide the results shown in Table 2.

Sensitivity for predicting death from cardiovascular disease for the seven risk factors in men ranges from 27% for smoking to 65% for low physical activity; the range in women is from 19% for smoking and an abnormal exercise test ECG to 77% for low physical

TABLE 2. Sensitivity, Specificity, and Predictive Accuracy of Various Screening Tests, Aerobics Center Longitudinal Study, Outcome = Cardiovascular Disease Mortality (284 Deaths in Men, 26 Deaths in Women),[a] 25,851 Men, 7,252 Women, 1970–1989

Risk factor[b]	Sensitivity (%)		Specificity (%)		Predictive accuracy (%)	
	Men	Women	Men	Women	Men	Women
Low fitness	58	58	78	80	2.9	1.0
High total cholesterol	46	46	76	82	2.1	0.9
High systolic BP	38	42	89	94	3.8	2.5
High diastolic BP	41	35	81	91	2.3	1.4
Current smoker	27	19	80	87	1.5	0.5
Positive exercise ECG	43	19	94	96	7.9	1.8
Physical inactivity	65	77	61	61	1.8	0.7

[a]Codes 390-448, ICD-9.
[b]Cut-points for high risk: fitness—least fit quintile; total cholesterol, ≥240 mg/dl; systolic blood pressure, ≥140 mm Hg; diastolic blood pressure, ≥90 mm Hg; smoking—currently smoking cigarettes; exercise ECG—coded abnormal by examining physician; physical activity—no reported leisure-time physical activity in the past month.
BP, blood pressure; ECG, electrocardiogram.

activity. The sensitivity of low physical fitness to identify individuals who later died from cardiovascular disease is 58% in men and women, and is higher than the values for the other major risk factors. Specificity ranges from moderate to high, with a low of 61% for low physical activity in both men and women to 94% for elevated systolic blood pressure in women. The specificity of low physical fitness is approximately 80% and is comparable to the other major risk factors in men. Specificity of low physical fitness in women is comparable to high cholesterol and somewhat lower than that for blood pressure and smoking.

The positive predictive accuracy of all screening tests is low. This is expected because of the relatively healthy population, average follow-up of 8 years, and cardiovascular disease mortality as the end point (some individuals may have extensive CHD, but are still alive). The positive predictive accuracy of an abnormal exercise test ECG is higher in men when compared with the other risk factors, but it is still quite low. Several sources recommend against exercise testing in asymptomatic populations because of low predictive accuracy and a high rate of false-positive results.[22,23]

The principal point of this discussion is to draw a distinction between the use of a test as a screening instrument and as a diagnostic tool. The use of diagnostic exercise testing is best limited to symptomatic populations. However, the importance of sedentary living habits in the etiology of cardiovascular disease warrants attention by the clinician. At the simplest level, this may involve questioning patients about their physical activity habits and counseling sedentary patients to become more active. The substantially elevated relative risk in low fitness level individuals compared with moderately fit individuals also may justify an exercise test to evaluate a patient's physical fitness. This provides another important bit of information regarding the patient's overall risk status. As discussed in the next section, we find that individuals who are low on other risk factors, but with low levels of physical fitness, are at increased risk. Thus, given current knowledge, a complete risk profile requires an evaluation of physical fitness, or at the very least, of physical activity habits.

An abnormal exercise test ECG in an otherwise healthy and asymptomatic patient should not be construed as a diagnosis of coronary artery disease, but it should be viewed as a risk factor for future coronary events. This is comparable to information from other screening tests such as blood pressure and cholesterol measurements. Current recommendations do not propose that an asymptomatic individual with an elevated blood pressure or cholesterol be sent for coronary arteriography; this same logic should apply to the 35 year-old man who is asymptomatic but has a positive exercise test ECG. This positive exercise test ECG should be presented in the context of overall risk factor counseling. Some may not agree with the rationale presented here, and may believe that a positive exercise test needs more aggressive follow-up. These persons may object to the use of the exercise test ECG in asymptomatic populations. We do not strongly disagree with this assertion, and recognize that false-positive exercise test ECG results do present some problems. However, we believe that the use of exercise testing in asymptomatic populations may be justified for the purpose of physical fitness evaluation. Screening physical fitness tests are widely offered in health clubs, YMCA and YWCA settings, and in worksite health promotion programs. We believe that such uses of low level–submaximal exercise testing are appropriate and provide benefits. These tests can be offered safely without medical supervision[24] and are relatively inexpensive. They are a useful addition to a comprehensive risk factor screening program.

Fitness Testing in Risk Stratification

Exercise testing can be used to determine physical fitness, instead of or in combination with diagnostic ECG exercise testing, as discussed in the preceding section. Here we present some additional data showing the importance of physical fitness in risk stratification. Physicians and other health professionals frequently counsel patients about their risk status. Many physicians tell apparently healthy patients who do not smoke, have low levels of blood pressure and cholesterol, and are not obese that they are at low risk for CHD and other health problems. This statement may not be true if these patients have low levels of physical fitness. For example, in our previously published data, men who have total cholesterol levels of 260 mg/dl or greater, but are physically fit, have a lower death rate (27/10,000 person-years of follow-up) than men with total cholesterol levels of 200 mg/dl or lower but are unfit (68/10,000 person-years of follow-up).[11]

We have extended mortality follow-up in the Aerobics Center Longitudinal Study through 1989, and some preliminary analyses are available. This extended follow-up is on a population of 26,980 men followed for 1 to 19 years after a baseline examination (average follow-up was approximately 8 years). There were 301 cardiovascular disease deaths during follow-up. We evaluated physical fitness by a maximal exercise test on a treadmill, and other risk factors were measured at the same examination. Men were considered at risk if they smoked, had resting systolic blood pressure of 140 mm Hg or greater, or had a total serum cholesterol of 240 mg/dl or greater. Men were classified as having 0, 1, 2, or 3 out of 3 risk factors, and age-adjusted cardiovascular disease death rates were calculated for low, moderate, and high levels of fitness within each of these risk factor groups. Results are shown in Table 3. Death rates illustrate a strong inverse gradient across fitness categories within each of the risk factor groups. For example, the death rate in the low fitness

TABLE 3. Age-adjusted Cardiovascular Disease Death Rates per 10,000 Person-years Across Physical Fitness Groups by Number of CHD Risk Factors, Aerobics Center Longitudinal Study, 26,980 men (301 cardiovascular disease deaths[a] over Approximately 8 Years of Follow-up), 1970–1989

Number of risk factors[b]	Physical fitness categories		
	Low	Moderate	High
None	22.8[c]	4.2	3.6
Any 1	23.9	10.2	6.5
Any 2	46.2	22.5	13.2
All 3	51.1	27.5	12.6

[a]Codes 390-448, ICD-9.
[b]Current smoker, systolic blood pressure >140 mm Hg, total serum cholesterol >240 mg/dl.
[c]Age-adjusted all-cause cardiovascular disease death rate/10,000 person-years of follow-up.
CHD, coronary heart disease.

level, no risk factor group is more than 6 times higher than the death rate in the high fitness level, no risk factor group. Low fitness level men who also had all three other risk factors were about 4 times more likely to die from cardiovascular disease than similar men who were in the high fitness level group. It is noteworthy that the low fitness level men with no risk factors had about the same death rate (22.8/10,000 person-years of follow-up) as moderately fit men with two risk factors (22.5/10,000). The low fitness level men in the no risk factor category had considerably higher death rates than the high fitness level men with either two (13.2/10,000) or three (12.6/10,000) risk factors.

The purpose of this chapter is not to diminish the importance of high blood pressure, high cholesterol, and cigarette smoking as risk factors for cardiovascular disease mortality. There is a clear increase in risk in these data with the number of risk factors, a finding demonstrated many years ago in earlier studies. We believe that these preliminary findings from extended follow-up in our population strongly support the value of assessing physical fitness in a comprehensive risk factor evaluation.

Summary

Several recent prospective population-based studies show a strong inverse gradient of cardiovascular disease mortality across physical fitness groups. The slope of this gradient, up to seven- to eightfold from low to high fitness categories, suggests that the data from studies on physical activity and cardiovascular disease mortality, which generally show about a doubling of risk in inactive individuals, may underestimate the importance of sedentary lifestyle as a risk factor. The difference between the studies on physical activity and the studies on physical fitness may be caused by less misclassification in the fitness studies because fitness measurements are more objective than activity measurements.

Exercise testing has several important clinical applications. There is, however, criticism of exercise testing in asymptomatic populations because of the high prevalence of false positive tests in these groups. This criticism applies to the use of exercise testing as a diagnostic tool, and we agree that exercise testing for diagnosis is best restricted to symptomatic individuals. An alternative view of exercise testing is to use it for risk factor screening, similar to blood pressure or cholesterol tests. The addition of physical fitness status appears to add important information regarding the risk of dying from cardiovascular disease, and clinical fitness testing is recommended as a useful tool.

Acknowledgment

We thank Laura Becker for manuscript preparation, proofreading, and producing the figures.

References

1. Cherry T: A theory of cancer. *Med J Aust* 1922;1:425–438
2. Sivertsen I, Dahlstrom AN: The relation of muscular activity to carcinoma. A preliminary report. *J Cancer Res* 1922;6:365–378
3. Morris JN, Heady JA, Raffle PAB, Roberts CG, Parks JW: Coronary

heart disease and physical activity of work. *Lancet* 1953;2:1053–1120

4. Hagberg JM: Exercise, fitness and hypertension, in Bouchard C, Shephard RJ, Stephens T, Sutton JR, McPherson BD (eds): *Exercise, Fitness, and Health: A Consensus of Current Knowledge*. Champaign, IL, Human Kinetics Books, 1990, pp 455–466

5. Tipton CM: Exercise, training and hypertension: an update, in Holloszy JO (ed): *Exercise and Sport Sciences Reviews: Volume 19, 1991*. Baltimore, Williams & Wilkins, 1991, pp 447–505

6. Powell KE, Thompson PD, Caspersen CJ, Kendrick JS: Physical activity and the incidence of coronary heart disease. *Annu Rev Public Health* 1987;8:253–287

7. Blair SN: Physical activity, fitness, and coronary heart disease. In: Bouchard C, Shepard RJ, Stephens T, (eds): *Physical Activity, Fitness, and Health 1992 Proceedings*. Champaign, IL, Human Kinetics Books.

8. Fletcher GF, Blair SN, Blumenthal J, Caspersen C, Chaitman B, Epstein S, Faus H, Sivarajan-Froelicher ES, Froelicher V, Pina IL: Statement on exercise: benefits and recommendations for physical activity programs for all Americans: a statement for health professionals by the Committee on Exercise and Cardiac Rehabilitation of the Council on Clinical Cardiology, American Heart Association. *Circulation* 1992;86:340–344

9. Caspersen CJ, Christenson GM, Pollard RA: Status of the 1990 Physical Fitness and Exercise Objectives—evidence from NHIS 1985. *Public Health Rep* 1986;101:587–592

10. Paffenbarger RS Jr, Hyde RT, Wing AL, Hsieh CC: Physical activity, all-caused mortality, and longevity of college alumni. *N Engl J Med* 1986;314:605–613

11. Blair SN, Kohl HW III, Paffenbarger RS Jr, Clark DG, Cooper KH, Gibbons LW: Physical fitness and all-cause mortality: a prospective study of healthy men and women. *JAMA* 1989;262:2395–2401

12. Hahn RA, Teutsch SM, Rothenberg RB, et al: Excess deaths from nine chronic diseases in the United States, 1986. *JAMA* 1990;264:2654–2659

13. Lie H, Mundal R, Erikssen J: Coronary risk factors and incidence of coronary death in relation to physical fitness. Seven-year follow-up study of middle-aged and elderly men. *Eur Heart J* 1985;6:147–157

14. Slattery ML, Jacobs DR Jr: Physical fitness and cardiovascular disease mortality: the U.S. Railroad Study. *Am J Epidemiol* 1988;127:571–580

15. Arraiz GA, Wigle DT, Mao Y: Risk assessment of physical activity and physical fitness in the Canada Health Survey Mortality Follow-up Study. *J Clin Epidemiol* 1992;45:419–428

16. Ekelund L-G, Haskell WL, Johnson JL, Whaley FS, Criqui MH, Sheps DS: Physical fitness as a predictor of cardiovascular mortality in asymptomatic North American men: the Lipid Research Clinics Mortality Follow-up Study. *N Engl J Med* 1988;319:1379–1384

17. Blair SN, Kohl HW III, Barlow CE, Gibbons, LW: Physical fitness and all-cause mortality in hypertensive men. *Ann Med* 1991;23:307–312

18. Kohl HW, Gordon NF, Villegas JA, Blair SN: Cardiorespiratory fitness, glycemic status, and mortality risk in men. *Diabetes Care* 1992;15:184–192

19. Peters RK, Cady LD Jr, Bischoff DP, Bernstein L, Pike MC: Physical

fitness and subsequent myocardial infarction in healthy workers. *JAMA* 1983;249:3052–3056

20. Sobolski J. Kornitzer M, De Backer G, Dramaix M, Abramowicz M, Degre S, Denolin H: Protection against ischemic heart disease in the Belgian Physical Fitness Study: physical fitness rather than physical activity? *Am J Epidemiol* 1987;125:601–610

21. Wilhelmsen L, Bjure J, Ekström-Jodal B, Aurell M, Grimby G, Svardsvadd K, Tildolin G, Wedel H: Nine years' follow-up of a maximal exercise test in a random population sample of middle-aged men. *Cardiology* 1981;68(suppl 2):1–8

22. Redwood DR, Borer JS, Epstein SE: Whither the ST segment during exercise? *Circulation* 1976;54:703–706

23. Council on Scientific Affairs: Indications and contraindications for exercise testing. *JAMA* 1981;246:1015–1018

24. American College of Sports Medicine: *Guidelines for Exercise Testing and Prescription*. 4th ed. Philadelphia, Lea & Febiger, 1991

25. Fletcher GF, Froelicher VF, Hartley H, Haskell WL, Pollock ML: Exercise standards: a statement for health professionals from the American Heart Association. *Circulation* 1990;82:2286–2322

26. Siscovick DS, Weiss NS, Fletcher RH, Lasky T: The incidence of primary cardiac arrest during vigorous exercise. *N Engl J Med* 1984;311:874–877

27. Chisholm D, Collis M, Kulak L, Davenport W, Gruber N: Physical Activity Readiness. *Br Columbia Med J* 1975;17:375–378

28. Blair SN, Kohl HW III, Gordon NF: Physical activity and health: a lifestyle approach. *Med Exerc Nutr Health* 1992;1:54–57

Chapter 18

Exercise, Lipoproteins, and Cardiovascular Disease

Marcia L. Stefanick, PhD

Considerable evidence has accumulated to support the hypotheses that high levels of total and/or low-density lipoprotein (LDL) cholesterol and low levels of high-density lipoprotein (HDL) cholesterol are each causally related to the development of coronary heart disease (CHD).[1,2] Elevated plasma triglycerides also may be causally related to CHD, but this remains to be demonstrated, partially because their strong associations with other major CHD risk factors, such as low HDL cholesterol and abnormal glucose metabolism make it difficult to detect their independent role.[2]

This chapter focuses predominantly on a progression of thought and line of inquiry underlying a series of training studies conducted in our laboratory at Stanford University, designed to determine whether the adoption of a physically active lifestyle results in changes in the plasma lipoprotein profile, which may lead to a reduced risk of CHD, in particular, to elevations in HDL cholesterol and reductions in plasma triglycerides. Previous reviews by Wood and coinvestigators[3–7] and meta-analyses by Tran and colleagues[8–10] provide a more comprehensive review of this literature, which is beyond the scope of this chapter; however, recent studies that were not included in these reviews are discussed where appropriate.

Supported by NIH grants HL 24462 and HL 45733, from the National Heart, Lung, and Blood Institute, for research in the area of exercise and lipoproteins.

From Fletcher GF, (ed): *Cardiovascular Response to Exercise*. Mount Kisco, NY, Futura Publishing Company, Inc., © 1994.

Epidemiologic Observations and Cross-sectional Studies

Before the 1975 publication of evidence of an inverse relationship between plasma HDL cholesterol and the development of ischemic heart disease,[11] Wood and coworkers determined fasting plasma lipid and lipoprotein concentrations, using the "standardized" methods of the Lipid Research Clinics (LRC), of 41 very active middle-aged men (defined as running >24 km/week) and a comparison group of 743 predominantly sedentary men of similar age, who were randomly selected from three northern California communities.[12] The runners had significantly lower mean concentrations of triglycerides (70 vs. 146 mg/dl; $p<0.001$) and total cholesterol (200 vs. 210 mg/dl; $p<0.05$) than the control group. Mean LDL cholesterol also was significantly lower in the runners (125 vs. 139 mg/dl; $p<0.01$) compared with a subset of 147 men randomly selected among the control men for these determinations. In contrast, mean HDL cholesterol was markedly higher in the runners than in this control subset (64 vs. 43 mg/dl; $p<0.001$). Despite no differences in self-reported weight at age 18 years, the runners weighed 10 kg less, on average, than men in the full control sample and they had significantly lower relative body weights (1.02), defined as the ratio of actual to ideal weight, based on the 1959 Metropolitan Life Insurance Company tables, compared with control men (1.22). The Bruce multistage treadmill test revealed an average endurance to maximal effort of 16 ± 3 minutes (mean$\pm$SD) in the runners, compared with a 9.4 ± 1.9 minutes for the controls, thereby confirming the anticipated high exercise capacity of the runners.

Similar fasting plasma lipid and lipoprotein comparisons were made between 43 active women (also selected for running >24 km/week) and 932 women randomly chosen from the same three California communities, for triglyceride and total cholesterol analyses, and a randomly selected subset of 101 of these women, for LDL and HDL cholesterol determinations.[13] As in men, the female runners had significantly ($p<0.5$) lower mean triglyceride (56 vs. 123 mg/dl) and total cholesterol (193 vs. 209 mg/dl) concentrations than female controls, and lower mean LDL cholesterol (113 vs. 124 mg/dl) than the subset of controls, whereas HDL cholesterol levels were higher in the runners versus women in this subset (75 vs. 56 mg/dl). Female runners were somewhat younger than the control women

$(42 \pm 8$ vs. 47 ± 7 years; $p < 0.05)$, introducing the possible confounder of menopausal status; however, similar differences between runners and controls persisted when women were divided into narrower age ranges (30–39, 40–49, 50–59). Although the female runners reported significantly greater weights at age 18 years than women in the full control group, the runners weighed approximately 8 kg less than controls at the time of testing and had significantly lower relative body weights (1.04 vs. 1.25).[12] Female runners averaged 13 ± 3 minutes on the Bruce treadmill test, whereas a sample of 85 women tested among the control subset averaged 6.7 ± 2.0 minutes.

Similar lipoprotein differences were seen between active and sedentary individuals when 25 men and 25 women, who reported regular tennis play as their exclusive aerobic activity, were subsequently recruited from the northern California cities and compared with 73 sedentary men and 49 sedentary women of the same age, who were randomly selected among participants of a CHD risk factor survey of Stanford faculty and staff.[14] In particular, plasma HDL cholesterol was significantly higher in the tennis players, who were considered above average, although not outstanding players, compared with sedentary men and women (58 vs. 46 mg/dl for men; 74 vs. 62 mg/dl for women), whereas triglyceride levels were much lower in the active men and women versus sedentary controls (84 vs. 156 mg/dl for men; 66 vs. 95 mg/dl for women). Total cholesterol and LDL cholesterol did not differ between active and sedentary men or women in this sample. As predicted, the tennis players had significantly $(p < 0.05)$ lower relative weights then sedentary controls (1.08 vs. 1.18 for men; 1.01 vs. 1.14 for women).

Among early confirmatory reports from other laboratories of a relationship between activity level and HDL cholesterol was a study by Nikkila et al. of 23 completely immobilized patients (14 men, 9 women) who were shown to have significantly $(p < 0.001)$ lower HDL cholesterol and apolipoprotein A-I levels than normally mobile paired controls.[15] Triglycerides were only slightly higher in patients, and significant only in women, and LDL cholesterol did not differ between groups.

Plasma lipoprotein determinations and treadmill exercise testing were performed on a larger epidemiologic sample of 2,319 white men and 2,067 white women, aged 20 years or older, who were randomly selected from population surveys by nine clinics of the LRC North American Prevalence Study.[16] Responses to two questions concerning performance of strenuous physical activity revealed that 64.5% of the men and 84% of the women were inactive, whereas 29% of men and 12% of women reported strenuous exercise or physical labor at least three times per week. Although neither treadmill exercise test duration nor heart rate response to submaximal exercise was significantly related to HDL cholesterol, participants who reported some strenuous physical activity generally had higher HDL cholesterol levels than those who reported none. Quetelet index (weight/height^2, as kg/cm^2 × 1,000) was slightly lower in physically active versus inactive participants (men, 2.58 vs. 2.64; women, 2.32 vs. 2.37). Frequency of alcohol use was similar for inactive and very active men, and only at ages 50 to 59 years did active women report a higher frequency of alcohol use than inactive women (67% vs. 55%), whereas active individuals smoked cigarettes less often than inactive men and women. The overall gonadal hormone usage by women was similar for inactive (27%) and very active (31%) women. When HDL cholesterol was adjusted for age, body mass index, alcohol use, cigarette smoking, and interclinic population variation, significantly higher levels were found in the more active men and women compared with their sedentary counterparts (47.1 vs. 45.2 mg/dl, $p = 0.0001$, for men; 59.6 vs. 57.7 mg/dl, $p = 0.02$, for women).

The observations in women prompted the question by other investigators of whether menopausal status may influence the relationship between habitual activity and HDL cholesterol level.[17] Hartung et al.[17] therefore recruited a group of women by mass media, running publications, and local races and running sites, who were not taking oral contraceptives or hormone replacement therapy, for a cross-sectional study of premenopausal (Pre-M) and postmenopausal (Post-M) long-distance runners (34 Pre-M, 10 Post-M), joggers (34 Pre-M, 13 Post-M), and inactive women (31 Pre-M, 14 Post-M). Higher HDL cholesterol levels were found in active versus inactive women, when women were grouped regardless of menopausal status, and HDL cholesterol levels differed significantly among Post-M groups, being highest in distance runners (79.8 mg/dl), intermediate in joggers (73.5 mg/dl), and lowest in inactive women (61.8 mg/dl), whereas a similar (but not significant) dose response was suggested in Pre-M groups, dropping from 72.1 mg/dl in long-distance women, to 69.9 mg/dl in joggers, and to 66.9 mg/dl in inactive volunteers. The tendency for HDL to be lower in inactive Post-M than inactive Pre-M women was balanced by an opposite trend for HDL to be higher in Post-M versus Pre-M distance runners and joggers, such that HDL did not differ between Pre-M and Post-M women overall, suggesting that HDL differences between pre- and postmenopausal women in larger population samples may reflect differences in activity level. Percent body fat, determined by four skinfold measurements, differed significantly between Pre-M and Post-M ($p<0.002$) and across the three activity groups ($p<0.001$), being lowest in long-distance runners (22.1%, Pre-M; 23.9%, Post-M), intermediate in joggers (26.7%; 26.2%), and highest in inactive women (28.3%; 33.1%).

To understand better the associations between lipoprotein concentrations and long-term exercise training, Williams et al.[18] examined lipoprotein subfraction concentrations, determined by analytical ultracentrifugation (ANUC), and postheparin lipoprotein and hepatic lipase activities in 12 male long-distance runners and 64 sedentary male nonsmokers who had volunteered for a 1-year training study and were, therefore, undergoing baseline measurements. The runners, who had significantly lower total cholesterol (190 vs. 217 mg/dl; $p = 0.02$), LDL cholesterol (116 vs. 147 mg/dl; $p = 0.004$) and triglyceride levels (71 vs. 123 mg/dl; $p = 0.001$), and higher HDL cholesterol levels (65 vs. 50 mg/dl; $p = 0.0001$) than the nonrunners, had significantly lower serum mass concentrations of the smaller, denser LDL particles of flotation rates $S_f 0-7$ ($p = 0.0001$) and VLDL particles of $S_f 20-400$ ($p = 0.001$), and higher concentrations of HDL particles with flotation rates between $F_{1.20} 2.0-9.0$ ($p = 0.0002$) than did the nonrunners. Postheparin lipoprotein lipase activity (which does not distinguish skeletal muscle LPL from adipose tissue LPL or LPL released from other tissues after heparin injection, nor does it specify LPL activity of any given skeletal muscle bed or adipose tissue site) was shown to be significantly higher in runners than nonrunners (5.0 vs. 3.6 mEq fatty acid/ml per hour; $p = 0.04$), whereas postheparin hepatic triglyceride lipase activity was lower in the runners (4.1 vs. 6.5 Eq fatty acid/ml per hour; $p = 0.02$). As expected, runners had a much lower mean body mass index (BMI; weight/height^2, as kg/m^2), than nonrunners (22.6 vs. 25.1; $p = 0.006$); however, LDL and HDL cholesterol and the ANUC lipoprotein variables listed above remained significantly different between runners and nonrunners after adjustment for body mass index. In contrast, this adjustment eliminated significant postheparin LPL and hepatic lipase activity differences between the active and inactive men.

Recent comparisons between master cross-country skiers (48

women, aged 30–57 years; 128 men, aged 30–78 years) at a time when they were at a high level of physical fitness and age-matched men and women from the LRC Population Studies confirmed that men and women who regularly engage in other (nonrunning) aerobic activities have significantly higher HDL cholesterol and lower triglycerides than people of comparable age and sex in the general population, and that these differences were significant for almost every 5-year age increment examined in both men and women, although the numbers were very small for older age intervals.[19] Serum LDL cholesterol and total cholesterol levels also were markedly lower in the male cross-country skiers and, to a lesser extent, in the women skiers, at each age, relative to the LRC population samples. As with the runners, the cross-country skiers were much leaner than the general public, differing significantly from LRC subjects in weight, Quetelet index, and triceps skinfold at nearly every age interval analyzed.

Training Studies

It is generally understood that one cannot conclude that a causal relationship exists simply because a variable is shown to differ between study samples in cross-sectional analyses, no matter how consistently the observation may be reported. Differences between active and inactive individuals in lipoproteins could arise primarily from genetic factors that predispose a person to both a more active lifestyle and to higher HDL cholesterol and lower triglyceride levels. For instance, a higher proportion of slow oxidative (red) muscle fibers, which are characterized by a high activity level of skeletal muscle lipoprotein lipase (LPL), which hydrolyzes the triglycerides in VLDLs, would make endurance activity easier to adopt, while also reducing circulating triglycerides and facilitating the metabolism of VLDL to HDL. Alternatively, or additionally, active individuals may be more likely to differ from inactive people in other behavioral factors that influence HDL cholesterol, such as smoking status, alcohol intake, or diet composition. To test the hypothesis that exercise itself raises fasting HDL cholesterol levels or lowers fasting triglycerides or affects other lipoproteins, independently of other factors that may differ between active and inactive people, such as body habitus, a randomized, controlled trial should be conducted and such a trial should be of sufficient length and sample size to ensure than an exercise effect can be detected. This argument resulted in the design of the first training study by our group, which we refer to as the Stanford Exercise Study.

Stanford Exercise Study

The Stanford Exercise Study involved randomization of 81 men, aged 30 to 55 years to either: 1) a 1-year supervised jogging program ($n = 48$), or 2) 1 year of no major change in activity level, that is, "control" ($n = 33$), specifically to determine the effect of increased regular physical activity on HDL cholesterol.[20] No instruction was given regarding diet. Neither initial body mass index nor percent body fat determined by hydrostatic weighing, differed between groups at baseline, averaging about 25 kg/m² and 21–22%, respectively. Fitness, assessed during a maximal graded exercise treadmill test, also was similar in the two groups, averaging a maximum of 35 ml oxygen consumed per kilogram of body weight per minute. Fasting triglycerides, total, LDL and HDL cholesterol, and apolipoproteins A-I, A-II, and B also were similar between exercisers and controls at the outset of the trial; however, HDL_2 mass was significantly ($p < 0.05$) greater in the men assigned to exercise versus control.

By 1 year, maximal oxygen consumption had increased by 9.0 ± 1.6 ml/kg per minute in exercisers versus controls ($p < 0.0001$), and work time on the treadmill increased by 2.4 ± 0.3 minutes versus controls ($p < 0.0001$); furthermore, despite no evidence of differences between groups in changes in caloric intake or percent of calories from any given food source, from 3-day food records, exercisers lost significant weight relative to controls (2.5 kg; $p < 0.001$), reducing percent body fat by 3.8% versus control ($p < 0.0001$). Data were analyzed as an "intention to treat" clinical trial, with all men who completed 1 year measurements included in primary analyses, whether they actually exercised during the year or not. No significant differences were detected between the 46 men assigned to exercise and the 32 controls who completed 1 year tests in any of the lipoprotein variables studied, including HDL cholesterol and its subfractions, triglycerides, total or LDL cholesterol, or apolipoproteins AI, AII, or B; however, secondary analyses, which separated exercisers into four treatment-dose groups according to mileage achieved (0–3.9, 4–7.9, 8–12.9, and 13+ miles/week), revealed significant treatment effects for HDL cholesterol (Spearman's rho = 0.48; $p = 0.0008$), total cholesterol ($r = -0.29$; $p = 0.05$), and LDL cholesterol ($r = -0.31$; $p = 0.04$). Only 25 men averaged at least eight miles (12.9 km) of running per week and these men increased their HDL cholesterol by 4.4 mg/dl ($p < 0.05$) compared with controls.

Further analyses revealed that men who started with higher baseline HDL cholesterol levels and lower plasma triglycerides achieved greater mileage, supporting the idea that cross-sectional studies are indeed biased by a self-selection effect.[21] Analyses on data collected at 3-month intervals also demonstrated that HDL and LDL cholesterol generally did not begin to change until a threshold exercise level (10 miles, or 16 km/week) was maintained for at least 9 months and that fitness increased and percent body fat decreased sooner and at lower exercise levels than required for the lipoprotein changes.[21]

Among the exercisers, quite a few men reported active dieting, including diets involving major changes in diet composition. When these men were excluded, secondary analyses on the 32 exercisers who did not report caloric restriction during the trial showed that kilometers run per week correlated significantly with changes in HDL cholesterol (Spearman's rho = 0.45; $p = 0.003$), but also with body fat changes ($r = -0.49$; $p = 0.002$), which in turn correlated with HDL cholesterol changes ($r = -0.47$; $p = 0.004$).[20] To determine whether weight changes may be responsible for the HDL changes seen in the exercisers, curve-fitting statistical procedures and regression analyses were applied to the data collected in a defined subset of the exercisers and sedentary controls, which suggested that processes associated with weight change produced much of the plasma HDL cholesterol change induced by moderate exercise; however, the interaction between weight change and plasma HDL concentration was significantly different ($p < 0.001$) in the exercisers and controls, suggesting that metabolic consequences of exercise-induced weight change differed from weight change in the sedentary state.[22] In view of consistent findings of greater leanness in active versus inactive men and women, in addition to higher HDL cholesterol and lower triglyceride levels, these observations raised the obvious question: does weight loss cause the exercise-induced increase in plasma high-density lipoproteins? This question led to the design of our first 1-year weight loss study.

First Stanford Weight Control Project

The first Stanford Weight Control Project (SWCP-I) randomized 155 moderately overweight men (20–50% above ideal body weight), aged 35 to 59 years, to 1-year interventions of 1) group instruction by a registered dietitian on moderate caloric restriction, without change in diet composition ($n = 51$), 2) supervised group walking or jogging sessions, with no dietary changes ($n = 52$), or 3) no change in caloric intake, diet, or physical activity.[23] No significant baseline differences were seen among the three groups for BMI (which averaged about 29 kg/m^2), body composition by hydrostatic weighting (which averaged about 28% body fat), caloric intake determined by 7 day food records (which averaged about 2,400 kcal/day), or cardivascular fitness level during a maximal graded exercise treadmill test (which averaged about 34 ml/kg per minute for maximal oxygen consumption). Lipoproteins also were similar among all groups.

Major measurements were repeated at 7 months and 1 year. Caloric reduction was significant in dieters versus controls at 7 months (about 335 kcal/day; $p<0.01$) and 1 year (about 240 kcal/day; $p<0.01$), whereas caloric intake did not differ between exercisers and controls at either period. Caloric reduction also was significant in dieters versus exercisers at 7 months, but not at 1 year, possibly because of a 6-week weight stabilization period before these tests. Maximal oxygen consumption was significantly improved in exercisers at 1 year compared with dieters (4.1 ml/kg per minute; $p<0.001$) and controls (6.5 ml/kg per minute; $p<0.001$). Seven months after baseline tests, exercisers had lost 2.9 kg of fat weight versus control ($p<0.001$), but only 0.3 kg of lean mass (n.s.) and by 1 year, fat mass loss averaged 3.8 kg versus control ($p<0.001$), with lean mass loss remaining insignificant. Dieters lost 2.9 kg more fat weight than exercisers by 7 months ($p<0.001$), but no significant differences were seen between dieters and exercisers in fat weight loss by 1 year, although both groups had lost significant fat weight versus controls; in contrast, lean mass loss was significantly greater in dieters relative to controls ($p<0.001$) and to exercisers ($p<0.01$) at both 7 months and 1 year.

HDL cholesterol levels were elevated significantly and triglycerides (TG) were reduced significantly in both dieters and exercisers, versus controls, at both major measurement points; these changes did not differ between the men who lost weight by caloric restriction alone and the men who lost weight by exercise alone at 7 months (HDL: 2.3 vs. 3.5 mg/dl; TG: -35.4 vs. -22.1 mg/dl) or 1 year (HDL: 4.2 vs. 4.6 mg/dl; TG: -23.9 vs. -14.2 mg/dl). HDL_2 and HDL_3 cholesterol subfractions also were increased significantly in the two weight loss groups versus control by 1 year, and these increases did not differ between the two weight loss groups. Plasma HDL_2 ($F_{1.20}$ 3.5–9.0) and HDL_3 ($F_{1.20}$ 0.0–3.5) mass concentrations, determined by ANUC, also were elevated significantly in both dieters and exercisers, with no differences between groups, whereas VLDL mass (S_f 20–400) was decreased only in the dieters versus control and did not differ between exercisers versus control or dieters.[24] LDL cholesterol was not changed in either weight loss group; however, small LDL mass (S_f 0–7) decreased significantly in dieters at both 7 months ($p<0.001$) and 1 year ($p<0.05$) and in exercisers at 7 months ($p<0.05$), versus controls. Decreases in small LDL mass in dieters were not significantly different from changes in exercisers at either time point, whereas LDL peak particle diameter increased significantly in both dieters (2.4 A) and exercisers (3.2 A) versus control, with no differences between dieters and exercisers.

Postheparin LPL activity was significantly elevated in exercisers versus control (0.62; $p<0.05$) at 7 months, whereas LPL increases were not significant in dieters (0.36; $p<0.10$)[25]; however LPL increases were not significant for exercisers at the 1-year point, possibly because of a reduction in exercise during the 6-week weight stabilization period, which may have altered the acute effects of exercise on LPL, nor was LPL activity changed in dieters at 1 year.[26] In contrast, postheparin hepatic triglyceride lipase (HTGL) activity was reduced significantly in both dieters and exercisers, versus control, at both 7 months (-0.84 and -0.59 mU/ml per minute, respectively) and 1 year (-0.97 and -0.70 mU/ml per minute), with no significant differences between dieters and exercisers at either time point.[25,26] These data suggest that exercise may have a unique effect on LPL activity, whereas weight loss may be the major factor affecting hepatic lipase activity. One-year changes in both postheparin HTGL and LPL activities were significantly ($p<0.01$) related in exercisers to changes in HDL cholesterol ($r=-0.42$ and $r=0.40$, respectively) and HDL_2 mass ($r=-0.40$ and $r=0.38$), as were changes in postheparin HTGL activity and HDL_2 cholesterol ($r=-0.41$) and changes in LPL activity and HDL_3 mass ($r=0.33$; $p<0.05$), whereas postheparin lipase activity changes were not significantly correlated with changes in HDL or its subfractions in dieters or controls.[26] Thus, it is reasonable to hypothesize that HDL changes after adoption of habitual activity involve both a direct effect of exercise and an indirect effect of exercise-induced weight loss.

Further evidence of a direct exercise (active muscle) effect was published by Kiens and Lithell,[27] who used a single leg (knee extension) training design, in which one leg served as the untrained control, to demonstrate that resting skeletal muscle LPL activity increased in the trained leg to 70% above that in the untrained leg and that there was a markedly higher arteriovenous (A-V) VLDL triglyceride difference (greater uptake) over the trained thigh, as well as a higher production of HDL cholesterol and HDL_2 cholesterol by the trained thigh.[27] Furthermore, positive correlations between muscle LPL activity and A-V differences of VLDL-TG were found only in the trained thigh. Further discussion of the multiple mechanisms that may underlie the effects of exercise on lipid and lipoprotein metabolism appear in our recent review of this literature.[28]

Second Stanford Weight Control Project

The second Stanford Weight Control Study (SWCP-II) involved randomization of 132 moderately overweight men (body mass index between 28 and 34 kg/m^2) and 132 moderately overweight, premenopausal women (body mass index between 24 and 30 kg/m^2) to 1-year interventions of 1) diet: group instruction by a registered dietitian on reduction of saturated fat and dietary cholesterol, with concomitant caloric restriction and a consistent message that women should not drop below 1,200 kcal/day or men below 1,500 kcal/day, 2) diet plus exercise: identical diet instruction combined with supervised group walking or jogging sessions, or 3) control: no change in caloric intake or activity.[29] Within each sex, the three study groups were well matched at baseline for age (men, 40 ± 6 years, women, 39 ± 6 years), body composition by hydrostatic weighing (men, 70.7 kg lean mass, 27.7 kg fat mass; women, 48.1 kg lean mass, 26.9 kg fat mass), aerobic capacity during a maximal graded exercise treadmill test (men, 34.1 ± 4.9 ml/kg per minute; women, 27.0 ± 4.2 ml/kg per minute); total calories assessed by 7-day food records (men, about

2,630 kcal/day; women, about 1,945 kcal/day), and the intake of most nutrients (men, 38.1% of calories from fat, 14.0% from saturated fat; women, 37.1% from fat, 13.6% from saturated fat).

One-year measurements were completed on 40 of 45 men and 31 of 42 women randomized to the hypocaloric reduced fat/reduced cholesterol diet; on 39 of 43 men and 42 of 47 women assigned to the diet-plus-aerobic exercise; and on 40 of 44 men and 39 of 43 women randomized to control. Caloric reduction was significant in both men and women assigned to diet-only or to diet-plus-exercise versus control and did not differ between men or women assigned to diet only versus diet plus exercise. Significant ($p<0.001$) reductions in percent of calories from total fat and saturated fat, versus control, did not differ between diet-only and diet-plus-exercise groups, with the exception of a significantly ($p<0.05$) greater reduction in total fat and increase in carbohydrate intake in men assigned to diet-plus-exercise compared with diet-only men. Both diet intervention groups closely achieved a National Cholesterol Education Program Step 1 diet (<30% of calories as total fat; <10% as saturated fat; <300 mg of dietary cholesterol per day).

Both diet-only and diet-plus-exercise women lost significant ($p<0.001$) fat weight versus controls (4.5 kg and 6.0 kg, respectively). Fat weight loss did not differ between women assigned to diet-plus-exercise versus diet-only, possibly because of the higher dropout rate in women assigned to diet-only; similarly, significant decreases versus control in percent body fat did not differ between exercising dieters (5.2%) and diet-only women (3.5%). Lean mass loss was negligible in women who lost weight by either diet-only or diet-plus-exercise and did not differ between groups. Women assigned to diet-plus-exercise improved their aerobic capacity significantly relative to diet-only women (6.4 vs. 1.4 ml/kg per minute improvement above baseline; $p<0.001$) and control, who made no change.

Both diet-only and diet-plus-exercise women significantly ($p<0.05$) and similarly decreased total cholesterol (-13.9 and -9.7 mg/dl, respectively), LDL cholesterol (-9.7 and -10.1 mg/dl) and apolipoprotein B (-5.8 and -6.0 mg/dl; $p<0.01$) versus control, but only the diet-plus-exercise women decreased triglyceride levels (-13.3 mg/dl; $p<0.05$). Contrary to an expected increase in HDL with weight loss, the women assigned to lose weight on the low-fat diet without exercise reduced HDL cholesterol about 3.9 mg/dl (n.s.) compared with controls, and also lowered HDL_2 cholesterol about 4.3 mg/dl ($p<0.5$). In contrast, diet-plus-exercise women raised HDL cholesterol about 2.7 mg/dl and HDL$_2$ cholesterol about 3.1 mg/dl, compared with controls (n.s.), such that diet-only had significantly ($p<0.01$) reduced HDL cholesterol (-6.6 mg/dl) and HDL$_2$ cholesterol (-7.3 mg/dl) compared with diet-plus-exercise women. Apolipoprotein A-I also was reduced significantly in diet-only women versus control (-8.8 mg/dl; $p<0.05$), whereas the increase in apolipoprotein A-I (1.9 mg/dl) in diet-plus-exercise compared with control was not significant.

In men, as in women, both diet-only and diet-plus-exercise groups lost significant ($p<0.001$) fat weight versus controls (5.5 kg and 9.0 kg, respectively), with loss of fat mass being significantly greater in men assigned to diet-plus-exercise versus diet-only ($p<0.001$). Percent body fat also decreased significantly ($p<0.001$) more in men who dieted and exercised (-7.0% vs. control) compared with men who only dieted (-3.8% vs. control). Lean mass loss in men assigned to either diet only or diet-plus-exercise was significant ($p<0.05$) versus control and averaged 1.3 kg and 1.4 kg, respectively, with no difference between groups. Men assigned to diet-plus-exercise improved their aerobic capacity significantly compared with diet-only men (8.6 vs. 1.6 ml/kg per minute above baseline; $p<0.001$) and control (-0.02 ml/kg per minute). When the weight and body composition changes of men in the SWCP-II were compared with those of SWCP-I, which comprised a similar sample of moderately overweight, sedentary, albeit slightly younger, men, it would appear that weight loss achieved by a low-fat diet may result in greater fat weight loss than one characterized by caloric restriction only.

Nonetheless, men assigned to lose weight on the low-fat diet without exercise failed to show significant elevations in HDL cholesterol (2.7 mg/dl) or HDL$_2$ cholesterol (0.0 mg/dl) versus control. In contrast, diet-plus-exercise men increased their HDL cholesterol about 7.3 mg/dl ($p<0.001$) and HDL$_2$ cholesterol about 3.9 mg/dl ($p<0.01$) versus control, and these increases were significant compared with HDL and HDL$_2$ cholesterol changes in diet-only men ($p<0.01$). Apolipoprotein A-I also was increased significantly ($p<0.01$) in diet-plus-exercise men versus control (7.2 mg/dl) and versus diet-only men (7.3 mg/dl). Largely because of decreases in total and LDL cholesterol at 1 year (-5.4 and -7.7 mg/dl, respectively) in male controls, who had significantly higher baseline levels than diet-only men and diet-plus-exercise men, decreases in the two male weight loss groups in total cholesterol (-16.2 and -15.0

mg/dl, respectively) and LDL cholesterol (-15.1 and -10.5 mg/dl) were not significant versus control. In contrast, apolipoprotein B was significantly reduced (-5.8 and -6.0 mg/dl; $p<0.01$) versus control. Diet-plus-exercise men showed profound decreases in triglyceride levels (-58.5 mg/dl vs. control, $p<0.001$; -31.9 mg/dl vs. diet-only, $p<0.05$).

These data suggest that the beneficial effects of the low-fat diet for LDL cholesterol and apolipoprotein B may be offset partially by its reducing effects on HDL cholesterol and apolipoprotein A-I. Men who adopted the diet appear to have an HDL-protective effect of weight loss; however, the substantial weight loss in diet-only women was not adequate to compensate for the HDL-lowering effect of the low-fat/increased-carbohydrate diet. Clearly, a large proportion of the population is overweight and could afford to (and should be encouraged to) lose weight as a compensatory strategy for the tendency of the low-fat diet to reduce HDL cholesterol; however, adoption of the low-fat diet by lean individuals could lead to even greater decreases in HDL cholesterol. Therefore, it would seem important to recommend that exercise be combined with the diet, to ensure the HDL-raising effect of exercise, as well as to increase the likelihood that weight loss will occur for those who need to lose weight.

One possible explanation for a greater protective or beneficial effect of weight loss in men versus women may lie in the predominance of an android (male-type) obesity pattern in men that is more likely to be improved by weight loss than the gynoid (female-type) pattern. It is likely that weight loss that is accompanied by a reduction of abdominal fat will have the greatest benefits to the lipoprotein profile, based on an ever-growing body of literature on regional adiposity, which consistently demonstrates that a lower waist to hip ratio or visceral fat compartment is associated with a healthier lipoprotein profile (particularly, higher HDL cholesterol),[30–34] including mass subfractions, as studied by the ANUC.[33,34] We have recently reviewed this literature, with a discussion of mechanisms that may underlie the interrelationships between exercise-induced changes in visceral and abdominal fat and lipoproteins.[28,35] The waist to hip girth ratio (WHR) was significantly reduced in SWCP-II men assigned to either diet-only or diet-plus-exercise, versus control, although significantly greater WHR reductions were seen in men assigned to diet-plus-exercise than diet-only.[29] In contrast, WHR was reduced significantly in SWCP-II women assigned to diet-plus-exercise, versus control, but did not reach significance in diet-only women versus control; on the other hand, WHR differences were not significant between diet-only and diet-plus-exercise women.

Questions Not Yet Addressed in Our Laboratory

Many obvious questions cannot be answered by these three 1-year training studies. One that is of particular interest to us is how effective exercise is in bringing about HDL changes in the absence of weight loss. Although this was the original intention of the Stanford Exercise Study, it was not emphasized and therefore not achieved. Other investigators have designed studies to look at this specific question, generally by increasing caloric intake and then struggling with the confounding effects of diet change, or by studying only lean individuals who have little weight to lose. Others have achieved this without trying, as exercise-only treatments are not always accompanied by major weight loss, particularly in women. Another (series of) question(s) relates to the intensity at which one must work to achieve HDL cholesterol or other lipoprotein benefits and whether this differs between younger and older persons or premenopausal versus postmenopausal women. Obviously, it would also be valuable to know whether racial differences exist in the effectiveness of exercise in bringing about improvements in the lipoprotein profile.

Cooper Institute for Aerobics Study of Women Walking

A recently published study, designed to address the role of intensity in bringing about HDL changes in women, randomized 102 sedentary premenopausal women, 20 to 40 years of age, into one of four treatment groups, but only 59 of the women completed the trial: 16 aerobic walkers (8.0 km/hr), 12 brisk walkers (6.4 km/hr), 18 strollers (4.8 km/hr), and 13 sedentary controls.[36] All intervention groups walked 4.8 km/day, 5 days per week, on a tartan-surfaced, 1.6-km track for 24 weeks and showed minor weight gain over the course of the study, presumably because of increased lean mass, as evidenced by a minor decrease in percent body fat, which was significant in strollers versus controls. Controls gained 4.2 kg over the 24-week period, apparently because of an increase of body fat, such that they differed significantly in weight change compared with brisk walkers, who gained only 0.1 kg. Maximal oxygen consumption increased significantly versus control in the three intervention groups ($p<0.0001$) in a dose-response manner (aerobic walkers, 5.0 ml/kg per minute; brisk walkers, 3.0 ml/kg per minute; strollers, 1.4 ml/kg per minute; controls, -1.7 ml/kg per minute). HDL cholesterol was increased significantly ($p<0.05$) versus control in strollers (2.3 mg/dl) and aerobic walkers (2.5 mg/dl), although not in brisk walkers (1.3 mg/dl), demonstrating that vigorous exercise is not necessary to increase HDL significantly in premenopausal women.

Stanford-Sunnyvale Health Improvement Program (SSHIP)

Another recently published study, also designed to address the question of intensity, recruited older individuals from Sunnyvale, California, by a combination of random-digit dialing and general media campaign for a 1-year, community-based exercise training study.[37] After baseline measurements, 197 men and 160 postmenopausal women, aged 50 to 65 years, were randomly assigned to control, high-intensity, group-based exercise, high-intensity, home-based exercise, or low-intensity home-based exercise, with the high-intensity program defined as three 60-minute training sessions per week, each containing a 40-minute training period at 73–88% peak treadmill heart rate, and the low-intensity program defined as five 30-minute sessions per week at 60–73% maximum heart rate. Men started with a fitness level in a treadmill test of 30 ml/kg per minute, with test duration around 12.5 minutes, whereas women started at a mean of about 23 ml/kg per minute and duration of 9.0 minutes). Eighty-five percent of randomized individuals completed 1-year assessments. Adherence measures indicated that participants engaged in exercise at a level considerably above baseline, with no major differences between group (supervised) and home-based programs. Among the participants randomized to the three exercise conditions, VO_2 max increased by approximately 5% ($p<0.03$ vs. control) and treadmill duration increased by 14% between baseline and 1 year ($p<0.001$ vs. control), with no differences detected among the high- and low-intensity groups. There were no significant weight loss or body composition changes, as assessed by hydrostatic weighing. Neither men nor women in any of the intervention groups showed significant changes versus control in any lipoprotein variable, including HDL cholesterol and triglycerides. Because a large proportion of participants were recruited through a random-digit dialing method, this study population may be more representative of the population and less biased by self-selection factors than most studies in the literature, although it is likely that the primary motivation of participants who volunteered for our two weight loss studies was weight loss rather than an exercise program. It is important to understand that HDL cholesterol may not be easily raised by the level of exercise that the average individual in the population can comfortably accommodate, *particularly if weight loss is not achieved,* so that we do not set up false expectations with respect to lipoprotein changes for patients and participants in community exercise programs. On the other hand, the SSHIP investigators have reported that significant HDL increases were seen at the 2-year follow-up visit,[38] suggesting that an even longer period of time and greater frequency of exercise bouts might be needed to achieve such changes in older adults.

Summary and Future Directions

Cross-sectional studies generally show that physically active men and women have much lower plasma triglyceride and higher HDL-cholesterol concentrations than sedentary, age-matched controls, whereas total- and LDL-cholesterol levels tend to be lower in active versus sedentary people. A series of training studies conducted in our laboratory and studies by other investigators have demonstrated that exercise training generally does lead to increases in the HDL cholesterol levels and decreases in triglycerides; however, there is little evidence to support a causal relationship between activity and LDL cholesterol change, with the possible exception of changes in small, dense (more atherogenic) LDL particles. Thus, a consensus is slowly developing that exercise will lead to an improved lipoprotein profile, at least in individuals who readily take up an exercise program. Because exercise often is accompanied by weight loss, which also can result in HDL increases, depending on the fat/carbohydrate composition of the diet and degree of weight loss, it has been difficult to tease apart the role of increased muscle activity from that of body fat loss; however, it is likely that both factors play a major and independent role in exercise-induced lipoprotein changes.

An extremely important question to answer is whether exercise can benefit men and women who may particularly need to raise HDL, because of very low initial levels of this protective lipoprotein, or who should be highly encouraged to adopt a Step II NCEP diet, characterized by even further reduction of saturated fat, because of an unhealthy LDL cholesterol level, regardless of what it does to the HDL cholesterol levels. To address this, we are currently conducting a large 1-year trial, called the Diet and Exercise for Elevated (CHD) Risk (DEER) trial, in postmenopausal women, aged 45 to 64 years and men, aged 30 to 64 years, who are being recruited on the basis of having HDL cholesterol values in the bottom half of the population, as well as elevated LDL cholesterol within the NCEP cut-offs for dietary (before drug) treatment, to determine the best nonpharmacological approach to their lipoprotein management. The four treatments are exercise only, exercise combined with a Step II NCEP diet, Step II NCEP diet only, and control; the trial will be completed in 1995. We are particularly eager to determine whether similar results will be seen in postmenopausal women as those seen in the premenopausal SWCP-II women and whether the large proportion of men with HDL levels below 35 mg/dl, an independent risk factor in the NCEP algorithm, can be treated in a hygienic manner.

Acknowledgment

I would like to express my sincere appreciation and gratitude to my good friend and colleague, Peter D. Wood, DSc, PhD, for carefully reviewing the manuscript and providing helpful suggestions for its revision, as well as continuous collaborative support.

References

1. Consensus Development Conference: Lowering blood cholesterol to prevent heart disease. *JAMA* 1985;253:2080–2086

2. NIH Consensus Conference: Triglyceride, high-density lipoprotein, and coronary heart disease. *JAMA* 1993;269:505–510
3. Wood PD, Haskell WL: The effect of exercise on plasma high density lipoproteins. *Lipids* 1979;14:417–427
4. Wood PD, Williams PT, Haskell WL: Physical activity and high-density lipoproteins, in Miller NE, Miller GJ (eds): *Clinical and Metabolic Aspects of High-Density Lipoproteins.* Amsterdam: Elsevier Science Publishers, 1984, pp 133–165
5. Haskell WL: The influence of exercise on the concentrations of triglyceride and cholesterol in human plasma. *Exerc Sports Sci Rev* 1984;12:205–244
6. Haskell WL, Stefanick ML, Superko R: Influence of exercise on plasma lipids and lipoproteins, in Horton ES, Terjung RL (eds): *Exercise, Nutrition and Energy Metabolism.* New York: MacMillan Publishing Co, 1988, pp 213–227
7. Wood PD, Stefanick ML: Exercise, fitness, and atherosclerosis, in Bouchard C, Shephard RJ, Stephens T, Sutton JR, McPherson BD (eds): *Exercise, Fitness, and Health: A Consensus of Current Knowledge.* Champaign, IL: Human Kinetics Books, 1990, pp 409–423
8. Tran ZV, Weltman A, Glass GV, Mood DP: The effects of exercise on blood lipids and lipoproteins: a meta-analysis of studies. *Med Sci Sports Exerc* 1983:15;393–402
9. Tran ZV, Weltman A: Differential effects of exercise on serum lipid and lipoprotein levels seen with changes in body weight: a meta-analysis. *JAMA* 1985:245;919–924
10. Lokey EA, Tran Zu: Effects of exercise training on serum lipid and lipoprotein concentrations in women: a meta-analysis. *Int J Sports Med* 1989:10;424–429
11. Miller GJ, Miller NE: Plasma high-density lipoprotein concentration and development of ischemic heart disease. *Lancet* 1975;1:16–19
12. Wood PD, Haskell WL, Klein H, Lewis S, Stern MP, Farquhar JP: The distribution of plasma lipoproteins in middle-aged male runners. *Metabolism* 1976;25:1249–1257
13. Wood PD, Haskell WL: Plasma lipoprotein distributions in male and female runners. *Ann NY Acad Sci* 1977;301:748–763
14. Vodak PA, Wood PD, Haskell WL, Williams PT: HDL-cholesterol and other plasma lipoprotein concentrations in middle-aged male and female tennis players. *Metabolism* 1980:29;745–752
15. Nikkila EA, Kuusi T, Myllynen P: High density lipoprotein and apolipoprotein A-I during physical activity. *Atherosclerosis* 1980;37:457–462
16. Haskell WL, Taylor HL, Wood PD, Schrott H, Heiss G: Strenuous physical activity, treadmill exercise test performance and plasma high-density lipoprotein cholesterol: the Lipid Research Clinics Program Prevalence Study. *Circulation* 1980;62(suppl IV):IV-53–61
17. Hartung GH, Moore CE, Mitchell R, Kappus CM: Relationship of menopausal status and exercise level to HDL cholesterol in women. *Exp Aging Res* 1984;10:13–18
18. Williams PT, Krauss RM, Wood PD, et al: Lipoprotein subfractions of runners and sedentary men. *Metabolism* 1986;35:45–52

19. Stray-Gundersen J, Denke MA, Grundy SM: Influence of lifetime cross-country skiing on plasma lipids and lipoproteins. *Med Sci Sports Exerc* 1991;23:695–702

20. Wood PD, Haskell WL, Blair SN, Williams PT, Krauss RM, Lindgren FT, Albers JJ, Ho PH, Farquhar JW: Increased exercise level and plasma lipoprotein concentrations: a one-year, randomized, controlled study in sedentary, middle-aged men. *Metabolism* 1983;32:31–39

21. Williams PT, Wood PD, Haskell WL, Vranizan KM: The effects of running mileage and duration on plasma lipoprotein levels. *JAMA* 1982;247:2674–2679

22. Williams PT, Wood PD, Krauss RM, Vranizan KM, Blair SN, Terry R, Farquhar JW: Does weight loss cause the exercise-induced increase in plasma high density lipoproteins? *Atherosclerosis* 1983;47:173–185

23. Wood PD, Stefanick ML, Dreon DM, Frey-Hewitt B, Garay S, Williams PT, Superko HR, Fortmann SP, Albers JJ, Vranizan KM, Ellsworth NM, Terry RB, Haskell WL: Changes in plasma lipids and lipoproteins in overweight men during weight loss through dieting as compared with exercise. *N Engl J Med* 1988;319:1173–1179

24. Williams PT, Krauss RM, Vranizan KM, Wood PD: Changes in lipoprotein subfractions during diet-induced and exercise-induced weight loss in moderately overweight men. *Circulation* 1990;81:1293–1304

25. Stefanick ML, Frey-Hewitt B, Hoover CA, Terry RB, Wood PD: The effect of active weight loss achieved by dieting versus exercise on postheparin hepatic and lipoprotein lipase activity, in Wurtman RJ, Wurtman JJ (eds): *Human Obesity.* Ann NY Acad Sci 1987;499:338–339

26. Stefanick ML, Terry RB, Haskell WL, Wood PD: Relationships of changes in postheparin hepatic and lipoprotein lipase activity to HDL-cholesterol changes following weight loss achieved by dieting versus exercise, in Gallo LL (ed): *Cardiovascular Disease: Molecular and Cellular Mechanisms, Prevention, and Treatment.* New York, Plenum Press, 1987, pp 61–68

27. Kiens B, Lithell H: Lipoprotein metabolism influenced by training-induced changes in human skeletal muscle. *J Clin Invest* 1989;83:558–564

28. Stefanick ML, Wood PD: Physical activity, lipid and lipoprotein metabolism, and lipid transport, in Bouchard C, Shephard RJ, Stephens T (eds): *Physical Activity, Fitness and Health: 1992 Proceedings.* Champaign, IL: Human Kinetics Publishers, 1993, *in press*

29. Wood PD, Stefanick ML, Williams PT, Haskell WL: The effects on plasma lipoproteins of a prudent weight-reducing diet, with or without exercise, in overweight men and women. *N Engl J Med* 1991;325:461–466

30. Despres JP, Allard D, Tremblay A, Talbot J, Bouchard C: Evidence for a regional component of body fatness in the association with serum lipids in men and women. *Metabolism* 1985;34:967–973

31. Anderson AJ, Sobocinski KA, Freedman DS, Barboriak JJ, Rimm AA, Gruchow HW: Body fat distribution, plasma lipids, and lipoproteins. *Arteriosclerosis* 1988;8:88–94

32. Terry RB, Wood PD, Haskell WL, Stefanick ML, Krauss RM: Regional

patterns in relation to lipids, lipoprotein cholesterol, and lipoprotein subfraction mass in men. *J Clin Endocrinol Metab* 1989;68:191–199

33. Terry RB, Stefanick ML, Haskell WL, Wood PD: Contributions of regional adipose tissue depots to plasma lipoprotein concentrations in overweight men and women: possible protective effects of thigh fat. *Metabolism* 1991;40:733–740

34. Wing RR, Matthews KA, Kuller LH, Meilahn EN, Plantiga P: Waist to hip ratio in middle-aged women: associations with behavioral and psychosocial factors and with changes in cardiovascular risk factors. *Arterioscler Thromb* 1991;11:1250–1257

35. Stefanick ML: Exercise and weight control. *Exerc Sports Sci Rev* 1993;21:363–396

36. Duncan JJ, Gordon NF, Scott CB: Women walking for health and fitness: how much is enough? *JAMA* 1991;266:3295–3299

37. King AC, Haskell WL, Taylor CB, Kraemer HC, DeBusk RF: Group- vs home-based exercise training in healthy older men and women: a community-based clinical trial. *JAMA* 1991;266:1535–1542

38. King AC, Young DR, Oka RK, Haskell WL: Effects of exercise format and intensity on two-year health outcomes in the aging adult (abstract). *Gerontologist* 1992;32:190

Chapter 19

Genetics of the Response to Exercise and Training

Claude Bouchard, PhD

This chapter provides a brief overview of the genetics of the cardiovascular and metabolic response to exercise and of the adaptation to exercise training based on human studies. In general, genetic issues can be considered from two different perspectives. The first is from the genetic epidemiology perspective. Here, the evidence is derived from samples of humans, particularly families, large pedigrees, relatives by adoption, or twins. The data can be epidemiologic in nature, but may also include molecular markers. As in many other fields, the search for the genetic basis of the cardiovascular response to exercise or training has begun with familial aggregation and heritability studies and is gradually evolving to segregation, association, and linkage analyses.

The second perspective is molecular and pertains to transcription, translation, and regulatory mechanisms and how they adapt or come into play in response to various forms of acute exercise and training. In this case, the tissue (generally heart muscle or skeletal muscle) is "perturbed" by an acute or chronic stress and the changes are monitored. The emphasis therefore is on the molecular mechanisms involved in the adaptation.

Both approaches are useful in delineating how important genes are for a given phenotype. However, they differ considerably in the type of information they can provide. The first approach asks whether individual differences for a given phenotype are caused by DNA sequence variation, gene–environment interaction and gene–gene interaction seen among humans and, ultimately, what are the genes involved and the DNA sequence variants accounting for the

From Fletcher GF, (ed): *Cardiovascular Response to Exercise.* Mount Kisco, NY, Futura Publishing Company, Inc., © 1994.

heterogeneity in phenotype. The second approach relies heavily on animal models with a focus on the role of various DNA sequences on regulatory mechanisms with no particular interest for the differences that may exist among the members of the strain or of the species.

Both perspectives are useful and progressively converging. They both can contribute to the understanding of the biological basis of the response to exercise and training. The genetic epidemiology approach is of particular interest to us because it deals with individual differences caused by DNA sequence variation. Results available from the genetic epidemiology perspective therefore will constitute most of this chapter.

Response to Exercise

An assessment of the importance of genetic variation in the response to exercise among sedentary but otherwise healthy people can be made from the data available on submaximal power output, maximal oxygen uptake, heart size, muscle fiber type distribution, glycolytic and aerobic-oxidative markers of skeletal muscle metabolism, lipid mobilization from adipose cells, indicators of substrates oxidized, and so forth. Heritability of these phenotypes is generally low (about 25% or less) and rarely exceeds 50%.[1,2] The genetic effect seems to be polygenic with no evidence to date for single gene effects. A weak maternal effect has been reported for only one phenotype, namely $\dot{V}O_2$max per kg body weight.[3] Table 1 summarizes the currently available data on familial resemblance and heritability levels as defined in a recent review on this topic.[1]

Response to Exercise Training

The participants in the studies reviewed thus far were mainly sedentary and thus unchallenged by the demands of regular exercise. Under a sedentary state, individual differences likely are influenced less by DNA variants that affect gene expression, as opposed to a situation in which people are under the stress of large increases in metabolic rate. Thus, it would seem reasonable to suggest that genetic differences may become more striking when sedentary persons are exposed to regular exercise.[4]

Research has amply demonstrated that aerobic performance, stroke volume, skeletal muscle oxidative capacity, and lipid oxidation are phenotypes that can adapt to training. For instance, the $\dot{V}O_2$max of sedentary persons increases, on the average, by about 25% after a few months of training. The skeletal muscle oxidative potential can easily increase by 50% with training and, at times, it may even double. However, if one is to consider a role for the genotype in such responses to training, there must be evidence of individual differences in trainability. There is now considerable support for this concept.[4,5] Some indications about the extent of individual differences in the response of maximal oxygen uptake to training are given in Table 2.[6] The same training program applied to 17 young men resulted in almost no change in $\dot{V}O_2$max for some, whereas others gained as much as 1 l of O_2 uptake. Such differences in trainability cannot be accounted for by age (all participants were young adults, 17–29 years of age) or gender. The initial (pretraining) level accounted for about 25% of the variance in the response of $\dot{V}O_2$ max; the lower the initial level the greater the increase with training.

Similar individual differences were observed for other relevant phenotypes such as indicators of endurance, oxidative markers of

TABLE 1. A Summary of Recent Research on Familial Resemblance and Heritability of Phenotypes of Interest

	Familial Resemblance[a]	Heritability[b]
PWC_{150}/kg	+	<10
$\dot{V}O_2$max/kg	+	<25[c]
Heart dimensions	+ +	<25
Max O_2 Pulse	+ +	>50
Skeletal muscle		
Fiber-type proportion	+ +	[d]
Oxidative potential	+ +	<50
Lipid oxidation rate	+ +	>25[e]
Lipid mobilization rate	+ +	>50

[a]Significant familial concentration = + ; very significant familial concentration = + + .
[b]Expressed as a percent of the age- and gender-adjusted phenotypic variance.
[c]Twin studies with small sample size have generally reported values of 50% and higher.
[d]Reported values are discordant with a range of 6–100%.
[e]At submaximal exercise, but zero at maximal exercise intensity.

TABLE 2.   Maximal O_2 Uptake in Liters Before Training and the Response to Training in Young Adult Men

	Pretraining phenotype		Changes in phenotype			
	Mean	SD	Mean	SD	Min	Max
Québec (n = 17)[a]	2.9	0.42	0.63	0.25	0.13	1.03
Arizona (n = 29)[b]	3.4	0.57	0.42	0.22	0.06	0.95

[a]Men were trained for 20 weeks following the procedures described earlier. See ref. 6.
[b]Men were trained for 12 weeks, 3 times per week, 40 minutes per session, at onset of blood lactate accumulation (OBLA) (about 70–77% of $\dot{V}O_2$max). See ref. 6.
SD, standard deviation; min, minimum; max, maximum.

skeletal muscle oxidative metabolism, adipose tissue lipolytic characteristics and lipoprotein lipase activity, relative ratio of lipid and carbohydrate oxidized, fasting glucose and insulin levels as well as their response to a glucose challenge, and fasting plasma lipids and lipoproteins.[1,4,7–9] In summary, all these phenotypes respond to regular exercise in young adults of both sexes. However, there are considerable individual differences in the response of these biological markers to exercise training: some exhibit a high responder pattern whereas others are almost nonresponders. There is a whole range of response phenotypes between these two extremes.

What is the main cause of the individuality in the response to training? We believe that it has to do with as yet unidentified genetic characteristics.[4] To test this hypothesis, we performed several different training studies with pairs of identical [monozygotic (MZ)] twins. Our rationale is that the response pattern can be observed for individuals who have the same genotype (within pairs) and for persons with differing genetic characteristics (between pairs). We have concluded from these studies that the individuality in trainability of cardiovascular fitness phenotypes and in response to exercise training of cardiovascular risk factors is highly familial and most likely genetically determined. Table 3 summarizes some of the evidence pertaining to the response to exercise training of several phenotypes relevant to this topic.[1,2] The data are expressed in terms of the ratio of the variance between genotypes to that within genotypes in the response to standardized training conditions. The

TABLE 3. Importance of the Between-genotypes Variance with Respect to the Within-genotype Variance in the Phenotype Response to Training.

Phenotype	Approximate F Ratio
Submaximal power output[b]	2:4
$\dot{V}O_2$max	6:9
Muscle fiber composition	1:2
Muscle oxidative potential	2:5
Lipid substrate oxidation	2:5
Lipid mobilization	5:10

[a]Summary based on several studies reported from our laboratory.
[b]Physical working capacity phenotypes or ventilatory threshold data.
The evidence is summarized in terms of F ratios of the two variance components.[a]

similarity of the training response among members of the same MZ pair is illustrated in Figure 1 for the $\dot{V}O_2$max phenotype.[10] In this case, 10 pairs of MZ twins were subjected to a fully standardized and laboratory controlled training program for 20 weeks; gains of absolute $\dot{V}O_2$max showed almost 8 times more variance between pairs than within pairs.

Over a period of several years, 26 pairs of MZ twins were trained in our laboratory with standardized endurance and high-intensity cycle exercise programs for periods of 15 or 20 weeks.[1] After 10 weeks of training, the twins were exercising 5 times per week, 45 minutes per session at the same relative intensity in each program. These training programs caused significant increases in $\dot{V}O_2$max and other indicators of aerobic performance. They also were associated with a decrease in the intensity of the cardiovascular and metabolic responses at a given submaximal power output. For instance, when exercising in relative steady state at 50 watts, there were decreases in heart rate, oxygen uptake, pulmonary ventilation, ventilatory equivalent of oxygen and in respiratory quotient with an increase in oxygen pulse. These various metabolic improvements were, however, all characterized by a significant within-pair resemblance.[1] The results are particularly interesting for the respiratory quotient. Thus, despite the fact that twins were subjected to similar training regimens, individuals with the same genotypes were more similar in the changes with training for the pattern of substrates oxidized at a low power output level than those with different

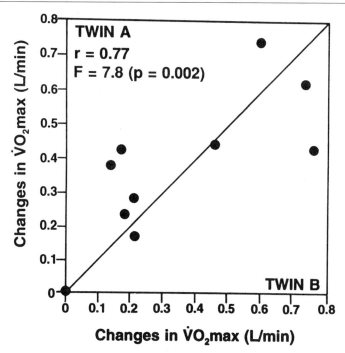

Changes in V̇O₂max (L/min)

FIGURE 1. *Intrapair resemblance (intraclass coefficient) in 10 pairs of MZ twins for training changes in V̇O₂max (liters of O₂/minute) after 20 weeks of endurance training. Constructed from the original data in Reference 10.*

genotypes. These results would seem to suggest that there may be an inherited tendency for some individuals to oxidize more lipid than carbohydrate substrates with training under similar conditions.[1]

The adipose tissue metabolism response to training has not been studied to any significant extent. Only one study has dealt with the isolated fat cell lipolysis from the suprailiac depot in eight pairs of MZ twins who took part in a 20-week endurance training program.[7] Changes with training in epinephrine-stimulated lipolysis were highly similar within MZ pairs, as shown by the intraclass coefficients ranging from 0.84 to 0.94. In addition, the changes brought about by regular endurance exercise in activities of key enzymes of skeletal muscle oxidative metabolism also have been hardly investigated.[8,9] We have shown that there were 2 to 5 times more variances between identical twin pairs than within pairs in the response of these enzymes assayed from biopsies of the vastus lateralis muscle before and after a standardized 15-week cycle ergometer training program.[9]

Response of Cardiovascular Risk Factors to Regular Exercise

Nonpharmacological interventions designed to improve the cardiovascular risk profile center around the cessation of smoking, weight loss by means of dietary restriction and at times regular physical activity, dietary modifications aimed at fat, sodium, and fiber intake, and regular exercise to improve health-related fitness. Among the expected changes associated with a regular exercise regimen, one finds in a group of sedentary and unfit adults a decrease in resting heart rate and blood pressure, a reduction in fasting plasma insulin level and in its response to a glucose load, a decrease in plasma triglycerides and, occasionally, in low-density lipoprotein (LDL) cholesterol and total cholesterol, and an increase in plasma high-density lipoprotein (HDL) cholesterol. Little is known about the individual differences in the response of these important clinical markers to regular exercise and about the role of genetic variation. We have used the MZ twin design to explore these issues in two studies. In one experiment, six pairs of young adult male MZ twins exercised on the cycle ergometer 2 hours per day for 22 consecutive days.[11] The mean intensity of training reached 58% of $\dot{V}O_2$max and the program was designed to induce an energy deficit of about 1,000 kcal/day. Baseline energy intake was assessed and prescribed for the 22 days of the training program. The diet prescription was fully enforced for each person in the metabolic ward where they lived for the duration of the experiment. The program induced a significant increase in $\dot{V}O_2$max and a significant decrease in body fat content. Significant changes were observed in fasting plasma insulin and in the insulin response to an oral glucose tolerance test.[12] Plasma triglycerides, total cholesterol, LDL cholesterol and apo B as well as the HDL cholesterol to total cholesterol ratio also were modified.[13] Moreover, significant within-MZ-pair resemblance was observed for the response of fasting plasma insulin, and LDL cholesterol, HDL cholesterol, and HDL cholesterol to total cholesterol ratio.

Given the above results, a more extensive investigation of the changes brought about by regular exercise and of the role of genetic variation in response was clearly warranted. To this end, seven pairs of male MZ twins completed a 100-day negative energy balance protocol during which they exercised on cycle ergometers to expend about 1,000 kcal/day above resting metabolic rate while energy intake was kept constant.[14] The participants had a day of rest from the exercise protocol every 10 days. Mean body weight loss was 5.0 kg and it was entirely accounted for by fat mass (4.9 kg from underwater weighing). Body energy content was reduced by about 46,000 kcal. $\dot{V}O_2$max was augmented significantly by the program. Considerable individual differences were observed in response to the negative energy balance and exercise protocol for resting heart rate, systolic and diastolic blood pressure, fasting insulin level and insulin action assessed from a euglycemic–hyperinsulinemic clamp procedure, and plasma lipids and lipoproteins. Indications of a significant MZ twin resemblance in response to the protocol were found for body weight, body fat mass, subcutaneous fat, abdominal visceral fat assessed by computerized tomography, glucose disposal rate at submaximal insulin levels, plasma triglyceride and total cholesterol levels, as well as for several markers of triglyceride and cholesterol transport. No twin resemblances, however, were found for resting heart rate, blood pressure, or fasting insulin level.

Conclusion

The role of inherited differences in the response to acute exercise and in the response to regular physical activity needs to be considered for a proper understanding of the role of exercise in preventive and therapeutic programs. Genetic epidemiology studies reported thus far reveal that the heritability level of many phenotypes relevant to cardiovascular health is significant and in the range of 25–50% of the age- and gender-adjusted variance. Exercise training experiments undertaken with MZ twins indicate that although there are large interindividual differences in response to regular exercise, persons with the same gene complement exhibit a more homogeneous response pattern than persons who are genetically unrelated. This genotype dependency is seen not only for the cardiovascular adaptation to exercise training but also for the modifications in several of the common cardiovascular risk factors. The major tasks that lie ahead are 1) to document further the phenomenon of the individual differences in response to exercise training, 2) to pursue the efforts aimed at establishing the familiarity of the responder phenotypes, and 3) to identify the genes that are responsible for the variation in response for the phenotypes of interest for cardiovascular health.

References

1. Bouchard C, Dionne FT, Simoneau JA, Boulay MR: Genetics of aerobic and anaerobic performances. *Exerc Sport Sci Rev* 1992;20:27–58
2. Bouchard C: Genetic determinants of endurance performance, in Astrand PO, Shephard RJ (eds): *The Olympic Book of Endurance in Sports*. Oxford, Blackwell Scientific Publications, 1992, pp 149–159
3. Lesage R, Simoneau JA, Jobin J, Leblanc C, Bouchard C: Familial resemblance in maximal heart rate, blood lactate and aerobic power. *Hum Hered* 1985;35:182–189
4. Bouchard C: Genetics of aerobic power and capacity, in Malina RM, Bouchard C (eds): *Sport and Human Genetics*. Champaign, IL, Human Kinetics, 1986, pp 59–88
5. Lortie G, Simoneau JA, Hamel P, Boulay MR, Landry F, Bouchard C: Responses of maximal aerobic power and capacity to aerobic training. *Int J Sports Med* 1984;5:232–236
6. Dionne FT, Turcotte, L, Thibault MC, Boulay MR, Skinner JS, Bouchard C: Mitochondrial DNA sequence-polymorphism, VO$_2$max, and response to endurance training. *Med Sci Sports Exerc* 1991;23: 177–185
7. Després JP, Bouchard C, Savard R, Prud'homme D, Bukowiecki L, Theriault G: Adaptive changes to training in adipose tissue lipolysis are genotype dependent. *Int J Obes* 1984;8:87–95
8. Hamel P, Simoneau JA, Lortie G, Boulay MR, Bouchard C: Heredity and muscle adaptation to endurance training. *Med Sci Sports Exerc* 1986;18:690–696
9. Simoneau JA, Lortie G, Boulay MR, Marcotte M, Thibault MC, Bouchard C: Inheritance of human skeletal muscle and anaerobic capacity adaptation to high-intensity intermittent training. *Int J Sports Med* 1986;7:167–171
10. Prud'homme D, Bouchard C, Leblanc C, Landry F, Fontaine E: Sensitivity of maximal aerobic power to training is genotype-dependent. *Med Sci Sports Exerc* 1984;16:489–493
11. Poehlman ET, Tremblay A, Nadeau A, Dussault J, Thériault G, Bouchard C: Heredity and changes in hormones and metabolic rates with short-term training. *Am J Physiol (Endocrinol Metab)* 1986;250:E711–E717

12. Tremblay A, Poehlman E, Nadeau A, Pérusse L, Bouchard C: Is the response of plasma glucose and insulin to short-term exercise-training genetically determined? *Horm Metab Res* 1987;19:65–67

13. Després JP, Moorjani S, Tremblay A, Poehlman ET, Lupien PJ, Nadeau A, Bouchard C: Heredity and changes in plasma lipids and lipoproteins after short-term exercise training in men. *Arteriosclerosis* 1988;8:402–409

14. Bouchard C, Tremblay A, Després JP, Thériault G, Nadeau A, Lupien PJ, Moorjani S: The response to exercise with constant energy intake in identical twins (abstract). *FASEB J* 1992;6:A1647

Part 6

Clinical Applications

Chapter 20

Role of Exercise Conditioning in Patients with Severe Systolic Left Ventricular Dysfunction

Martin J. Sullivan, MD

Research in cardiac rehabilitation over the past 3 decades has focused primarily on patients with coronary artery disease with preserved left ventricular (LV) systolic function who are either status post–myocardial infarction or have chronic stable angina. In this group, exercise conditioning leads to an increased work rate at the angina threshold,[1,2] favorable alterations in blood lipids,[1,3] improved peak $\dot{V}o_2$,[4–7] and a potential decrease in mortality and reinfarction rates.[8] Recent studies combining diet and exercise[9] or diet, exercise, and stress management[10] have demonstrated a delay in the progression of atherosclerosis and a reduction in exercise-induced ischemia[9] and angina,[10] highlighting the potentially important role of exercise and risk factor modification in treating this disorder. Because it has been traditionally held that exercise was contraindicated in patients with severe LV systolic dysfunction and congestive heart failure (CHF), it has been only in the last decade that the effects of exercise training have been examined in these patients. The results of numerous studies now indicate that stable patients with CHF caused by systolic LV dysfunction can safely participate in cardiac rehabilitation programs and can improve peak

Supported by Grant HL-17670 from the National Heart, Lung and Blood Institute, Bethesda, Maryland, by General Medical Research Funds from the Veterans Administration Medical Center, Durham, North Carolina, and by Grant M01-RR-30, Division of Research Resources, General Clinical Research Centers Program, NIH. Dr. Sullivan is supported by a Grant-in-Aid and Established Investigator award from the American Heart Association.

From Fletcher GF, (ed): *Cardiovascular Response to Exercise*. Mount Kisco, NY, Futura Publishing Company, Inc., © 1994.

$\dot{V}o_2$ and symptoms after exercise training.[11–21] This chapter focuses on the physiology of exercise training in patients with severe systolic LV dysfunction and examines current issues in the clinical application of cardiac rehabilitation in this high-risk subset of patients.

Training in Normal Persons

Long-term aerobic conditioning is associated with a number of important physiological adaptations in normal persons[22–24] that may be beneficial in patients with cardiac diseases. Exercise training leads to an improvement in both submaximal[25] and maximal[22–24] exercise performance in normal persons, favorably affects blood lipid levels,[26] and may act to delay the development of coronary artery disease.[27] Improved exercise tolerance in normal persons is mediated through both central hemodynamic changes including increased stroke volume and peripheral adaptations. During submaximal exercise after training, cardiac output is unchanged whereas blood lactate levels are reduced. This is associated with increased aerobic enzyme content, glycogen content and capillary density in skeletal muscle,[28] and decreased circulating catecholamine levels during submaximal exercise.[29] At peak exercise in normal persons some,[23,24] but not all,[22] studies report an increase in cardiac output mediated through an increase in stroke volume without a change in peak heart rate. This increase in stroke volume is caused by an increase in LV end-diastolic volume (EDV), as indices of LV systolic performance such as ejection fraction do not increase with training. Although strenuous exercise training in elite athletes may lead to cardiac hypertrophy,[30] it appears that many of the effects on LV volumes after training reflect the use of the Frank-Starling mechanism. It is likely that most of the increase in stroke volume after training is caused by an increased plasma volume and total body hemoglobin coupled with a more efficient "muscle pump" to facilitate venous return during intense exercise. This concept is supported by the rapid decrease in stroke volume that is noted after deconditioning in normal persons,[31] which is not accompanied by changes in cardiac wall thickness.

Training in Patients with Coronary Artery Disease

Studies have demonstrated that exercise training in patients with coronary artery disease leads to an increase in peak oxygen consumption, a training bradycardia, and an increase in peak arteriovenous oxygen difference.[4–7] Although exercise stroke volume may improve in selected patients after 12 months of intense exercise training,[14] most studies have not demonstrated an improvement in stroke volume, LV ejection fraction, or intracardiac filling pressures after training.[4–7,11,12] Thus, peripheral adaptations that lead to more efficient oxygen extraction including an increase in peak muscle blood flow[7] and increased aerobic enzyme content in skeletal muscle[32] play an important role in the response to training in patients with coronary artery disease and preserved systolic LV function. Although patients with coronary artery disease may achieve a relative improvement in peak exercise performance that is similar to that seen in age-matched normal persons, this has not been the primary goal of exercise training in these patients. Much of the research in this group of patients has been aimed at reducing risk factors, increasing anginal threshold, and potentially decreasing mortality and reinfarction rates.[1,3,8–10] In contrast, in ambulatory patients with chronic heart failure, exertional dyspnea and fatigue are important causes of morbidity and loss of work, making improved submaximal and maximal exercise tolerance the primary end point of exercise training in these patients.

Exercise Physiology in Patients with Severe Systolic LV Dysfunction

Recent studies in patients with severe systolic LV dysfunction suggest that exercise intolerance is due primarily to the early onset of anaerobic metabolism in skeletal muscle.[33–39] Two factors have been identified that may contribute to this response in patients: reduced muscle perfusion during exercise[33,35] and alteration in skeletal muscle histology and biochemistry, which include decreased aerobic enzyme content,[36,38,39] decreased Type I fiber content,[36,39] reduced mitochondrial volume density,[39] and decreased capillarization.[36,39]

Previous studies using ^{31}P-MRI have demonstrated that early anaerobic metabolism occurs independent of reduced blood flow[40,41] and is not due solely to skeletal muscle atrophy.[42,43] Studies in our laboratory have demonstrated that lactate appearance at a given submaximal work rate in patients with severe LV systolic dysfunction and CHF is not closely related to muscle blood flow but is inversely related to aerobic enzyme content in skeletal muscle ($r = -0.74$, $p = 0.02$) (Figure 1). These data suggest that intrinsic alteration in skeletal muscle histology and biochemsitry play an important role in determining exercise tolerance in this disorder.

Although increased intrapulmonary pressures may be impor-

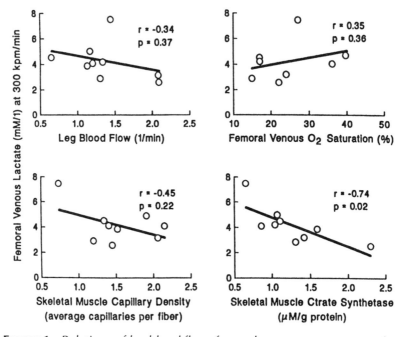

FIGURE 1. *Relations of leg blood flow, femoral venous oxygen saturation, skeletal muscle capillary density, and citrate synthetase to femoral venous blood lactate at 300 kpm/min in patients with chronic heart failure. r = correlation coefficient. Reproduced from Reference 37 with permission.*

tant in producing dyspnea in acute heart failure, several lines of evidence indicate that this is not the primary factor limiting exercise in stable ambulatory patients with chronic heart failure. Massie et al.[35] have demonstrated no relationship between peak exercise pulmonary capillary wedge pressure and peak $\dot{V}o_2$ in patients with chronic heart failure. In examining ventilatory control in this disorder,[44] we have demonstrated that during short-term maximal exercise in patients with CHF that 70% are limited by leg fatigue and that increased pulmonary dead space and ventilation during exercise are related to decreased cardiac output and not to increased pulmonary wedge pressures. As illustrated in Figure 2, pulmonary wedge pressures are not higher in patients limited by dyspnea versus those limited by fatigue, suggesting that exertional dyspnea is not due primarily to pulmonary venous congestion in this disorder. The concept that the skeletal muscle metabolic response to exercise plays the primary role in determining exercise tolerance in this disorder provides a physiological rationale for using exercise train-

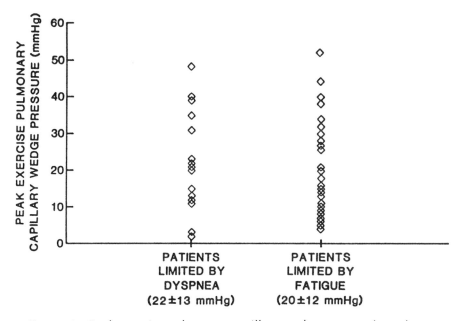

FIGURE 2. *Peak exercise pulmonary capillary wedge pressure in patients limited by dyspnea versus those limited by fatigue. Data from Sullivan et al.[18]*

ing as a potential means to improve exertional symptoms in patients with chronic heart failure.

Exercise Training in Patients with Severe LV Dysfunction

Although a small number of patients with severe systolic LV dysfunction have been included in earlier training studies,[12,14] it has been in only the last 10 years that research has been directed specifically at examining the training response in this group of patients. Lee et al.[13] were the first to report the effects of exercise training in patients with impaired LV dysfunction caused by coronary artery disease. Eighteen patients with LV ejection fractions less than 0.40 underwent exercise testing and cardiac catheterization before and after 12 to 42 months of physical conditioning. Peak exercise capacity increased significantly, and there were no changes in LV dimensions or intracardiac pressures after exercise training. Studies from our institution by Conn et al.[15] demonstrated an increase in peak exercise capacity in patients with LV ejection fractions of 13% to 25% after 4 to 37 months of exercise conditioning, which was accompanied by an increase in peak exercise oxygen pulse with no exercise-related complications. Studies by Kellerman et al.[45] and Hoffman et al.[46] also have demonstrated an increase in peak exercise performance after training in patients with LV dysfunction and have noted no change in LV ejection fraction or alterations in wall motion abnormalities with no exercise-related morbidity.

Recent studies in our laboratory[17,18] have examined the effects of 4 to 6 months of exercise conditioning in patients with Class I–III CHF caused by systolic LV dysfunction (LV ejection fraction $24 \pm 10\%$). Before and after training, patients underwent maximal graded bicycle exercise with measurement of expired gases. Before exercise a catheter was introduced into the right pulmonary artery for measurement of central hemodynamics, a thermodilution catheter was positioned in the femoral vein for measurement of leg blood flow, and a cannula was introduced into the brachial artery. At rest and at each work load, blood was drawn for determination of oxygen content and lactate. Hemodynamic measurements included right atrial pressure, pulmonary, and pulmonary wedge pressures, leg blood flow by thermodilution, and cardiac output by the direct Fick technique. Radionuclide angiography was performed at rest and at each work load using a gated equilibrium technique to determine LV ejection fraction. Left ventricular end-diastolic volume (EDV) and end-systolic volume (ESV) were calculated from the Fick stroke volume and the radionuclide ejection fraction.

Four patients did not complete the exercise training program and were excluded from analysis, one had sudden death unrelated to exercise, and one had worsening heart failure. Patients exercised for 4.1 ± 0.6 hours per week and improved both functional class from 2.4 ± 0.6 to 1.3 ± 0.7 ($p<0.01$) and peak exercise work load from 520 ± 105 to 613 ± 119 kpm/min ($p = 0.02$). Peak $\dot{V}o_2$ (Figure 3A) increased from 1.11 ± 0.33 l/min (16.8 ± 3.7 ml/kg per minute) to 1.40 ± 0.40 l/min (20.6 ± 4.7 ml/kg per minute) (both $p<0.01$) after training. Cardiac output was unchanged during submaximal exercise (Figure 3B), but demonstrated a tendency to increase at maximal exercise from 8.9 ± 2.9 to 9.9 ± 3.2 l/min ($p = 0.13$). Heart

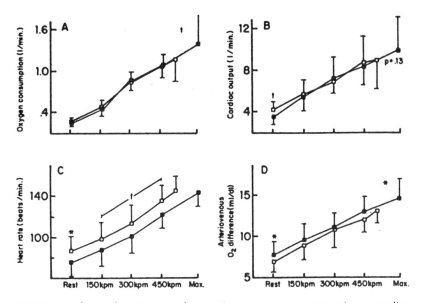

FIGURE 3. *Plots of resting and exercise oxygen consumption, cardiac output, heart rate, and systemic arteriovenous oxygen difference in patients before (open boxes) and after (closed boxes) training. *p<0.05; +p<0.01 by Wilcoxon signed rank test. Reproduced from Reference 17 with permission.*

rate (Figure 3C) was reduced at rest and during submaximal exercise but did not change at maximal exercise. Systemic arteriovenous oxygen ($A\dot{V}O_2$) difference (Figure 3D) was increased at rest, unchanged during submaximal exercise, and increased at peak exercise from 13.1 ± 1.4 to 14.6 ± 2.3 ml/dl ($p<0.05$). Resting and exercise arterial, right atrial, pulmonary capillary wedge, and pulmonary artery pressures were unchanged after training. Stroke volume was unchanged at rest but tended to increase during exercise, although these changes did not reach statistical significance ($p = 0.12$). Resting and exercise LV ejection fraction, LVESV, and LVEDV were not altered significantly by training, and there were no changes in rest or exercise wall motion abnormalities.

Leg blood flow, leg oxygen delivery, leg vascular resistance, and leg $A\dot{V}O_2$ difference (Figure 4) did not change at rest or during submaximal exercise after training. Blood flow to the single leg (Figure 4A) increased at peak exercise from 2.5 ± 0.7 to 3.0 ± 0.8 l/min ($p<0.01$), as did leg oxygen delivery (Figure 4B). There was a

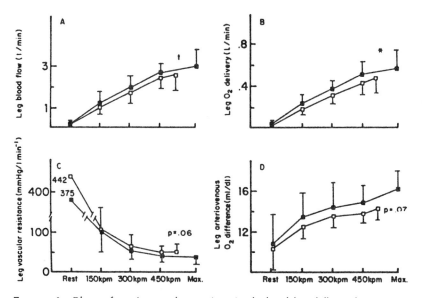

FIGURE 4. *Plots of resting and exercise single leg blood flow, leg oxygen delivery, leg vascular resistance, and leg $A\dot{V}O^2$ difference in patients before (open boxes) and after (closed boxes) training.* $^*p<0.05$; $^+p<0.01$ *by Wilcoxon signed rank test. Reproduced from Reference 17 with permission.*

tendency for leg vascular resistance (Figure 4C) to decrease ($p = 0.06$) and leg A$\dot{\text{V}}\text{o}_2$ difference (Figure 4D) to increase at peak exercise (14.5 ± 1.3 vs. 16.1 ± 1.9 ml/dl; $p = 0.07$). Thus, single-leg $\dot{\text{V}}\text{o}_2$, determined using the Fick principle, increased from 0.36 ± 0.11 to 0.47 ± 0.13 l/min ($p < 0.01$) at peak exercise.

Arterial and femoral venous lactate concentrations were reduced markedly during submaximal exercise (Figures 5A and 5B) but were unchanged at rest or maximal exercise after training. Similarly, training decreased femoral arteriovenous lactate difference and leg lactate production during submaximal exercise (Figures 5C and 5D) without changing these variables at rest or maximal exercise. The $\dot{\text{V}}\text{o}_2$ at which the ventilatory anaerobic threshold occurred, assessed by blinded inspection of breath-by-breath data using the ventilatory equivalents method, increased from 10.1 ± 1.2 to 12.1 ± 2.6 ml/kg per minute ($p < 0.01$) (Figure 6). This was accompanied by an increase in exercise time at a fixed submaximal work

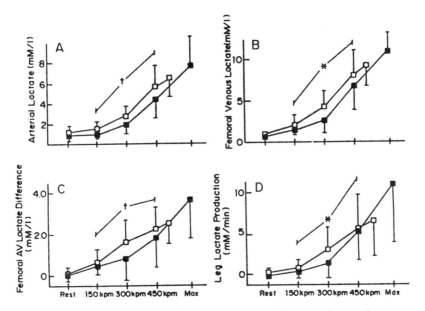

FIGURE 5. *Plots of resting and exercise arterial lactate, femoral venous lactate, femoral arteriovenous lactate difference, and leg lactate production in patients before (open boxes) and after (closed boxes) training. *$p < 0.05$; $^+p < 0.01$ by Wilcoxon signed rank test. Reprinted from Reference 17 with permission.*

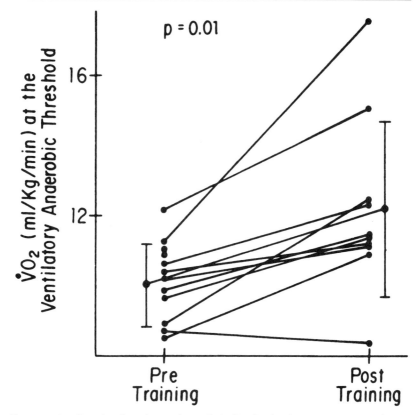

FIGURE 6. *Graph showing plot of individual changes in ventilatory anaerobic threshold with exercise training in 12 patients with chronic heart failure. Reproduced from Reference 18 with permission.*

rate from 938 ± 410 to $1,429 \pm 691$ seconds. During this submaximal endurance fixed work rate protocol there was a decrease in heart rate (Figure 7A) with no change in $\dot{V}O_2$ (Figure 7B). Ventilatory variables including $\dot{V}CO_2$, RER, ventilation and $VE/\dot{V}CO_2$ were all decreased during this fixed work rate protocol after training (Figures 7C–7F). There was no relationship between the change in peak $\dot{V}O_2$ after exercise training and any hemodynamic variable measured during the baseline exercise study. Specifically, the rest and peak exercise LV ejection fraction, stroke volume, cardiac output, $\dot{V}O_2$, systemic $A\dot{V}O_2$ difference, leg $A\dot{V}O_2$ difference, and femoral vein oxygen saturation were all unrelated to the response to training.

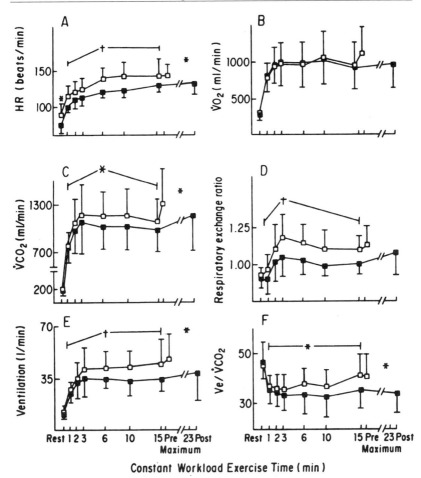

Constant Workload Exercise Time (min)

FIGURE 7. *Plots of resting and exercise heart rate, $\dot{V}O^2$, $\dot{V}CO^2$, respiratory exchange ratio, ventilation, and ventilation to $\dot{V}CO^2$ ratio before (open square) and after (blackened square) exercise training in nine patients with chronic heart failure during the constant workload exercise study. HR, heart rate; Ve, ventilation. *$p<0.05$; +$p<0.01$ by the Wilcoxon's signed rank test. Reproduced from Reference 18 with permission.*

Although our study was uncontrolled, the results indicate that exercise training may improve both submaximal and maximal exercise capacity in patients with mild to moderate heart failure and systolic LV dysfunction. Improved peak cardiac output contributed to improved peak $\dot{V}O_2$ in some patients, although peripheral adaptations including increased skeletal muscle vascular conductance and oxygen extraction and decreased skeletal muscle lactate production were primarily responsible for the training effect in our patients. Previous studies have identified markedly reduced aerobic enzyme content in skeletal muscle in patients with this disorder;[36,38,39] it is possible that exercise training may act, in part, by reversing these biochemical alterations and increasing aerobic enzyme activity in skeletal muscle.[32]

This concept is supported by a recent study by Minotti et al.,[34] which examined forearm metabolism by ^{31}P-NMR before and after one-arm training in five patients with chronic heart failure. The slope of the increase in the ratio of inorganic phosphate to phosphocreatine during exercise was lower after training, thus indicating a delay in anaerobic metabolism. This was accompanied by no changes in forearm muscle mass or blood flow, suggesting that biochemical alterations in skeletal muscle led to improved exercise performance. An important recent study by Coats et al.[19] also has examined exercise training in patients with chronic heart failure (LV ejection fraction $16 \pm 8\%$) employing a crossover design with the investigators blinded to training status. Patients demonstrated a significant improvement in peak $\dot{V}O_2$ and a decrease in heart rate during submaximal exercise after training. Sympathetic nervous system activation as indicated by power spectral analysis and radiolabeled norepinephrine spillover studies at rest was decreased after training. Symptom scores, assessed by a modified Likert questionnaire, also were improved in patients after training. In addition, these authors demonstrated a decrease in peak $\dot{V}O_2$ back to baseline after a period of detraining, indicating that improved peak $\dot{V}O_2$ was not due solely to familiarization with the exercise protocol. The finding that neuroendocrine activation is reduced in patients with CHF suggests that long-term exercise actually may decrease afterload and thereby delay progressive LV dysfunction in this disorder.

Previous studies in our laboratory[12,17] and by others[11,45,46] have demonstrated no change in LV ejection fraction or resting wall motion abnormalities after exercise training in patients with severe LV systolic dysfunction. Although Jugdutt et al.[47] have suggested that ventricular dilation and shape distortion may occur with exercise in patients with recent anterior myocardial infarction, Gianuzzi et al.[20] in a controlled trial found no adverse effects of exercise in this high-risk subgroup of patients. This group examined LV geometry by two-dimensional echocardiography in 49 patients after anterior myocardial infarction. Patients were randomized to aerobic exercise training or a nonexercising control group 4 to 10 weeks after infarction and followed for 6 months. Patients in the training group significantly improved both peak $\dot{V}o_2$ and the $\dot{V}o_2$ at which the anaerobic threshold occurred. In both treatment and control groups patients with LV ejection fractions <0.40 demonstrated an increase in EDV with a worsening of percent of diameter with wall motion abnormalities and shape distortion index after 6 months of follow-up. It is important to note that there were no differences in changes in ventricular geometry in the two groups, indicating that ventricular dilation occurs after extensive anterior myocardial infarction, which is not adversely affected by exercise conditioning.

Arvan[48] examined the exercise training response in 85 patients with coronary artery disease and subdivided them into four groups based on high or low LV ejection fraction (> or <0.40) and the presence or absence of a positive exercise treadmill test for ischemia. Patient groups with an LVEF >0.40 with or without ischemia and those with an LVEF <0.40 without ischemia all demonstrated a training effect as indicated by an increase in peak $\dot{V}o_2$ and a decrease in submaximal exercise heart rate. Patients with severe LV systolic dysfunction and ischemia did not demonstrate a training effect, although 5 of 11 had angina on the post-training exercise test, which may have limited the utility of peak $\dot{V}o_2$ measurements. These results suggest that high-risk patients with a reduced LV ejection fraction and significant ongoing ischemia may not achieve a benefit from exercise training.

Summary

Based on recent studies and the experience at our institution[12,15,17,18] and others,[13,16–21,45,46,49] it appears that medically stable patients with moderate heart failure and severe systolic LV dysfunction may benefit from participation in long-term aerobic exercise conditioning programs. Patients with persistent rales and uncontrolled edema on maximal medical therapy with digoxin, diuretics, and vasodilators have not been included in most previous studies, and generally do not participate in exercise programs at the Duke Center for Living. However, a preliminary report by Kavanagh et al.[21] has demonstrated that patients with functional class III–IV CHF can achieve important benefits from a progressive walking program including improved peak $\dot{V}O_2$ and anaerobic threshold and a decrease in symptoms. The results of this study suggest that even selected patients with severe CHF may benefit from moderate exercise conditioning. Patients with active ischemia and severe LV dysfunction probably should undergo angiography and, if possible, myocardial revascularization before exercise training. Previous studies have indicated that this group may accrue the largest absolute mortality reduction from surgical (or possibly angioplasty) intervention[50,51] and may not achieve a marked training benefit if they undergo training with ongoing severe ischemia.[48] A recent meta-analysis study in patients with coronary artery disease suggests a benefit of exercise training on long-term morbidity and mortality.[8] However, most of these patients have preserved LV systolic function and these results may not apply to patients with severe systolic dysfunction. Although patients with LV systolic dysfunction, especially in the setting of ischemia, have a higher risk for exercise-related complications, it appears that this risk is relatively small when compared with the high incidence of non–exercise-related sudden death reported in clinical series in these patients.[52] Analogous to the coronary artery bypass grafting experience,[50,51] it is possible that patients with severe LV systolic dysfunction may achieve a benefit in terms of morbidity or mortality from exercise training precisely because they are at highest risk. However, studies examining the long-term effects of exercise training on morbidity and mortality in patients with LV dysfunction are currently unavailable and are needed in this area. In light of recent studies,[11-20,45,46,52] it appears that patients with severe LV dysfunction and stable Class I–III heart failure controlled on medical therapy achieve a clinically important improvement in exercise performance and symptoms through exercise conditioning that is comparable to that achieved by vasodilator therapy. At present it appears that exercise conditioning may represent a valuable therapeutic adjunct to the pharmacological management of patients with CHF.

References

1. Thompson PD: The benefits and risks of exercise training in patients with chronic coronary artery disease. *JAMA* 1988;259(10):1537–1540

2. Laslett LJ, Paumer L, Amsterdam EA: Increase in myocardial oxygen consumption indexes by exercise training at onset of ischemia in patients with coronary artery disease. *Circulation* 1985;71:958–962
3. Wenger NK: Rehabilitation of the coronary patient in 1989. *Arch Intern Med* 1989;149:1504–1506
4. Clausen JP: Circulatory adjustments to dynamic exercise and effect of physical training in normal subjects and patients with coronary artery disease. *Prog Cardiovasc Dis* 1976;18:459–495
5. Varnauskas E, Bergman H, Houk P, Bjorntorp P: Hemodynamic effects of physical training in coronary patients. *Lancet* 1966;2:8–12
6. Detry JM, Rousseau M, Vandenbroucke G, Kusumi F, Brasseur LA, Bruce RA: Increased arteriovenous oxygen difference after physical training in coronary heart disease. *Circulation* 1971;44:109–118
7. Clausen JP, Trap-Jensen J: Effects of training on the distribution of cardiac output in patients with coronary artery disease. *Circulation* 1970;42:611–624
8. O'Connor GT, Buring JE, Yusuf S, Goldhaber SZ, Olmstead EM, Paffenbarger RS, Hennekens CH: An overview of randomized trials of rehabilitation with exercise after myocardial infarction. *Circulation* 1989;80:234–244
9. Schuler G, Hambrecht R, Schlierf G, Niebauer J, Hauer K, Neumann J, Hoberg E, Drinkmann A, Bacher F, Grunze M: Regular physical exercise and low-fat diet: effects on progression of coronary artery disease. *Circulation* 1992;86:1–11
10. Ornish D, Brown SE, Scherwitz LW, Billings JH, Armstrong WT, Ports TA, McLanahan SM, Kirkeeide RL, Brand RJ, Gould KL: Can lifestyle changes reverse coronary heart disease? The Lifestyle Heart Trial. *Lancet* 1990;336:129–33
11. Letac B, Cribier A, Desplanches JF: A study of left ventricular function in coronary patients before and after physical training. *Circulation* 1977;56:375–378
12. Cobb FR, Williams RS, McEwan P, Jones RH, Coleman RE, Wallace AG: Effects of exercise training on ventricular function in patients with recent myocardial infarction. *Circulation* 1982;66:100–108
13. Lee AP, Ice R, Blessey R, Sanmarco ME: Long-term effects of physical training on coronary patients with impaired ventricular function. *Circulation* 1979;60:1519–1526
14. Hagberg JM, Ehsani AA, Holloszy JO: Effect of 12 months of intense exercise training on stroke volume in patients with coronary artery disease. *Circulation* 1983;67:1194–1199
15. Conn EH, Williams RS, Wallace AG: Exercise responses before and after physical conditioning in patients with severely depressed left ventricular function. *Am J Cardiol* 1982;49:296–300
16. Coats AJS, Adamopoulos S, Meyer TE, Conway J, Sleight P: Effects of physical training in chronic heart failure. *Lancet* 1990;335:63–66
17. Sullivan MJ, Higginbotham MB, Cobb FR: Exercise training in patients with severe left ventricular dysfunction: hemodynamic and metabolic effects. *Circulation* 1988;78:506–515
18. Sullivan MJ, Higginbotham MB, Cobb FR: Exercise training in patients

with chronic heart failure delays ventilatory anaerobic threshold and improves submaximal exercise performance. *Circulation* 1989;79:324–329

19. Coats AJS, Adamopoulos S, Radaelli A, et al: Controlled trial of physical training in chronic heart failure: exercise performance, hemodynamics, ventilation, and autonomic function. *Circulation* 1992;85:2119–2131
20. Giannuzzi P, Temporelli PL, Tavazzi L, Curra U, Gattone M, Imparato A, Gioroano A, Schweiger C, Sala L, Malinnerwi MD, ANO the EAMY Study Group, Cami-exercise training in anterior myocardial infarction: An ongoing multicenter randomized trial *Chest* 101 1972;(10):3155–3225
21. Myers MG, Baigrie RS, Kavanagh T, Guyatt GH: Benefits of physical training in patients with heart failure. *Circulation* 1992;86:(Suppl I):1595
22. Seals DR, Hagberg JM, Hurley BF, Ehsani AA, Hollszy JO: Endurance training in older men and women I: cardiovascular responses to exercise. *J Appl Physiol* 1984;57:1024–1029
23. Blomqvist CG, Saltin B: Cardiovascular adaptations to physical training. *Annu Rev Physiol* 1983;45:169–189
24. Scheuer J, Tipton CM: Cariovascular adaptations to physical training. *Annu Rev Physiol* 1977;39:221–251
25. Henriksson J: Training induced adaptation of skeletal muscle and metabolism during submaximal exercise. *J Physiol* 1977; 270:661–675
26. Wood PD, Haskell WL, Blair SM: Increased exercise level and plasma liproproteins. *Metabolism* 1983;32:31
27. Peters PK, Cady LD, Bischoff DB: Physical fitness and subsequent myocardial infarction in healthy workers. *JAMA* 1983;249:3052
28. Saltin B, Gollnick PD: Skeletal muscle adaptability: significance for metabolism and performance, in Peachey LD (ed): *The Handbook of Physiology. The Skeletal Muscle System.* Bethesda, MD: American Physiological Society, 1982, pp 555–631
29. Peronnet F, Cleroux J, Perrault H, Cousineau D, de Champlain J, Nadeau R: Plasma norepinephrine response to exercise before and after training in humans. *J Appl Physiol (Respirat Environ Exercise Physiol)* 1981;51(4):812–815
30. Fagard R, Aubert A, Lysens R, Staessen J, Vanhees L, Amery A: Noninvasive assessment of seasonal variations in cardiac structure and function in cyclists. *Circulation* 1983;67(4):896–901
31. Sullivan MJ, Binkley PF, Unverferth DV, Ren JH, Boudulas H, Bashore TM, Merola AJ, Leier CV: Prevention of bedrest-induced physical deconditioning by daily dobutamine infusions: implications for drug-induced physical conditioning. *J Clin Invest* 1985;76:1632–1642
32. Ferguson RJ, Taylor AW, Cote P, Charlebois J, Dinelle Y, Peronett F, De Champlain J, Bourassa MG: Skeletal muscle and cardiac changes with training in patients with angina pectoris. *Am J Physiol* 1982;243:H830–H836
33. Sullivan MJ, Knight JD, Higginbotham MB, Cobb FR: Relation between central and peripheral hemodynamics during exercise in patients with

chronic heart failure: muscle blood flow is reduced with maintenance of arterial perfusion pressure. *Circulation* 1989;80:769–781

34. Minotti JR, Johnson EC, Hudson TL, Zuroske G, Murata G, Fukushima E, Cagle TG, Chick TW, Massie BM, Icenogle MV: Skeletal muscle response to exercise training in congestive heart failure. *J Clin Invest* 1990;86:751–758

35. Massie BM: Exercise tolerance in congestive heart failure: role of cardiac function, peripheral blood flow, and muscle metabolism and effect of treatment. *Am J Med* 1988;84(suppl 3A):75–82

36. Sullivan MJ, Green HJ, Cobb FR: Skeletal muscle biochemistry and histology in ambulatory patients with long-term chronic heart failure. *Circulation* 1990;81:518–527

37. Sullivan MJ, Green HJ, Cobb FR: Altered skeletal muscle metabolic response to exercise in chronic heart failure: relationship to hemodynamics and skeletal muscle aerobic enzyme activity. *Circulation* 1991;84:1597–1607

38. Mancini DM, Coyle E, Coggan A, Beltz J, Ferraro N, Montain S, Wilson JR: Contribution of intrinsic skeletal muscle changes to ^{31}P NMR skeletal muscle metabolic abnormalities in patients with chronic heart failure. *Circulation* 1989;80:1338–1346

39. Drexler H, Riede U, Münzel T, König H, Funke E, Just H: Alterations of skeletal muscle in chronic heart failure. *Circulation* 1992;85:1751–1759

40. Wilson JR, Fink L, Maris J, Ferraro N, Power-Vanwart J, Eleff S, Chance B: Evaluation of energy metabolism in skeletal muscle of patients with heart failure with gated phosphorus-31 nuclear magnetic resonance. *Circulation* 1985;71:57–62

41. Massie BM, Conway M, Rajagopalan B, Yonge R, Frostick S, Sleight P, Ledingham J, Radda G: Skeletal muscle metabolism during exercise under ischemic conditions: evidence for abnormalities unrelated to blood flow. *Circulation* 1988;78:320–326

42. Mancini DM, Walter G, Reichek N, Lenkinski R, McCully KK, Mullen JL, Wilson JR: Contribution of skeletal muscle atrophy to exercise intolerance and altered muscle metabolism in heart failure. *Circulation* 1992;85:1364–1373

43. Sullivan MJ, Charles HC, Negro-Villar R, Kennedy JE, Cobb FR: Early skeletal muscle anaerobic metabolism occurs independent of muscle atrophy in heart failure. *Circulation* 1991;84(suppl II):II–7

44. Sullivan MJ, Higginbotham MB, Cobb FR: Increased exercise ventilation in chronic heart failure: intact ventilatory control despite hemodynamic and pulmonary abnormalities. *Circulation* 1988;77(3):522–559

45. Kellermann JJ, Ben-Ari E, Fisman E, Hayet M, Drory Y, Haimovitz D: Physical training in patients with ventricular impairment. *Adv Cardiol* 1986;34:131–147

46. Hoffmann A, Duba J, Lengyel M, Majer K: The effect of training on the physical working capacity of MI patients with left ventricular dysfunction. *Eur Heart J* 1987;8:43–49

47. Jugdutt BI, Michorowski BL, Kappagoda CT: Exercise training after

anterior Q wave myocardial infarction: importance of regional left ventricular function and topography. *J Am Coll Cardiol* 1988;12:362–372

48. Arvan S: Exercise performance of the high risk acute myocardial infarction patient after cardiac rehabilitation. *Am J Cardiol* 1988;62:197–201

49. Squires RW, Gau GT, Miller TD, Allison TG, Lavie CJ: Cardiovascular rehabilitation: status, 1990. *Mayo Clin Proc* 1990;65:731–755

50. Alderman EL, Fisher LD, Litwin P, Kaiser GC, Myers WO, Maynard C, Levine F, Schloss M: Results of coronary artery surgery in patients with poor left ventricular function (CASS). *Circulation* 1983;68:785

51. Vigilante GJ, Weintraub WS, Klein LW, Schneider RM, Seelaus PA, Parr GVS, Lemole G, Agarwal JB, Helfant RH: Improved survival with coronary bypass surgery in patients with three-vessel coronary disease and abnormal left ventricular function. Matched case-control study in patient with potentially operable disease. *Am J Med* 1987;82:697

52. Van Camp SP, Peterson RA: Cardiovascular complications of outpatient cardiac rehabilitation programs. *JAMA* 1986;256:1160–1163

Chapter 21

Magnetic Resonance Methods to Assess Physiological Exercise of the Cardiovascular System

Gerald G. Blackwell, MD, Louis J. Dell'Italia, MD, and Gerald M. Pohost, MD

Magnetic resonance methods are increasingly being applied in the clinical and research evaluation of the cardiovascular system. The unique potential of magnetic resonance imaging (MRI) and magnetic resonance spectroscopy (MRS) to provide anatomical, functional, and biochemical information in a single examination is responsible for much of the interest in this technology. The first part of this chapter briefly introduces the information that can be obtained from MRI and MRS. The second part discusses the potential of these methods for assessing physiological exercise of the cardiovascular system.

Cardiovascular Magnetic Resonance Methods

Assessment of Morphology and Function

Magnetic resonance imaging permits tomographic assessment of the cardiovascular system in any desired imaging plane. These tomographic slices are acquired using electrocardiographic gating to functionally freeze cardiac motion and can be reconstructed to allow a high-resolution, three-dimensional evaluation of both anat-

From Fletcher GF, (ed): *Cardiovascular Response to Exercise*. Mount Kisco, NY, Futura Publishing Company, Inc., © 1994.

omy and function. Conventional imaging is limited to hydrogen nuclei, which are distributed widely in the human organism.[1] Static spin-echo images typically are acquired for evaluating structure. These images depict the blood pool as a signal void (black blood) and discrimination between vascular structures and the blood pool is quite good. Spin-echo images are used occasionally to depict cardiac function, but constraints of the acquisition pulse sequence limit temporal resolution. The gradient-echo pulse sequence, alternatively, produces images in which the blood pool appears bright (white blood, cine MRI). A temporal resolution of 25 to 30 sec is easily obtainable and multiple cardiac phases can be formatted as an endless loop cine movie of cardiac function.[2] Animal and human studies have shown the accuracy of magnetic resonance methods for assessing cardiac volumes, mass, and function.[3] The data are so strong that a persuasive argument can be made that MRI now represents the gold standard for in vivo assessment of these clinically important parameters.[4,5]

Noninvasive Assessment of Cardiac Biochemistry

Magnetic resonance spectroscopy provides biochemical information noninvasively in the intact organism. Oxidative phosphorylation provides living cells with their most efficient source of energy in the form of adenosine triphosphate (ATP). Myocardial oxygen consumption (MVo_2) is determined primarily by cardiac energy use, which is reflected in the concentration and kinetics of reactions involving high-energy phosphate compounds.[6] Accordingly, most data to date have focused on phosphorous-31 MRS. Insight into cellular energetics and viability can be obtained by observing compounds such as phosphate esters, phosphocreatine (PCr), and ATP. Figure 1 is a typical human cardiac magnetic resonance phosphorous spectra. Carbon-13 and hydrogen-rich lipid compounds also are nuclear magnetic resonance (NMR) "visible" and can be interrogated to provide unique spectroscopic data. Subsequently, this chapter will focus on the use of the above magnetic resonance methods to assess physiological exercise.

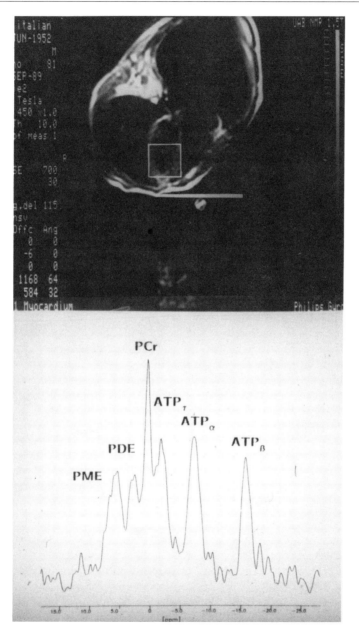

FIGURE 1. *Volume-localized phosphorous-31 spectrum from a normal human heart.* **Top:** *The volume of interest as a box localized over the heart.* **Bottom:** *The resultant spectrum. Note the three separate phosphorous resonances of ATP. PCr, phosphocreatine; ATP, adenosine triphosphate; PDE, phosphodiesters; PME, phosphomonoesters.*

Assessment of Physiological Exercise by Magnetic Resonance Methods

Magnetic Resonance Imaging

Cardiovascular fitness is determined by cardiac as well as peripheral factors and the cardiovascular response to chronic exercise depends on the nature and duration of the exercise. A person performing largely isometric exercise training (ie., weight lifting) forces the ventricle to adapt to an intermittent pressure overload. Alternatively, a highly trained distance runner forces his/her heart to adapt to intermittent demands for a very high cardiac output. Whatever the physiological stress, the ventricle must "remodel" to optimize its chamber geometry for the required task. At the chamber level, there must be either an increase in myocardial mass, chamber diameter, or both. In the adult heart, the adaptive mechanism to increase myocardial mass involves an increase in myocyte size.[7,8] Accompanying this increase in myocyte size are ultrastructural changes involving the interstitial collagen and capillary density as well as myocyte biochemistry.[9] The adaptive mechanism to increase resting ventricular diastolic dimension (preload) may involve an increase in circulating blood volume. The ultimate goal is to match the intermittent demand for increased oxygen delivery with an adequate oxygen supply at both the myocyte level and organism level.

Comprehensive evaluation of ventricular function by MRI includes an assessment of three major determinants of MVO_2, namely, preload, afterload, and contractility.[10,11] Preload is estimated easily by measurement of end-diastolic dimensions or, more precisely, end-diastolic volume. Work in our laboratory and in others has demonstrated the ability of magnetic resonance to measure, accurately and reproducibly, ventricular volumes and mass.[12–19]

Afterload, defined as the force opposing shortening of myocardial fibers, usually is estimated clinically by measuring blood pressure. A more accurate approximation of true afterload at the myocyte level, however, is given by wall stress. The mathematical expression is shown in the LaPlace relationship:

wall stress~(pressure * radius)/wall thickness

From this equation it can be seen that the accuracy of wall stress as a measure of afterload is derived from the incorporation of factors both internal (radius and wall thickness) and external (pressure) to the ventricle.[12] The physiological response of a pressure overloaded ventricle (isometric exercise) is to increase wall thickness and reduce chamber radius to normalize afterload. A marathon runner, alternatively, more closely resembles a volume overloaded ventricle (Figure 2). In these patients marked chamber dilatation is the primary adaptation with chamber hypertrophy occurring as required to normalize the radius to wall thickness ratio.

Contractility is a difficult parameter to measure in vivo because of the dependence on ventricular loading conditions. The limitations of an ejection phase index such as ejection fraction are well known but when correctly interpreted remain clinically useful. Ejection

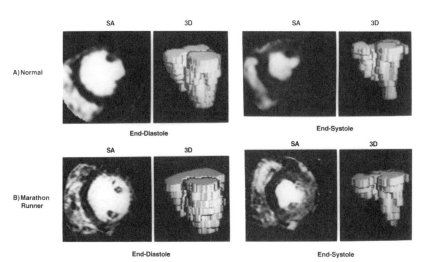

FIGURE 2. **A:** *Normal volunteer.* **B:** *Marathon runner. The left side of each panel shows a short axis slice at the tip of the papillary muscle; the right side demonstrates a three-dimensional reconstruction of the entire serial short axis cine MRI study. Note the excellent resolution of both the right and left ventricular blood pools. In the marathon runner ventricular volumes are markedly increased but chamber geometry remains intact. The three-dimensional reconstructions were obtained using an automated edge detection algorithm designed by H. Ross Singleton in our laboratory. SA, short axis; 3-D, three-dimensional reconstruction.*

fraction is obtained easily using MRI.[17,19] More complicated physiological constructs such as end-systolic pressure-volume and stress-volume relations also have been used to assess contractility. Animal work from our laboratory and preliminary human data have shown the ability of MR methods to derive these parameters accurately, although clinical utility remains to be proven.[20,21]

In summary, MRI methods can provide important morphologic and functional information regarding adaptation to both isometric and isotonic types of exercise. The noninvasive, inherently three-dimensional data set permits a comprehensive assessment of both the left and right ventricle. Automated edge detection and computer-based three-dimensional reconstruction algorithms are areas of intense research and will be important for the advancement of both clinical and research applications because of the enormous amount of data available for analysis from even a single examination. Data from Singleton et al. in our laboratory provide a promising automated technique to routinely identify blood pool (Figure 2) and ventricular myocardium.[22]

Although well suited for assessing the chronic myocardial effects of physiological exercise, current magnetic resonance instruments are poorly suited for assessing the acute effects of exercise. There is limited room within the bore of commercial instruments and any mode of exercise must make use of equipment that is nonferromagnetic. A further complicating factor is the motion involved in all forms of exercise. Motion severely degrades image quality in MRI. Instruments have been devised that permit both lower extremity[23] and upper extremity exercise[24] in the magnetic resonance instrument. Although ingenious and perhaps effective, the technical obstacles are significant, and in the near future it seems unlikely that there will be widespread use. It is possible that implementation of ultrafast techniques and near "real-time" MRI sequences such as echo-planar may permit acute studies.

Magnetic Resonance Spectroscopy

Magnetic resonance spectroscopy has been applied most extensively to assess high-energy phosphate metabolism in skeletal muscle of patients with congestive heart failure postexercise. Specialized surface coils are used to increase signal-to-noise ratios and cardiac gating is not required, thus making the technique easier to apply. Unfortunately, data to date using phosphorus magnetic resonance of skeletal muscle have been inconclusive.[25,26] It is possible that higher field strength instruments and interrogation of other MR-visible compounds such as lactate may provide additional insight.

The best data regarding physiological stress in cardiac spectroscopy come from the work of Weiss et al.[24] at the Johns Hopkins University. This group studied patients with known left anterior descending coronary artery disease using isometric handgrip exercise. Patients were stressed to approximately 30% of their maximal effort and phosphorous MRS performed before and after this exercise. The protocol caused minimal problems with motion and patients were able to satisfactorily perform this task. In the study group, exercise caused a drop in the ratio of PCr to ATP, a finding suggestive of ischemia. In a subset of patients retested after revascularization, the PCr:ATP ratio did not fall with exercise, suggesting relief from ischemia.

Summary

Magnetic resonance imaging and magnetic resonance spectroscopy offer clinicians and basic scientists an excellent tool for studying adaptation and de-adaptation to exercise in both the normal and failing ventricle. The methods are well suited for the study of long-term myocardial effects of chronic exercise. Simultaneously assessing the geometry and function of both the right ventricle and left ventricle noninvasively is a major advantage. The ability to look at metabolic parameters with MRS makes this the only technique to date capable of doing such extensive evaluation in a single examination. Equipment to facilitate stress within the magnet has not been developed for use on a wide scale and is not anticipated in the near future. The influence of ultrafast imaging sequences and use of higher field spectrometers remains speculative at present.

References

1. Doyle M, Blackwell G: Basic principles of MRI, in Blackwell G, Cranney G, Pohost G (eds): *MRI: Cardiovasular System*. New York, Gower Medical Publishing, 1992

2. Blackwell G, Doyle M, Cranney G: Cardiovascular MRI techniques, in Blackwell G, Cranney G, Pohost G (eds): *MRI: Cardiovascular System.* New York, Gower Medical Publishing, 1992

3. Blackwell G, Cranney G, Lotan C: Ventricular volume, function, and mass, in Blackwell G, Cranney G, Pohost G (eds): *MRI: Cardiovascular System.* New York, Gower Medical Publishing, 1992

4. Weiss JL, Shapiro EP, Buchalter MB, Beyar R: Magnetic resonance imaging as a noninvasive standard for the quantitative evaluation of left ventricular mass, ischemia, and infarction. *Ann NY Acad Sci* 1990;601:95–106

5. Higgins CB: Which standard has the gold? *J Am Coll Cardiol* 1992;19:1608–1609

6. Katz LA, Swain JA, Portman MA, Balaban RS: Relation between phosphate metabolites and oxygen consumption of heart in vivo. *Am J Physiol* 1989:256;H265–H274

7. Weber KT, Clark WA, Janicki JS, Shroff SG: Physiologic versus pathologic hypertrophy and the pressure-overloaded myocardium. *J Cardio Pharm* 1987;10:S37–S49

8. Meerson FZ: A mechanism of hypertrophy and wear of the myocardium. *Am J Cardiol* 1965;15:755–760

9. Swynghedauw B: Remodelling of the heart in response to chronic mechanical overload. *Eur Heart J* 1989;10:935–943

10. Baller D, Bretschneider HJ, Hellige G: A critical look at currently used indirect indices of myocardial oxygen consumption. *Basic Res Cardiol* 1981;76:163–181

11. Sonnenblick EH, Ross J, Braunwald E. Oxygen consumption of the heart newer concepts of its multifactorial determination. *Am J Cardiol* 1968;22:328–336

12. Dell'Italia L, Blackwell G, Thorn B, Pearce D, Pohost G: Time-varying wall stress: an index of ventricular-vascular coupling. *Am J Physiol* 1992;H597–H605

13. Pearce DJ, Dell'Italia LJ, Blackwell GG, Cranney GB, Pohost GM: Simultaneous evaluation of the right and left ventricular pressure-volume relationship in an intact canine model. *Soc Mag Res Med,* New York, August 18–24, 1990

14. Rehr RB, Malloy CR, Filipchuk NG, Peshock RM: Left ventricular volumes measured by MR imaging. *Radiology* 1985;156:717–719

15. Sechtem U, Pflugfelder PW, Gould RG, Cassidy MM, Higgins CB: Measurement of right and left ventricular volumes in healthy individuals with cine MR imaging. *Radiology* 1987;163:697–702

16. Florentine, MS, Grosskreutz CL, Chang W, Hartnett SA, Dunn VD, Ehrhardt JC, Fleagle SR, Collins SM, Marcus ML, Skorton DJ: Measurement of left ventricular mass in vivo gated nuclear magnetic resonance imaging. *J Am Coll Cardiol* 1986;8:107–112

17. Cranney GB, Lotan CS, Dean L, Baxley W, Bouchard A, Pohost GM: Left ventricular volume measurement using cardiac axis nuclear magnetic resonance imaging—validation by calibrated ventricular angiography. *Circulation* 1990;82:154–163

18. McDonald KM, Parrish T, Wennberg P, Stillman AE, Francis GS,

Cohn JN, Hunter D: Rapid, accurate and simultaneous nonivasive assessment of right and left ventricular mass with nuclear magnetic resonance imaging using the snapshot gradient method. *J Am Coll Cardiol* 1992;19:1601–1607

19. Benjelloun H, Cranney GB, Kirk KA, Blackwell GG, Lotan CS, Pohost GM: Interstudy reproducibility of biplane cine nuclear magnetic resonance measurements of left ventricular function. *Am J Cardiol* 1991;67:1413–1410

20. Blackwell G, Dell'Italia L, Pearce D, Cranney G, Webb E, Hefner L, Pohost G: The End-Systolic Stress Volume Relationship Derived From Cine NMR and High Fidelity Left Ventricular Pressures *Circulation* 1990;82:III–124.

21. Auffermann W, Wagner S, Holt WW, Buser PT, Kircher B, Schiller NB, Lim TH, Wolfe CL, Higgins CB: Noninvasive determination of left ventricular output and wall stress in volume overload and in myocardial disease by cine magnetic resonance imaging. *Am Heart J* 1991:121:1750

22. Singleton HR: Automatic image segmentation using edge detection by tissue classification in local neighborhoods. *Proc IEEE, Southeastcon* 1992;1:286–290

23. Schaefer S, Peshock RM, Parkey RW, et al: A new device for exercise MR imaging. *AJR* 1986;147:1289–1290

24. Weiss RG, Bottomley PA, Hardy CJ, Gerstenblith G: Regional myocardial metabolism of high-energy phosphates during isometric exercise in patients with coronary artery disease. *N Engl J Med* 1990;323:1593–1600

25. Wilson JR, Fink L, Maris J, Ferraro N, Power-Vanwart J, Eleff S, Chance B: Evaluation of energy metabolism in skeletal muscle of patients with heart failure with gated phosphorus-31 nuclear magnetic resonance. *Circulation* 1985;71:57–62

26. Mancini DM, Coyle E, Coggan A, Beltz J, Ferraro N, Montain S, Wilson JR: Contribution of intrinsic skeletal muscle changes to ^{31}P NMR skeletal muscle metabolic abnormalities in patients with chronic heart failure. *Circulation* 1989;80:1338–1346

Chapter 22

Effects of Aging on the Cardiovascular Response to Exercise

Jerome L. Fleg, MD

The widespread application of exercise testing and training to many thousands of older Americans over the past decade has necessitated a greater understanding of how age per se changes the cardiovascular response to exercise. Elucidating the pure effects of aging on the cardiovascular exercise response is a formidable task. This response is influenced by the exercise modality (*ie*, treadmill vs. ergometer), body position (supine or upright), level of effort, gender, physical conditioning status, and the presence or absence of cardiovascular disease, which often is clinically silent. Thus, apparent discrepancies between studies often can be accounted for by methodological differences. In this chapter, the effect of age on maximal aerobic capacity, left ventricular pump performance, and cardiac arrhythmias during exercise is discussed.

Maximal Aerobic Capacity

The most widely accepted measurement of aerobic exercise performance is maximal oxygen consumption ($\dot{V}O_2$max), usually measured during treadmill or bicycle exercise. $\dot{V}O_2$max is the product of cardiac output (central) and arteriovenous oxygen difference (peripheral) components at maximal effort; to compare individuals of different body use, $\dot{V}O_2$max is characteristically expressed as ml O_2/kg body weight per minute. $\dot{V}O_2$max is highly reproducible

From Fletcher GF, (ed): *Cardiovascular Response to Exercise*. Mount Kisco, NY, Futura Publishing Company, Inc., © 1994.

and is not altered by the involvement of additional muscle once 50–60% of total muscle mass is exercised.

Numerous studies over the past half century have demonstrated an age-associated decline in $\dot{V}O_2$max, approximating 8–10% per decade in sedentary populations.[1-8] This decline in $\dot{V}O_2$max parallels the decrease in maximal work capacity, indicating that it is not secondary to greater metabolic efficiency of older persons. In fact, at a given external work load, the elderly may demonstrate a slightly higher oxygen consumption than the young, probably because of reduced mechanical efficiency.[9] Although the percentage decline in $\dot{V}O_2$max with age is similar in men and women,[4] men have a higher $\dot{V}O_2$max than women at any given age, probably reflecting their greater muscularity and higher blood hemoglobin. Given that muscle mass declines with age and that exercising muscles consume more than 90% of the oxygen during maximal exercise, it is plausible that the former accounts for a sizeable proportion of the age-related decline in $\dot{V}O_2$max. In a recent study in the Baltimore Longitudinal Study of Aging (BLSA) volunteers, the decrease of $\dot{V}O_2$max explicable by age was reduced from 60% to 14% in men and from 50% to 8% in women when $\dot{V}O_2$max was normalized to muscle mass rather than body weight (Figure 1).[4] This normalization also abolished the gender difference in $\dot{V}O_2$max.

Ogawa et al.[10] observed a similar attenuation of the age-associated decline (as well as the gender difference) in $\dot{V}O_2$max, after normalizing $\dot{V}O_2$max for fat-free mass in sedentary individuals. In this study a three- to four-decade age increment was associated with a 40% lower $\dot{V}O_2$max. A smaller stroke volume accounted for almost half of this decrease in $\dot{V}O_2$max with age, while a blunted maximal heart rate and arteriovenous oxygen difference contributed about equally to the remainder. These investigators also have observed a strong direct relationship between $\dot{V}O_2$max and maximal hyperemic calf conductance, an index of peripheral vasodilatory capacity.[11]

Additional evidence of the importance of peripheral factors in the age-associated decline in $\dot{V}O_2$max are derived from training studies. When healthy sedentary men 60 to 79 years old (mean $\dot{V}O_2$max of 30 ml/kg per minute) were compared with age-matched endurance trained athletes (mean $\dot{V}O_2$max of 50 ml/kg per minute), about two thirds of the difference in $\dot{V}O_2$max was explained by an augmented arteriovenous oxygen difference in the athletes.[12] Similarly, an increase in $\dot{V}O_2$max from 25.4 to 32.9 ml/kg per minute after

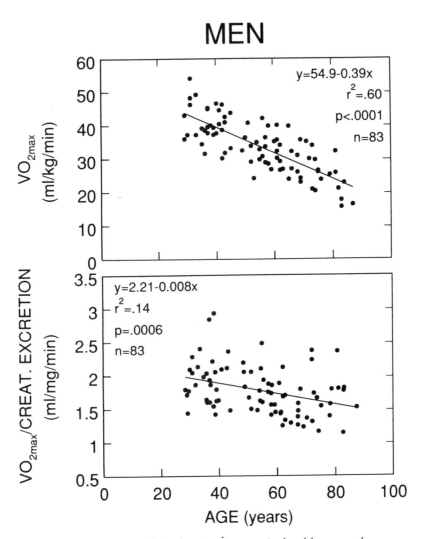

FIGURE 1. *Age-associated decline in V̇O₂max in healthy, nonobese men expressed in the usual ml/kg body weight (top panel) and normalized per mg urinary creatinine as an index of total muscle mass (bottom panel). The decline in V̇O₂max attributable to aging is markedly attenuated after normalization for muscle mass. Adapted from Reference 4.*

1 year of endurance training was accomplished by only a 6% augmentation of cardiac output but a 16% increase of arteriovenous oxygen difference (Table 1).[13]

The age-associated decline in $\dot{V}O_2$max appears to be attenuated with regular intensive endurance training. For example, the $\dot{V}O_2$max of endurance-trained men 50 to 72 years old averaged only 15% less than in young athletes 19 to 27 years old with similar current training habits and prior peak running performances.[5] If one assumes similar $\dot{V}O_2$max levels for the two groups in the third decade, the extrapolated decline of $\dot{V}O_2$max in these older athletes is 5% per decade, a rate of decline approximately half that of sedentary populations. A similar trend was observed by Ogawa et al., who noted a 7% $\dot{V}O_2$max decline per decade in trained men compared with 11% per decade in their sedentary counterparts.[10] Longitudinal studies of older runners have corroborated these results.[14,15] In one study of 24 male runners aged 52 to 62 years, half the men maintained their average running speed over the next decade whereas the other half reduced their pace by 1.5 min/mile; running distance was maintained in both groups. Whereas the men who reduced training intensity experienced a 13% loss of $\dot{V}O_2$max, those who maintained a high training intensity lost only 2% of $\dot{V}O_2$max over the decade (Figure 2).[14] These compelling data suggest that much of the age-associated decline in aerobic capacity may be secondary to declines in activity patterns that accompany aging.

TABLE 1. Central and Peripheral Responses to Exercise Training in Older Individuals

	Before training	After training
$\dot{V}O_2$max (ml/kg per minute)	25.4±4.6	32.9±7.6[a]
$\dot{V}O_2$max (l/min)	1.91±0.4	2.39±0.6[a]
Maximal cardiac output (l/min)	17.6±3.2	18.7±2.9
Maximal heart rate (beats per minute)	174±10	174±7
Maximal stroke volume (ml)	101±18	108±16[b]
Maximal arteriovenous O_2 difference (ml O_2/dl)	11.0±3.0	12.8±2.5[a]

[a] $p<0.01$; [b] $p<0.05$.
Adapted from Reference 11.

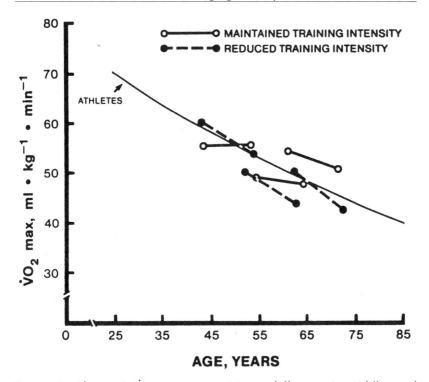

FIGURE 2. *Change in V̇O₂max over a 10-year follow-up in middle-aged male endurance athletes who maintained or reduced their training intensity. The solid curve for athletes is from Reference 5. Reproduced from Reference 14 with permission.*

Left Ventricular Response to Exercise

The decrease in V̇O₂max observed with aging has been attributed to declines in both central and peripheral components. The magnitude and mechanisms of the decline in the central component (*ie,* cardiac output) have varied widely between studies. Early invasive studies during supine cycle ergometry described a decrease in both maximal heart rate and maximal stroke volume with age.[6,16] Resultant declines in cardiac output have generally approached 30–35% for the third to the eighth decades in these studies. For example, when 17 clinically healthy Scandinavian men 61 to 83 years old were compared with young men in their 20s, during supine bicycle exercise the older men were found to have a lower maximal heart rate (130 vs. 151 beats/min) stroke volume (101 vs. 118 ml), cardiac output (13.1 vs. 18.5 1/mm), and $\dot{V}o_2max$ (1.46 vs. 2.06 1/min).[16] However, systolic blood pressure was 39 mm Hg higher and pulmonary artery wedge pressure 6.5 mm Hg higher in the elderly group.

More recent studies also consistently demonstrate age-associated declines in maximal heart rate with lesser declines or no change in stroke volume. Hossack and Bruce performed invasive Fick measurements of cardiac output during treadmill exercise in 12 normal men and 11 women aged 20 to 64 years and developed regression equations to extrapolate cardiac index from $\dot{V}o_2max$; these were then applied to 98 men and 104 women who underwent noninvasive measurement of $\dot{V}o_2max$.[17] Maximal cardiac index declined with age in both sexes ($r = -0.66$ in each sex), but the slope of the decline was greater in men than women (0.082 vs. 0.053 1/min per year) because of a steeper decline in maximal heart rate in men (1.07 vs. 0.60 beats/min per year); stroke volume index decreased slightly with age in both sexes.

Younis et al. measured left ventricular (LV) performance by radionuclide ventriculography in 18 young (17–25 years) and 17 older (51–61 years) men and women during upright cycle ergometry;[18] volunteers were screened with exercise electrocardiograms (ECGs) and thallium scans to exclude coronary artery disease. Age-associated decreases in $\dot{V}o_2max$, cardiac index, and heart rate were observed at normal effort. Although not analyzed statistically, stroke volume index was higher in older than younger volunteers of both sexes at maximum work load, because of higher end-diastolic volume indices. Older volunteers, however, were not able to reduce their end-systolic volumes, resulting in a blunted exercise ejection fraction compared with their younger counterparts. Mean arterial pressure was higher throughout exercise in older volunteers.

In 61 BLSA volunteers 25 to 79 years old screened by exercise ECG and thallium scan to exclude coronary artery disease, maximal cardiac index measured by radionuclide ventriculography declined only nominally with age ($r = 0.14$, $p = NS$) despite the expected decrease of approximately one beat per minute per year in maximal heart rate ($r = -0.66$, $p < 0.001$) during upright cycle exercise.[19] Cardiac index was preserved during exercise in these older volunteers by an augmented stroke volume, mediated by a greater end-diastolic volume compared with the younger volunteers (Figure 3). However, maximal ejection fraction and the augmentation of ejection fraction from rest (Figure 4) were blunted with age because of a lesser reduction of end-systolic volume in older individuals. The extension of the initial sample to 145 volunteers (95 men and 50 women) has elicited certain gender differences: maximal heart rate declines with age more slowly in women (0.63 vs. 1.05 beats per min per year, respectively) whereas maximal stroke volume is better preserved with age in men. Although maximal exercise ejection fraction declines with age similarly in both sexes, the augmentation of ejection fraction from rest is less in women than men at any age.[20]

Higginbotham et al.[21] performed right heart catheterization, radionuclide ventriculography, and expired gas analyses of 24 apparently healthy men 20 to 50 years old during upright cycle ergometry. Over this 3-decade age range, the authors observed a 25% decrease in $\dot{V}O_2$ and cardiac index at maximal effort and a 20% decline in maximal heart rate. No age relationship was seen for exercise stroke volume, end-diastolic volume, or end-systolic volume indices or ejection fraction. The inclusion of nine regular joggers and the exclusion of volunteers older than 50 years must be considered when interpreting these results.

Mann et al.[22] examined the effect of age on LV performance by radionuclide ventriculography during submaximal supine cycle exercise in six young men (37 ± 4 years) and eight older (59 ± 2 years) volunteers (6 men and 2 women) without apparent heart disease. At fixed external work loads of 200 to 600 kpm, older volunteers demonstrated higher cardiac outputs, mediated by higher end-diastolic and stroke volumes with similar heart rates; ejection fraction responses also were greater in the older groups. It must be recognized, however, that the 600-kpm work load represented only 55% of maximal effort for the young but 89% of maximum for the older groups.

In addition to the above studies, which examined the cardiac output responses to exercise across age, other studies have concentrated on the effect of age on the ejection fraction response to maximal cycle exercise. Using radionuclide ventriculography, Port et al.[23] measured ejection fraction during maximal upright cycle ergometry in 77 volunteers 20 to 95 years old without apparent heart disease. These investigators were the first to document an age-associated decline in maximal ejection fraction and in the change of ejection fraction from rest. Of note, in 24 of the 29 individuals older than 60 years, ejection fraction increased <5 units, the generally accepted

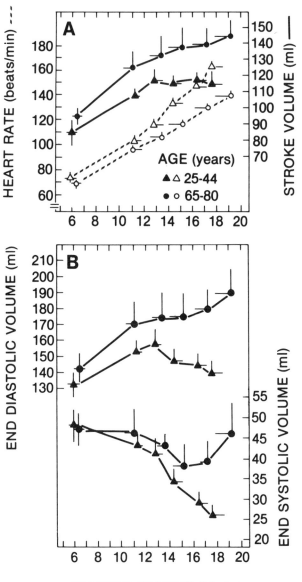

FIGURE 3. *Hemodynamic variables plotted as a function of cardiac output during upright cycle ergometry in healthy volunteers rigorously screened to exclude cardiovascular disease. In* **A,** *heart rate (○) is lower and stroke volume (●) higher in men aged 65 to 80 years than heart rate (△) and stroke volume (▲) higher in men 25 to 44 years old, at a given level of cardiac output.* **B** *demonstrates that in older individuals, both end-diastolic volume (●) and end-systolic volume (●) are higher at any given cardiac output during exercise than in the young (▲). Adapted from Reference 19.*

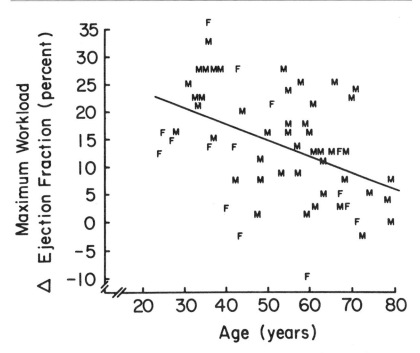

FIGURE 4. *Effect of age on the augmentation of ejection fraction from rest to maximal effort during upright cycle ergometry in healthy men (M) and women (F). The ejection fraction response decreases with age (p<0.001) and tends to be lower in women than men. Reproduced from Reference 19 with permission.*

lower limit of normal. Furthermore, exercise-induced regional wall motion abnormalities were not seen in volunteers younger than 50 years but were present in 44% of those aged 70 years and older. Since such wall motion normalities are generally considered specific evidence for coronary artery disease, it is possible that many of these older volunteers, screened only for the clinical absence of cardiovascular disease, actually had undetected coronary artery disease.

Kuo et al.[24] performed maximal supine cycle ergometry on 27 men and 30 women 30 to 79 years old with normal coronary arteriograms; most were individuals with chest pain syndromes and most were receiving cardiac medications. Those volunteers younger than 50 years (mean, 43 years) exercised longer and had greater augmentation of ejection fraction with exercise (10.6 vs. 4.8 units) than older volunteers (mean, 58 years). Men achieved higher work loads than women as well as larger increments of ejection fraction (9.8 vs. 5.3 units). By multivariate analysis, maximal work load achieved, but not age or gender, was a significant determinant of the ejection fraction response to exercise. Interpretation of these results must be tempered by the unusual selection criteria for these individuals and the fact that most were receiving cardioactive medications.

Adams et al.[25] examined the radionuclide ventriculographic responses of 55 healthy men and women 18 to 56 years old during supine cycle exercise. Both peak LV ejection fraction (78% vs. 72%) and the augmentation of ejection fraction from rest (14 vs. 8 units) were significantly greater in men; these differences were due to a greater decline of end-systolic volume in men than women (− 47% vs. − 24%). Age, however, did not predict the change in ejection fraction with exercise ($r = -0.18$), perhaps because of the limited age range studied.

Taken together, the radionuclide exercise studies above indicate several age-associated changes in the response to aerobic exercise. Maximal work load and $\dot{V}O_2$max, maximal heart rate ejection fraction, and cardiac output all decline with advancing age. Stroke volume at maximal effort declines with age in some studies but not others. It is noteworthy that in the two studies that employed rigorous screening with exercise ECG and thallium scanning to exclude latent coronary artery disease,[18,19] stroke volumes actually tended to increase with age because of greater increases in end-diastolic volume in older persons. Thus, the decline in exercise stroke volume with age observed in some studies may be secondary to undetected coronary artery disease.

Ehsani et al.[26] recently provided evidence that the blunted ejection fraction response to exercise in older men can be improved by intensive endurance training. In 10 healthy men 64 ± 3 years old, $\dot{V}O_2$max improved 26% over 12 months of training. Before training, LV ejection fraction during supine cycle ergometry increased only modestly from 66% at rest to 71% at peak effort; after training, however, LV ejection fraction increased from 67% at rest to 78% at peak, an augmentation twice that observed before training and similar to that seen in young sedentary men.

The hemodynamic profile of healthy older persons during strenuous aerobic exercise, a blunted maximal heart rate and ejection fraction response with prescreened or augmented stroke volume, resembles that seen during β-adrenergic blockade of younger individuals (Figure 5). The figure demonstrates that acute

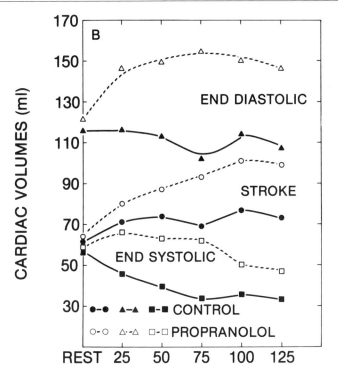

FIGURE 5. *Effect of acute administration of propranolol (0.15 mg/kg) intravenously on LV volumes during upright cycle ergometry. All volumes increased, whereas ejection fraction and heart rate decreased, at matched work loads after propranolol.*

administration of intravenous propranolol to a young person results in an impairment of LV emptying (*ie,* higher end-systolic volume thus before β-blockade). However, stroke volume actually is augmented after propranolol because of a large increase in end-diastolic volume.[27] A further similarity between normative aging and β-blockade is the augmentation of plasma catecholamines during exercise in both settings. A prior study of normal BLSA men documented an exaggerated plasma norepinephrine response to maximal treadmill exercise in older men despite resting levels similar to those in young and middle-aged individuals (Figure 6).[28] These findings also are consistent with the blunted chronotropic response to infused boluses of the beta agonist isoproterenol in older versus younger men.[29] Similarities between age changes in the

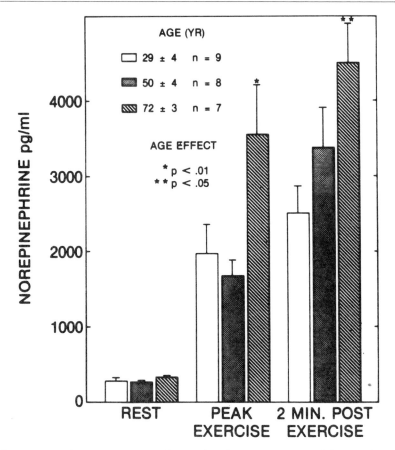

FIGURE 6. *Plasma norepinephrine levels in young middle-aged and elderly men at rest, at maximal treadmill effort, and during recovery from exercise. Although similar at rest among the three groups, norepinephrine values were significantly higher in the elderly men at maximal effort and in recovery. Adapted from Reference 28.*

response to exercise and those seen during β-adrenergic blockade are shown in Table 2.

Another contributor to the blunted ejection fraction response to exercise with advancing age may be the greater afterload seen in older persons, measured clinically by an exaggerated blood pressure response.[11,16,18] Furthermore, age-associated increases in characteristic aortic input impedance may cause increases in afterload not

TABLE 2.   Similarities Between Aging and β-adrenergic Blockade in Response to Exercise

	Aging	β-blockade
Maximal heart rate	↓	↓
Maximal ejection fraction	↓	↓
Maximal end-diastolic volume	↑	↑
Maximal cardiac output	↓	↓
Maximal plasma catecholamines	↑	↑

apparent from blood pressure measurements alone. Characteristic impedance describes instantaneous pressure–flow relationships throughout the cardiac cycle and requires simultaneous measurement of aortic pressure and flow. In beagle dogs, resting LV stroke volume and characteristic impedance were not age-related.[30] At low exercise work loads, young adult beagles had no change in impedance from rest and showed a stepwise increase in stroke volume with incremental work loads. By contrast, senescent animals demonstrated a marked augmentation of impedance during exercise and minimal increase of stroke volume. These differences persisted through maximal effort but were abolished by acute β-adrenergic blockade, which increased impedance in the young dogs (Figure 7).[30] Thus, the higher afterload imposed by the arterial tree of older persons during exercise may limit systolic emptying and thence ejection fraction response. This increased afterload with age may represent a deficit in arterial vasodilation in response to endogenous catecholamines. Similar reductions in the ability of exogenous β-adrenergic stimulation to relax older human forearm vessels[31] and isolated aortic muscle strips from senescent animals[32] have been documented.

Exercise-induced Arrhythmias

Another characteristic age-associated difference in the response to aerobic exercise is an increase in exercise-induced arrhythmias in older persons, both supraventricular and ventricular. In clinically healthy BLSA volunteers, isolated premature atrial complexes during treadmill exercise increased in prevalence from 7% below age

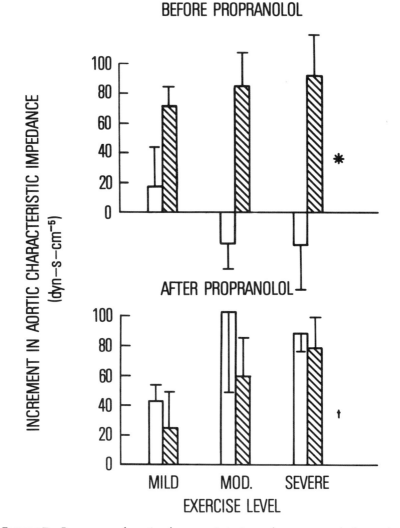

FIGURE 7. *Response of aortic characteristic impedance to graded exercise in young adult (□) and senescent (▨) beagle dogs. Before propranolol administration (top panel), impedance increased during exercise in the old but not the young animals. After propranolol (bottom panel), impedance increased similarly with exercise in both groups. Reproduced from Reference 30 with permission.*

30 years to 43% over 60 years. Exercise-induced paroxysmal supraventricular tachycardia (PSVT) has been detected in 3.5% of more than 3,000 maximal treadmill exercise tests in apparently healthy BLSA volunteers. PSVT increased in incidence from 0% in the 20s to about 10% over age 80 years; two thirds of these episodes were asymptomatic three- to five-beat salvos.[33] Although no increase in subsequent coronary events was seen over a mean follow-up of 5.5 years, 10% of the group with PSVT later developed a spontaneous atrial tachyarrhythmia compared with only 2% of age-matched controls without exercise-induced PSVT.

Exercise-induced ventricular arrhythmias, like their supraventricular counterparts, increase both in frequency and complexity with advancing age.[34-39] In apparently healthy BLSA volunteers, isolated premature ventricular complexes (PVCs) during or after maximal treadmill exercise increased in prevalence fivefold, from 11% to 57% between the third and ninth decades. Asymptomatic exercise-induced runs of ventricular tachycardia (VT), all ≤6 beats in duration, were found in 4% of apparently healthy individuals aged 65 years and older, a rate 25 times that of younger persons.[38] Perhaps more important, over a mean follow-up of about 2 years, none of these elderly persons with nonsustained VT during exercise testing developed angina, myocardial infarction, syncope, or cardiac death.

In a more recent BLSA analysis, 80 of 1,160 volunteers developed frequent PVCs (≥10% of beats in any minute) or nonsustained VT during maximal treadmill exercise testing (an average of 2.4 tests per individual were performed).[39] These 80 individuals were older than those free of such arrhythmia (64 vs. 50 years). Of note, the striking age-associated increase in the prevalence of these complex exercise-induced PVCs was limited to men (Figure 8). The prevalence of coronary risk factors and exercise-induced ischemia by ECG and thallium scanning did not differ between the 80 cases and a group of 80 age- and sex-matched controls. Furthermore, the incidence of cardiac events (angina pectoris, nonfatal infarction, cardiac syncope, and cardiac death) was nearly identical in cases and controls (10% vs. 12.5%, respectively) over a mean follow-up of 5.6 years without antiarrhythmic drug therapy.[39] Thus, the limited data available in older persons without apparent heart disease support a striking age-related increase in the prevalence and complexity of exercise-related PVCs; however, even frequent or repetitive PVCs induced by exercise do not appear to increase cardiac morbidity or mortality in these older volunteers.

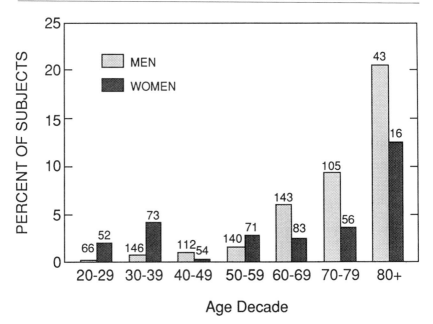

FIGURE 8. *Age-associated increase in frequent or repetitive ventricular premature complexes during a maximal treadmill test in asymptomatic volunteers. From Reference 39.*

References

1. Astrand I: Aerobic work capacity in men and women with special reference to age. *Acta Physiol Scand* 1960; 169:1–92
2. Conway J, Wheeler R, Sannerstedt R: Sympathetic nervous activity during exercise in relation to age. *Cardiovasc Res* 1971;5:577–581
3. Dehn MM, Bruce R: Longitudinal variations in maximal oxygen intake with age and activity. *J Appl Physiol* 1972;33:805–807
4. Fleg JL, Lakatta EG: Role of muscle loss in the age-associated reduction in Vo_2max. *J Appl Physiol* 1988;65:1147–1151
5. Heath GW, Hagberg JW, Ehsani AA, Holloszy JO: A physiological comparison of young and older endurance athletes. *J Apply Physiol* 1981;51:634–640
6. Julius S, Amery A, Whitlock LS, Conway J: Influence of age on the hemodynamic response to exercise. *Circulation* 1967;36:222–230
7. Robinson S: Experimental studies of physical fitness in relation to age. *Arbeitsphysiologie* 1938;10:252–323
8. Strandell T: Heart rate, arterial lactate concentration and oxygen

uptake during exercise in old men compared with young men. *Acta Physiol Scand* 1964;60:197–216

9. McConnell AK, Davies CTM: A comparison of the ventilatory responses to exercise of elderly and younger humans. *J Gerontol (Biol Sci)* 1992;47:B137–B141

10. Ogawa T, Spina RJ, Martin WH III, et al: Effects of aging, sex, and physical training on cardiovascular responses to exercise. *Circulation* 1992;86:494–503

11. Martin WH III, Ogawa T, Kohrt WM, et al: Effects of aging, gender, and physical training on peripheral vascular function. *Circulation* 1991;84:654–664

12. Fleg JL, Schulman S, Gerstenblith G, et al: Central versus peripheral adaptations in highly trained seniors. *Physiologist* 1988;31:A158

13. Seals DR, Hagberg JM, Hurley BF, Ehsani AA, Holloszy JO: Endurance training in older men and women: I. Cardiovascular responses to exercise. *J Appl Physiol* 1984;57:1024–1029

14. Pollock ML, Foster C, Knapp D, Rod JL, Schmidt DH: Effect of age and training on aerobic capacity and body composition of master athletes. *J Appl Physiol* 1987;62:725–731

15. Rogers MA, Hagberg JM, Martin WH III, Ehsani AA, Holloszy JO: Decline in $\dot{V}O_2$max with aging in master athletes and sedentary men. *J Appl Physiol* 1990;68:2195–2199

16. Granath A, Johnson B, Strendell T: Circulation in healthy old men studied by right heart catheterization at rest and during exercise in supine and sitting position. *Acta Med Scand* 1964;176:425–446

17. Hossack KF, Bruce RA: Maximal cardiac function in sedentary normal men and women: comparison of age-related changes. *J Appl Physiol* 1982;54:799–804

18. Younis LT, Melin JA, Robert AR, Detry JM: Influence of age and sex on left ventricular volumes and ejection fraction during upright exercise in normal subjects. *Eur Heart J* 1990;11:916–924

19. Rodeheffer RJ, Gerstenblith G, Becker LC, Fleg JL, Weisfeldt ML, Lakatta EG: Exercise cardiac output is maintained with advancing age in healthy human subjects: cardiac dilatation and increased stroke volume compensate for a diminished heart rate. *Circulation* 1984;64:203–213

20. Fleg JL, Gerstenblith G, Becker LC, et al: Independent effects of age and gender on specificity of ejection fraction response to upright cycle exercise. *Circulation* 1990;(supp III):III–137

21. Higginbotham MB, Morris KP, Williams RS, Coleman RE, Cobb FR: Physiologic basis for the age-related decline in aerobic work capacity. *Am J Cardiol* 1986;57:1374–1379

22. Mann DL, Denenberg BS, Gash AK, Makler PT, Bove AA: Effect of age on ventricular performance during graded supine exercise. *Am Heart J* 1986;111:108–115

23. Port S, Cobb FR, Coleman RE, Jones RH: Effect of age on the response of the left ventricular ejection fraction to exercise. *N Engl J Med* 1980;303:1133–137

24. Kuo LC, Bolli R, Thornby J, Roberts R, Verani MS: Effects of exercise tolerance, age, and gender on the specificity of radionuclide angiography: sequential ejection fraction analysis during multistage exercise. *Am Heart J* 1987;113:1180–1189

25. Adams KF, Vincent LM, McAllister SM, el-Ashmawy H, Sheps DS: The influence of age and gender on left ventricular response to supine exercise in asymptomatic normal subjects. *Am Heart J* 1987;113:732–742

26. Ehsani AA, Ogawa T, Miller TR, Spira RJ, Jilka SM: Exercise training improves left ventricular systolic function in older men. *Circulation* 1991;83:96–103

27. Fleg JL, Schulman S, O'Connor F, et al: Effect of propranolol on age-associated changes in left ventricular performance during exercise. *Circulation* 1991;84(suppl II):II–187

28. Fleg JL, Tzankoff SP, Lakatta EG: Age-related augmentation of plasma catecholamines during dynamic exercise in healthy males. *J Appl Physiol* 1985;59:1033–1039

29. Lakatta EG: Alterations in the cardiovascular system that occur in advanced age. *Fed Proc* 1979;38:163–167

30. Yin FCP, Weisfeldt ML, Milnor WR: Role of aortic input impedance in the decreased cardiovascular response to exercise with aging in dogs. *J Clin Invest* 1981;68:28–38

31. Van Brummelen P, Buhler FR, Kiowski W, Amann FW: Age-related decrease in cardiac and peripheral vascular responsiveness to isoprenaline; studies in normal subjects. *Clin Sci* 1981;60:571–577

32. Godfraind T: Alternative mechanisms for the potentiation of the relaxation evoked by isoprenaline in aortae from young and aged rats. *Eur J Pharm* 1979;53:272–279

33. Maurer MS, Fleg JL, Shefrin EA: Exercise-induced supraventricular tachycardia in apparently healthy volunteers. *J Am Coll Cardiol* 1992;19:35A

34. McHenry PL, Morris SN, Kavalier M, Jordan JW: Comparative study of exercise-induced ventricular arrhythmias in normal subjects and patients with documented coronary artery disease. *Am J Cardiol* 1976;37:609–616

35. Froelicher VF, Thomas MM, Pillow C, Lancaster MC: Epidemiologic study of asymptomatic men screened by maximal treadmill testing for latent coronary artery disease. *Am J Cardiol* 1974;34:770–776

36. Faris JV, McHenry PL, Jordan JW, Morris SN: Prevalence and reproducibility of exercise-induced ventricular arrhythmias during maximal exercise testing in normal men. *Am J Cardiol* 1976;37:617–622

37. Ekblom B, Hartley LH, Day WC: Occurrence and reproducibility of exercise-induced ventricular ectopy in normal subjects. *Am J Cardiol* 1979;43:35–40

38. Fleg JL, Lakatta EG: Prevalence and prognosis of exercise-induced nonsustained ventricular tachycardia in apparently healthy volunteers. *Am J Cardiol* 1984;54:762–764

39. Busby MJ, Shefrin EA, Fleg JL: Prevalence and long-term significance of exercise-induced frequent or repetitive ventricular ectopic beats in apparently healthy volunteers. *J Am Coll Cardiol* 1989;14:1659–1665

Chapter 23

Exercise Echocardiography

Steven M. Rosenthal, MD, and
Navin C. Nanda, MD

Exercise electrocardiography is limited by its low sensitivity and specificity and hence predictive value in evaluating myocardial ischemia. However, coupling it with noninvasive digital imaging of the heart provides useful clinical data concerning prognosis and the detection, localization, and determination of the extent of myocardial ischemia and damage. Radiochemical digital imaging techniques have been the cornerstone for this in clinical practice; an abundance of data have been accumulated attesting to its clinical use. Radionuclide angiography, which provides wall motion information but has been supplanted by planar and single photon computed tomographic imaging (SPECT), which uses thallium and the newer technetium-labeled agents, provides excellent sensitivity, specificity, and predictive value for the evaluation of myocardial perfusion (in contrast to wall motion) and the detection and localization of ischemic and infarcted regions. Despite its widespread use and considerable power, radiochemical cardiac imaging requires expensive machinery and maintenance contracts, and the acquiring, handling, and administration of expensive, heavily regulated radiochemicals that expose patients to at least low levels of radiation.

Improved echocardiographic technology implemented over the past decade provides high-resolution, real-time ultrasonic imaging of myocardial wall motion. When coupled with simple computer-generated image acquisition and display technology, echocardiography provides a convenient, relatively inexpensive means to detect exercise-induced ischemic, abnormal myocardial wall motion with

From Fletcher GF, (ed): *Cardiovascular Response to Exercise.* Mount Kisco, NY, Futura Publishing Company, Inc., © 1994.

sensitivity, specificity, and predictive value directly comparable to that of the radiochemical perfusion techniques.

In contrast to the direct myocardial perfusion data provided by thallium and the newer technetium-labeled perfusion agents, echocardiography highlights regional and global wall function as a marker of significant coronary artery disease hypoperfusion. It provides information about abnormal global and regional myocardial function, and can be adapted easily to provide information about ischemic mitral regurgitation.[1]

Exercise echocardiography can be used as a screening test in patients with nondiagnostic exercise electocardiograms, for locating and sizing myocardial perfusion abnormalities and identifying the culprit artery, for assessing success of revascularization procedures, for postmyocardial infarction prognostication, and for evaluation of myocardial viability (Table 1).

Background and Description of Exercise Echocardiography

Acute ischemia rapidly produces abnormal wall function that can be detected with echocardiography[2]; myocardial dysfunction actually precedes the appearance of electrical abnormalities that may partially contribute to the greater sensitivity of echocardiography over electrocardiography for detecting coronary ischemia.

TABLE 1.   Indications for Performing Exercise Echocardiography

1. Screening for ischemic heart disease in intermediate risk patients with nondiagnostic ECG (baseline ST-T or conduction abnormalities or LVH)
2. Identification of ischemic territory and its size
3. Identification of "culprit" coronary stenosis lesion
4. Post–myocardial infarction prognostication/risk stratification
5. Evaluation for residual or new ischemia post–coronary artery bypass grafting
6. Evaluation for residual or new ischemia post–percutaneous transluminal coronary angioplasty or other interventional procedure
7. Identification of viable myocardial tissue in the setting of hibernation or stunning

ECG, electrocardiogram; LVH, left ventricular hypertrophy.

Technology

M-mode echocardiography with its excellent temporospatial resolution was the first ultrasound technique used for this purpose in clinical research settings but proved to be clinically impractical because it failed to image large portions of the myocardium. By virtue of its ability to yield tomographic visualization of the heart in three anatomical dimensions, all in real time (the fourth dimension), two-dimensional echocardiography can image each of the left ventricular walls and apex. It was limited originally by the inadequate resolving properties of the early machines and to impaired transmission of ultrasound through the chest wall and cavity; transmission is impaired further by increased respiratory motions produced by exercise. With the demonstration that wall motion abnormalities usually persist for at least 60 seconds and for even longer than 30 minutes,[3] immediate postexercise imaging was shown to be superior to the limited images obtained during exercise,[1] although it should be completed within 90 seconds before mildly ischemic areas improve. Immediate postexercise imaging has led to significant improvement in the application and practicality of exercise echocardiography. Furthermore, significant improvements in the machinery[4] and the development of simple general purpose computer technology and video analogue-to-digital conversion boards (frame grabbers) have facilitated its use for investigating myocardial function in a manner suitable for clinical practice.

Real-time images of entire cardiac cycles are introduced into computer memory for visual display and comparison and can be recorded on digital media (magnetic or optical disk drives). The cardiac images can be acquired from preexisting images already acquired on conventional videotape and then converted to digital format, or they can be captured in real time during imaging to avoid the inevitable loss of resolution with videotape recording. If acquired from videotape, the operator can choose the best technical cycles from the videotape, whereas in the later setting, the computer might capture several cardiac cycle images in real time and allow the operator to choose the best image with the least respiratory motion artifact. Finally, playback at a standardized heart rate allows comparisons of pre- and immediate postexercise images.

Usually, four pre-exercise and their corresponding immediate postexercise views are examined; these include the parasternal long (interventricular septum and posterior walls) and parasternal short axes (septum, anterior, lateral, and inferior walls) and the apical four- (apical, septum, and lateral walls) and two-chamber views (apical, inferior, and anterior walls) (Figure 1). After arranging the pre- and postexercise views in side-by-side fashion, most laboratories find that simple visual comparisons of the views are adequate. The data can be evaluated semiquantitatively with a global wall motion score index[5–8]; in this setting, a numerical grade is determined subjectively for each segment of myocardium evaluated and a total global wall motion index calculated. Alternatively, it is possible to quantify directly the amount of segmental wall motion by manually tracing the pre– and post–end-diastolic and end-systolic ventricular contours and have the computer complete the calculations. Wall stress, which can be estimated directly if the wall thicknesses are measured, may increase the sensitivity of the technique.[9] Shapiro and Ginzton have had considerable experience with this technique using bicycle exercise with subxiphoid views.[10] These techniques are sophisticated and require very high-quality imaging and are not yet performed in most clinical laboratories.

Albunex, an injectable albumen–air bubble contrast agent, which has been approved recently by the Food and Drug Administration, may improve visualization of segmental wall motion and facilitate measurement of the endocardial surface. Automatic edge detection would facilitate cardiac cycle regional wall motion measurements but cannot yet reliably detect the ventricular epicardial surfaces in the general clinical exercise echocardiography setting.[11] Therefore, it is not yet possible to measure continuously the extent and rate of wall thickening and thinning, but this may develop further with the use of the contrast agents.

Exercise Methods and Level of Function

The production of wall motion abnormalities depends on the induction of ischemia. Therefore, exercise echocardiography is likely most sensitive at full levels of exertion; 85% to 90% predicted, age-adjusted heart rates should be achieved with an accompanying significant rise in systemic blood pressure and double product. Submaximal heart rate exercise testing has been performed success-

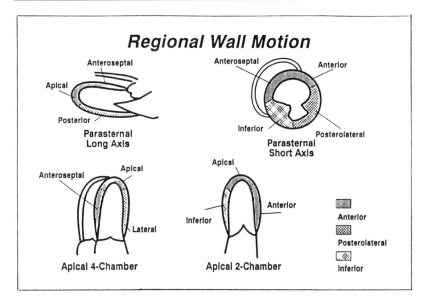

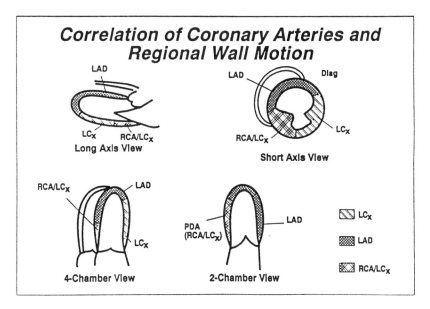

FIGURE 1: Top: *Distribution of anatomical walls for which motion is evaluated and assigned.* **Bottom:** *Correlation of coronary artery vascular territories with the anatomical walls they supply. Diag, diagonal; LAD, left anterior descending artery; LC$_X$, left circumflex artery; PDA, posterior descending artery; RCA, right coronary artery. Reproduced from Reference 14 with permission.*

fully but diagnosis and prognostication is specific to the maximum double product achieved and not beyond; it would seem fruitful at least to reach submaximal heart rates, or 70% of predicted, age-adjusted maximum heart rate when performing the test. In fact, in a report of 150 consecutive patients undergoing stress echocardiography and cardiac catheterization at the Cleveland Clinic (sensitivity = 84%, specificity = 86%), the major causes of false negative results related to single-vessel disease, submaximal exercise, and moderate stenosis (50–70%).[12]

Echocardiography can be combined with traditional treadmill or bicycle (supine or upright) exercise. Each has its inherent strengths and weaknesses and its own application to echocardiography as well. For instance, upright or supine bicycle testing produces reasonable images during testing at each level of exercise; imaging from the subxiphoid position can be performed in most patients, but may fail to visualize the apex. Furthermore, there is a tendency to fatigue earlier on the bicycle than on the treadmill, which results in the achievement of lower levels of oxygen consumption.[13] On the other hand, treadmill exercise precludes adequate imaging during exercise because of impaired chest wall transmission in that position; instead, the images are obtained immediately postexercise and can rival the images obtained during bicycle exercise,[13] but must be completed rapidly, as noted, by well-trained technologists because of possible lack of wall motion abnormality persistence. It is reported that rapid resolution of wall motion abnormalities reflects either mild ischemia or a well-collateralized ischemic territory. Most American cardiologists probably use treadmill testing because of the general familiarity with it and the higher sensitivity of detecting myocardial ischemia, whereas bicycle testing is more widespread in Europe.

Interpretation of Wall Motion Response

Interpretation of the cardiac response to exercise centers on the actual degree and rate of wall thickening, endocardial inward motion,[6] and, finally, the extent of left ventricular cavity narrowing.

The normal response to exercise is characterized by increased extent and rate of wall thickening and a decrease in end-systolic left ventricular diameter; any response less than hyperdynamic is abnormal. Exercise-induced ischemia is characterized by a segmental reduction from normal wall motion or a failure to increase motion. An akinetic wall that remains fixed is infarcted, stunned, or hibernating; improvement of a previously akinetic region probably reflects uncompromised circulation.[14] An area of uncertainty relates to interpreting the significance of a preexisting hypokinetic segment that remains unchanged versus the one that worsens.[15] The evaluation of wall motion is one of the more difficult aspects of performing and interpreting echocardiograms; a significant amount of baseline echocardiographic training in this technique as part of a fellowship or other extensive postgraduate training is important.[5] Guidelines already exist for the performance and interpretation of echocardiography.[16] The technologist should be well trained in exercise echocardiography and in performing the views needed and should review the results with the interpreting physician to ensure development of adequate images, whereas the physician should be well versed in the diagnosis and management of cardiac and coronary artery disease and its interpretation and correlation with echocardiography; the technologist cannot interpret the echocardiogram for the physician.

Accuracy of Exercise Echocardiography

The sensitivity of exercise echocardiography for detecting coronary artery disease is significantly greater than that for exercise electrocardiography. Over the years, these values have ranged from the mid-70s to 90s; recent, large studies have demonstrated sensitivities in the 90% range.[17,18] In one of these large studies, sensitivity ranged from 85% for those patients with a 70% or greater angiographic stenosis of a single vessel to 94% for triple-vessel disease. Specificity ranges from the low 60s to approximately the 90% range and varies with the source of patients. Finally, exercise echocardiography is reproducible.[8]

Determinations for sensitivity may be artificially lowered if, when using coronary arteriography as the "gold standard," 50%- rather than 70%-coronary artery lesions are considered to be clinically significant. There would be no ischemia and abnormal wall motion if some stenoses in this range were not hemodynamically significant (depending on a variety of factors including vessel caliber, stenosis length, cross-sectional area, and presence of collateralization). For instance, one study[7] found that only one half of 12 patients with single-vessel 50% stenoses demonstrated exercise-induced wall motion abnormalities whereas the remaining patients did not. In contrast, 11 of 11 patients with at least a 75% stenosis demonstrated exercise-induced wall motion abnormalities and 10 of 11 patients with less than 25% stenoses demonstrated normal motion. Quantitative coronary angiography revealed that the presence of ischemic wall motion abnormalities correlated with minimal lumen diameters, minimal cross-sectional areas, percent diameter stenosis, and percent area stenosis, and that these values were significantly different from those without ischemic wall motion abnormalities. Another study of 57 patients with single-vessel disease and normal resting left ventricular motion, which used quantitative echocardiography and quantitative coronary angiography, also revealed that the measurements for the stenoses were different in those patients who developed exercise-induced wall motion abnormalities.[19]

Kloner et al.[3] have reported that sensitivity might be improved by imaging for several minutes postexercise because several patients appeared to develop wall motion abnormalities 15 minutes after exercise where none had been present before. Only 16 of 22 patients (almost all had known coronary artery disease) demonstrated immediate postexercise wall motion abnormalities, whereas an additional 6 patients demonstrated initially normal postexercise wall motion that worsened by 15 minutes postexercise. All 6 had experienced prior myocardial infarction and 5 had previously undergone coronary artery bypass grafting. The cause of this finding is uncertain but further investigation of this phenomenon would be warranted.

Bayesian Probability Theory

An exercise test must be chosen, performed, and interpreted with Bayesian probability theory in mind.[20] Briefly, Bayes' theorem states that whereas test reliability is determined by its sensitivity and specificity, its predictive value can be determined only when referencing the prevalence of the disease in the population under study. Exercise echocardiography is used most efficiently and appropriately in those patients with nondiagnostic, or seemingly false positive or negative resting or exercise electrocardiograms. This should be combined with the information provided by the patient's clinical and electrocardiograpic response to exercise to achieve the best predictive value.

Comparison of Exercise Echocardiography with Nuclear Imaging Techniques

Radionuclide Angiography

There is a paucity of data comparing exercise echocardiography and radionuclide angiography. The studies were preliminary and performed 10 years ago using older echocardiographic machinery; the echocardiograms were all read without the benefit of modern frame-grabbing technology and so side-by-side comparisons of pre- and postexertional images could not be performed. The studies were small and echocardiographic and radionuclide angiographic imaging were never compared on the same exercise run. Three studies demonstrated no difference,[21] better radionuclide angiographic sensitivity and specificity,[22] and better echocardiographic sensitivity and specificity.[6]

The largest study, involving 73 patients who underwent treadmill exercise echocardiography, was compared with bicycle exercise radionuclide angiography peformed in 41 of the 73 patients[6]; ejection fraction and regional wall motion scores were calculated. The sensitivity and specificity for echocardiography were 91% and 88%, respectively, but the sensitivity was only 71% for radionuclide angiography. Furthermore, radionuclide angiography failed to detect any single-vessel disease and also was less sensitive for double- and triple-vessel disease (sensitivity for echocardiography vs. radionuclide angiography 100% vs. 80% for double-vessel disease and 100% vs. 90% for triple-vessel disease).

Exercise radionuclide angiography has been replaced by myocardial perfusion scanning for several reasons. First, the fall in ejection fraction attributed to coronary artery disease is now recognized to be less sensitive than originally believed because with only single- or double-vessel disease adequate remaining nonischemic muscle compensates for loss of function and maintains ejection fraction. Second, the usually single left anterior oblique view obtained with exercise radionuclide angiography is insufficient to evaluate each of the wall segments. Third, 2 minutes of imaging are required for each view and ischemia occurring at peak exercise at the very end of testing may be missed. Echocardiographically obtained ejection fraction is beset by a similar problem, but with its instantaneous beat-to-beat tomographic imaging of each of the myocardial segments, exercise echocardiography surpasses this problem.

Planar Thallium

Few studies have directly compared exercise echocardiography and planar thallium perfusion studies; most were small, performed in the earlier years of exercise echocardiography without the benefit of digital video acquisition boards, and were essentially pilot studies designed to determine the feasibility and usefulness of echocardiography.[1,23,24] One study[23] achieved adequate echocardiography in 71% of 28 patients suspected of having ischemic heart disease; 10 patients developed reversible wall motion abnormalities and of these, 6 who underwent planar thallium imaging demonstrated reversible perfusion defects.

In the first attempt to examine systematically the viability of immediate post-treadmill exercise echocardiographic imaging (to permit coupling of echocardiographic imaging to treadmill exercise), Maurer and Nanda[1] directly compared treadmill echocardiography with planar thallium on the same exercise study in 41 of 48 patients in whom adequate echocardiographic images could be obtained. The two techniques not only correlated well but echocardiography also allowed right ventricular imaging and the demonstration of detecting isolated right ventricular dysfunction in the presence of normal thallium scans.

Heng et al.[24] in 54 patients and Gentile et al. as reported by Roldan and Crawford[25] in 50 patients showed high sensitivity and specificity (100% and 93%, and 86% and 100% for the studies, respectively) and both demonstrated significant agreement and comparability between the two techniques.

Single Photon Emission Computed Tomography (SPECT)

Vasey et al.[26] presented preliminary data suggesting comparability between exercise echocardiography and SPECT using thallium.

Pozzoli et al.[27] compared echocardiography and SPECT using the new radionuclide perfusion agent, technetium-99m sestamibi in 75 patients with suspected coronary artery disease. They noted that only 45% of their patients reached 85% predicted maximum heart rate. They found sensitivities of 71% and 84% and specificities of 96% and 88%, respectively, for echocardiography and the SPECT studies; SPECT was more sensitive for the detection of single-vessel disease (82% vs. 61%).

By far, Quinones et al.[17] have produced the largest and most comprehensive comparison of exercise echocardiography and thallium SPECT. They performed the two procedures simultaneously on each of 292 patients who had completed treadmill exercise with almost identical sensitivities for the two imaging modalities. The sensitivity for exercise echocardiography and SPECT were 58% and 61%, respectively, for single-vessel disease, 86% for both methods for double vessel disease, and 94% for both methods for triple-vessel disease; specificity was 88% and 81%, respectively. Adequate echocardiographic studies were obtained in 289 (99%) patients and tests were normal in 137 and abnormal in 118 with 88% agreement. Discordant results were obtained in only 34 patients; 17 patients with normal SPECT examination demonstrated abnormal echocardiograms (16 of 17 actually demonstrated coronary artery disease by angiography or previous myocardial infarction), while 17 patients with normal exercise echocardiograms demonstrated abnormal SPECT examination (11 of 16 patients demonstrated coronary artery disease angiographically or by evidence of previous myocardial infarction). There was partial agreement (ie, normal vs. abnormal findings) in 88% of 867 myocardial regions analyzed and complete agreement (ie, exact findings) in 711 (82%). SPECT demonstrated more ischemic abnormalities (reversible or partially reversible reperfusion) than echocardiography (120 vs. 74) while echocardiography detected more fixed abnormalities than SPECT (128 vs. 84). Perhaps the most interesting findings related to the differentiation of ischemic regions from scar. Interestingly, ischemia was only slightly more frequently detected in areas of normal motion at rest with thallium SPECT while ischemia, characterized by areas of partial redistribution, was clearly more apparent with SPECT in areas of preexisting wall motion abnormalities. Although fixed radiochemical perfusion defects are thought classically to reflect infarction, it has become recognized that a nonreperfusing defect in the delayed images might reflect hibernation; of note, 30% of those patients with fixed defects actually demonstrated the presence of normal or decreased wall motion at rest with echocardiography, which worsened with exercise suggestive of ischemia.

Applications of Exercise Echocardiography (See Table 1)

Screening Test for Coronary Artery Disease

The sensitivity and specificity of exercise echocardiography has been described. Many of the reported findings with exercise echocardiographic studies were performed with populations with high disease prevalence, well over 50%. Ryan et al.[28] specifically evaluated exercise echocardiography in 64 previously undiagnosed patients with normal resting wall motion and found a sensitivity and specificity of 78% and 100%, respectively. The inclusion of only normal baseline wall function ensured that a diagnosis could not be established on the basis of an abnormal resting segmental wall motion and therefore would provide realistic values in a general undiagnosed population; this helps explain the relatively low sensitivity. A second explanation likely rests with underlying β-blockade that had not been discontinued. Sawada et al.,[29] also addressing this problem, studied 57 previously undiagnosed women who proved to have a 49% or moderate prevalence and found sensitivity and specificity values of 86% for each. Most studies have included patients with a higher prevalence of coronary artery disease and motion abnormalities and measures of increased sensitivity performed in these populations are valid in this type of population only. Crouse and Kramer[30] performed exercise echocardiography on 228 patients referred for evaluation who were not previously diagnosed to have coronary artery disease and found an overall sensitivity of 97% and specificity of only 64%. The presence and number of patients with resting wall motion abnormalities was not provided. Exercise echocardiography was abnormal in 19 patients with otherwise normal coronary arteries, and in 15 of these, there were resting wall motion abnormalities that accounted for the low specificity.

Post–Myocardial Infarction Prognostication

Exercise echocardiography has been used effectively for post–myocardial infarction prognostication.[13,31] Jaarsma et al.[32] used symptom-limited exercise echocardiography within 3 weeks of a first myocardial infarction in 43 patients with adequate images obtained in 88%. Each patient demonstrated a resting segmental wall motion abnormality but 18 also demonstrated transient remote asynergy, of which 17 (94%) demonstrated significant double- or triple-vessel obstruction. All seven patients with triple-vessel disease demonstrated transient remote segmental abnormalities; conversely, there were no additional exercise-induced remote wall motion abnormalities in the remaining 25 patients of whom 20 had only single-vessel disease; the remaining 5 with falsely negative findings had double-vessel disease, but only 2 of these 5 had obstruction of a major artery whereas the remaining 3 had small branch obstruction. In this manner, exercise-induced transient wall motion abnormalities yielded a sensitivity and specificity of 77% and 95%, respectively, for detecting multivessel disease. Over the following 16 weeks, 16 of the original 43 patients (37%) experienced further complications, with only 12 having had demonstrated transient remote asynergy yielding a sensitivity of 75% and specificity of 78% for predicting new events; seven of these events were reinfarctions.

Ryan et al.[33] performed low-level post–myocardial infarction treadmill exercise testing in 40 patients with a sensitivity and specificity of 82% and 88%, respectively, for the detection of multivessel disease. Over the next 10-month follow-up period, exercise echocardiography demonstrated a sensitivity and specificity of 80% and 95% for predicting future coronary artery complications; the test was positive for each of the six patients who experienced further infarction or death. These authors failed to describe patient selection and exclusion as well as echocardiographic imaging success rate.

Applegate et al.[34] screened 90 post–myocardial infarction patients and measured ejection fraction and segmental wall motion quantitatively with a success rate of 74%, entirely consistent with the difficulty in measuring these parameters with echocardiography. The sensitivity and specificity for the detection of important coronary artery disease were not reported but the sensitivity and specificity for prediction of future complication were 63% and 80%, respectively. Exertionally reduced ejection fraction predicted 44% of future cardiac events but was not as sensitive as the appearance of new or worsened wall motion abnormalities, which predicted 63% of new events.

Evaluation of Regional Myocardial Perfusion Post–Coronary Artery Bypass Grafting

One of the most important benefits of exercise echocardiography lies in its ability to localize the culprit vascular territory stenosis and it has been reported to be clinically useful for predicting the adequacy of regional myocardial perfusion in patients who have received coronary artery bypass grafting.[14,35] Swada et al.,[35] using upright bicycle exercise echocardiography, detected exercise-induced wall motion abnormalities in 94% of patients with nonrevascularized vessels while localization was possible in approximately 90% of them. Crouse et al.[14] have performed treadmill exercise echocardiography in 125 patients seen either in routine post–bypass surgery follow-up or for symptoms. Excluding infarct-related akinetic regions, very high sensitivity (98%) and specificity (92%), with very high positive (99%) and negative predictive values, were obtained. The extremely high sensitivity reflects the high-risk population, although in contrast to electrocardiography, post-exercise echocardiography maintained a very high specificity and negative predictive value.

Evaluation of Regional Myocardial Perfusion Postangioplasty or Other Interventional Revascularization Procedure

Exercise echocardiography can provide significant data on the success of angioplasty.[30,36] Broderick et al.[36] demonstrated improvement or resolution in inducible ischemic wall motion abnormalities in 29 of 31 patients. In another group of 35 patients who underwent exercise echocardiography preangioplasty, 40% demonstrated resting wall motion abnormalities; 71% of these improved to normal postangioplasty.[30] Conversely, three patients demonstrated renewed wall motion abnormalities postangioplasty that reflected artery restenosis. In a much larger extension study of 185 patients who were successfully angioplastied, exercise echocardiography demonstrated high sensitivity, specificity, and positive- and negative-predictive values (95%, 82%, 95%, and 82%, respectively).

In our laboratory, exercise echocardiography also has been applied to evaluation of restenosis after intracoronary stenting with a high sensitivity and specificity (90–95%, respectively).[37]

Advantages and Limitations

Exercise echocardiography in appropriately trained hands is practical, accurate, inexpensive, and convenient relative to other comparable techniques, provides rapid results without the need for delayed imaging, and does not produce radiation exposure (Table 2). Excellent information is provided concerning global and segmental wall motion and myocardial viability.

It has its limitations as well. Transthoracic echocardiographic imaging is affected by noise and impaired ultrasound transmission, which results in reduced resolution that necessitates the use of well-trained technologists and interpreters, and evaluation of quality control. Even so, the rate of successful exercise echocardiographic procedures varies from about 85% to as high as 99% in excellent national level laboratories, leaving a small number of patients in whom it cannot be performed. Exercise thallium studies can be performed in almost every patient.

Exercise echocardiography detects wall motion, which we use as an indirect rather than a direct measure of myocardial perfusion.

Conclusion

Exercise echocardiography is a cost-effective tool with sensitivity and specificity comparable to radionuclide perfusion imaging. It

TABLE 2.   Attributes of Exercise Echocardiography and Radionuclide Perfusion Scanning

Echocardiography	Radionuclide perfusion scanning
Examines myocardial wall motion as a marker of perfusion	Examines myocardial perfusion directly
Relatively new technique; capable of higher (1 mm) resolution	Long-standing use; much greater experience and background accumulated; lower resolution device
Portable; more versatile; provides information on valvular, pericardial, and myocardial function also	Provides information only on myocardial perfusion
Relatively inexpensive; inexpensive computer package required in addition to already existing good quality echocardiographic machine	More expensive, very specialized machinery necessary; SPECT scanner is more expensive than planar scanner
No injectates required	Expensive radioisotopes involved; nuclear regulatory site license and operator's license required for operation and handling radioisotopes
Immediate results available	4–24-hr delayed scanning and possible reinjection required
Imaging attempts unsuccessful in 2–5% of patients	Imaging attempt almost always successful
High degree of technologist and physician training required for competent performance and interpretation	Well-trained technologist and physician training are necessary

is a convenient, relatively inexpensive imaging test that provides clinically useful information concerning the presence of coronary artery stenoses, identification and size of the vascular territory at risk, and the viability of the muscle. It can be used in a variety of settings including post–myocardial infarction prognostication and for evaluating the success of revascularization procedures.

References

1. Maurer G, Nanda NC: Two dimensional echocardiographic evaluation of exercise-induced left and right ventricular asynergy: correlation with thallium scanning. *Am J Cardiol* 1981;48:720–727

2. Goldstein S, de Jong JW: Changes in left ventricular wall dimensions during regional myocardial ischemia. *Am J Cardiol* 1974;34:56–62

3. Kloner RA, Allen J, Cox TA, Zheng Y, Ruiz CE: Stunned left ventricular myocardium after exercise treadmill testing in coronary artery disease. *Am J Cardiol* 1991;68:329–334

4. Robertson WS, Feigenbaum H, Armstrong WF, Dillong JC, O'Donnell J, McHenry PW: Exercise echocardiography: a clinically practical addition in the evaluation of coronary artery disease. *J Am Coll Cardiol* 1983;2:1085–1091

5. Armstrong WF, O'Donnell J, Dillon JC, McHenry PL, Morris SN, Feigenbaum H: complementary value of two-dimensional exercise echocardiography to routine treadmill exercise testing. *Ann Intern Med* 1986;105:829–835

6. Limacher MC, Quinones MA, Poliner LR, Nelson JG, Winters WL Jr, Waggoner AD: Detection of coronary artery disease with exercise two-dimensional echocardiography. Description of a clinically applicable method and comparison with radionuclide ventriculography. *Circulation* 1983;67:1211–1218

7. Sheikh KH, Bengston JR, Helmy S Juarez C, Burgess R, Bashore TM, Kisslo J: Relation of quantitative coronary lesion measurements to the development of exercise-induced ischemia assessed by exercise echocardiography. *J Am Coll Cardiol* 1990;15:1043–1051

8. Oberman A, Fan PH, Nanda NC, Lee JY, Huster WJ, Sulentic JA, Storey OF: Reproducibility of two-dimensional exercise echocardiography. *J Am Coll Cardiol* 1989;14;923–928

9. Ginzton LE, Conant R, Brizendine M, Lee F, Mona I, Laks MM: Exercise subcostal two-dimensional echocardiography: a new method of segmental wall motion analysis. *Am J Cardiol* 1984;53:805–811

10. Shapiro SM, Ginzton LE: Quantitative stress echocardiography. *Echocardiography* 1992;9:85–96

11. Sher D, Revankar, Rosenthal SM: Computer methods in quantitation of cardiac wall parameters from two dimensional echocardiograms: a survey. *Int J Cardiac Imaging* 1992;8:11–26

12. Marwick TH, Nemec JJ, Haluska B, Pashkow FJ, Stewart WJ, Salcedo EE: Assets and limitations of exercise echocardiography in day-to-day practice. Noninvasive and invasive methods of cardiovascular diagnosis. *J Am Coll Cardiol* 1992;9:55–65

13. Crawford MF: Risk stratification after myocardial infarction with exercise and doppler echocardiography. *Circulation* 1991;84:I-163–I-166

14. Crouse LJ, Vacek JL, Beauchamp GD, Porter CB, Rosamond TL, Kramer PH: Exercise echocardiography after coronary artery bypass grafting. *Am J Cardiol* 1992;70:572–576

15. Feigenbaum H: Evolution of stress testing. Editorial. *Circulation* 1992;85:1217–1218

16. Pearlman AS, Gardin JM, Martin RP, Parisi A, Popp RL, Quinones MA, Stevenson JG: Guidelines for optimal physician training in echocardiography. Recommendations of the American Society of echocardiography committee for physician training in echocardiography. *Am J Cardiol* 1987;60:158–163

17. Quinones MA, Verani MS, Haichin RM, Mahmarian JJ, Suarez J, Zoghbi WA: Exercise echocardiography versus ^{201}Tl single-photon emission computed tomography in evaluation of coronary artery disease. Analysis of 292 patients. *Circulation* 1991;85:1026–1031

18. Crouse LJ, Harbrecht JJ, Vacek JL, Rosamond TL, Kramer PH: Exercise echocardiography as a screening test for coronary artery disease and correlation with coronary arteriography. *Am J Cardiol* 1991;67: 1213–1218

19. Agati L, Arata L, Luongo R, Iacoboni C, Renzi M, Vizza CD, Penco M, Fedele F, Dagianti A: Assessment of severity of coronary narrowings by quantitative exercise echocardiography and comparison with quantitative arteriography. *Am J Cardiol* 1991;67:1201–1207

20. Gibson RS, Beller GA: Should exercise electrocardiographic testing be replaced by radioisotope methods? in Rahimtolla SH, Brest AN (eds): *Controversies in Coronary Artery Disease, Cardiovascular Clinics.* Philadelphia: FA Davis Co, 1983, pp 1–31

21. Crawford MH, Petru MA, Amon W, Sorensen SG, Vance WS: Comparative value of 2-dimensional echocardiography and radionuclide angiography for quantitating changes in left ventricular performance during exercise limited by angina pectoris. *Am J Cardiol* 1984;53:42–46

22. Visser CA, van der Wieken RL, Kan G, Lie KI, Busemann-Sokele E, Meltzer RS, Durrer D: Comparison of two-dimensional echocardiography with radionuclide angiography during dynamic exercise for the detection of coronary artery disease. *Am Heart J* 1983;106:528–534

23. Wann LS, Faris JV, Childress RH, Dillon JC, Weyman AE, Feigenbaum H: Exercise cross-sectional echocardiography in ischemic heart disease. *Circulation* 1979;60:300–308

24. Heng MK, Simard M, Lake R, Udhoji VH: Exercise two-dimensional echocardiography for the diagnosis of coronary artery disease. *Am J Cardiol* 1984;54:502–507

25. Roldan CA, Crawford MH: Stress echocardiography versus radionuclide stress techniques. *Echocardiography* 1992;9:199–209

26. Vasey CG, Noblett T, Allen SM: Assessment of segmental wall motion by exercise echocardiography: comparison with single photon emission computed tomographic (SPECT) thallium immaging. *Circulation* 1989;80:II–66

27. Pozzoli MMA, Fioretti PM, Sallustri A, Reijs AEM, Roelandt JRTC: Exercise echocardiography and technetium-99m MIBI single photon emission computed tomography in the detection of coronary artery disease. *Am J Cardiol* 1991;67:350–355

28. Ryan T, Vasey CG, Presti CF, O'Donnell JA, Feigenbaum H, Armstrong WF: Exercise echocardiography: detection of coronary artery disease in patients with normal left ventricular wall motion at rest. *J Am Coll Cardiol* 1988;11:993–999

29. Sawada SG, Ryan T, Fineberg NS, Armstrong WF, Judson WE, McHenry PL, Feigenbaum H: Exercise echocardiographic detection of coronary artery disease in women. *J Am Coll Cardiol* 1989;14: 1440–1447

30. Crouse LJ, Kramer PH: Clinical applicability of echocardiographically

detected regional wall motion abnormalities provoked by upright treadmill exercise. *Echocardiography* 1992;9:97–106

31. O'Rourke RA: Risk stratification after myocardial infarction. *Circulation* 1991;84:I177–I181

32. Jaarsma W, Visser CA, Funke Kupper AJ, Res JCJ, Van Eenige MJ, Roos JP: Usefulness of two-dimensional exercise echocardiography shortly after myocardial infarction. *Am J Cardiol* 1986;57:86–90

33. Ryan T, Armstrong WF, O'Donnell JA, Feigenbaum H: Risk stratification after acute myocardial infarction by means of exercise two-dimensional echocardiography. *Am Heart J* 1987;114:1305–1316

34. Applegate RJ, Dell'Italia LJ, Crawford MH: Usefulness of two-dimensional echocardiography during low-level exercise testing early after uncomplicated acute myocardial infarction. *Am J Cardiol* 1987;60:10–14

35. Sawada SG, Judson WE, Ryan T, Armstrong WF, Feigenbaum H: Upright bicycle exercise echocardiography after coronary artery bypass grafting. *Am J Cardiol* 1989;64:1123–1129

36. Broderick T, Sawada S, Armstrong WF, Ryan T, Dillon JC, Bourdillon PD, Feigenbaum H: Improvement in rest and exercise-induced wall motion abnormalities after coronary angioplasty: an exercise echocardiographic study. *J Am Coll Cardiol* 1990;15:591–599

37. Hsiung MC, Roubin GS, Nanda NC: Usefulness of exercise echocardiography in the assessment of restenosis after intracoronary stenting (abstract). *Circulation* 1992;86:I789

Chapter 24

Practical Guidelines for Exercise in Patients with Normal Left Ventricular Function

Gary J. Balady, MD

Exercise training, like medications, should be tailored to meet individual needs and designed to maximize effectiveness at a minimal risk. Exercise therapy for patients with heart disease can thus be prescribed only after a thorough patient evaluation, taking into account any limitations that may be incurred from cardiac or other pre-existing diseases. Using information derived from medical screening and a baseline exercise test, an exercise program can be formulated and decisions can be made regarding the appropriate level of supervision and monitoring required to safely reach reasonable goals. A diverse training program should include a regimen of arm and leg exercises in both static and dynamic effort. Designing an enjoyable and effective program for the heterogeneous population of patients with heart disease is by no means a rote process, but rather a medical art that is founded on science and perpetuated by creativity.

Fundamental Exercise Physiology

To interpret and use guidelines for exercise training, a working knowledge of exercise physiology is essential. Exercise intervention should be likened to the application of controlled amounts of sympathetic stimulation triggered by the metabolic needs and

From Fletcher GF, (ed): *Cardiovascular Response to Exercise.* Mount Kisco, NY, Futura Publishing Company, Inc., © 1994.

by-products of moving muscle. Skeletal muscle contraction and subsequent relaxation are energy-dependent processes that use adenosine triphosphate (ATP). As fuel metabolism for the generation of ATP is primarily an oxygen-dependent process, the body's oxygen consumption (VO_2) must increase from resting levels in response to muscle contraction during exercise. VO_2 is directly related to cardiac output and arteriovenous oxygen difference (AVO_2 difference), which reflects the extraction of oxygen from the blood by the peripheral tissues, where:

$$VO_2 = \text{cardiac output} \times AVO_2 \text{ difference}$$
$$= \text{stroke volume} \times \text{heart rate} \times AVO_2 \text{ difference}[1]$$

Hence, the oxygen requirements of any given muscular activity will necessitate changes in any one or all of these factors. Myocardial oxygen demand increases in response to rises in heart rate, blood pressure, left ventricular contractility, and left ventricular wall stress.[2] Accordingly, a rise in total body oxygen demand during exercise will lead to concomitant increases in myocardial oxygen demand. The physiological responses during active exercise will manifest as changes in VO_2, heart rate, and blood pressure. These responses are specific to the type of exercise being performed, particularly in regard to the limbs used, the body position, and the predominant type of muscle contraction (static or dynamic) during exercise. Dynamic exercise involves a high repetition movement against low resistance and fosters an increase in blood flow to the working muscles with a concomitant increase in venous return of blood being pumped back to the heart from exercising muscles. Pure static exercise, which involves isometric contractions without muscle shortening, is not used in the exercise routine of cardiac patients. However, resistance exercise in which a limited dynamic component is added to static-type work (such as weight lifting) elicits a restriction in muscle blood flow during contraction as well as a centrally mediated pressor response.[3]

Energy costs during exercise are assessed most easily by using measurements of VO_2, in which for each liter of oxygen consumed, approximately 5 kcal of energy are expended.[4] VO_2 is directly related to the amount of work that is performed per unit time (termed work rate or power output). It can either be measured directly or it can be estimated from previously validated regression formulas.[5] As work rate is product of force, distance, and the reciprocal of time, the calculation of work rate for a weight-bearing exercise (*eg*, walking, stair climbing) differs from that of non–weight-bearing exercise (arm or leg cycle ergometry). During walking activity, body weight is the major component of the force moving through a given distance per unit time. At the same work rate, individuals of different body weights will have relatively similar VO_2 (in ml/kg body weight per minute). However, during cycle ergometry, the work rate is the product of the force of an external weight exerted on a flywheel, moving through the distance of the flywheel circumference per unit time. As most of the body weight is supported during this activity, it is much less of a factor in VO_2. Since VO_2 (expressed in ml/kg per minute) at a given work rate of cycle ergometry is greater in the lighter individual than the heavier person, body weight must be known to estimate this term correctly. This distinction is important since the heart rate, blood pressure, and cardiac output during exercise are directly related to VO_2.[4]

Moreover, the maximum oxygen uptake of an individual, termed VO_2max, is the best indicator of aerobic work capacity and fitness. A convenient method of expressing VO_2 at a given work rate is by use of the MET system. One MET is defined as the VO_2 of an awake resting individual, and equals 3.5 ml/kg of body weight per minute. Thus, the VO_2 during any given activity can be indexed against resting VO_2 by dividing that VO_2 (ml/kg per minute) by 3.5.

Guidelines for Exercise

Patient Evaluation/Risk Stratification

Any patient with ischemic heart disease who is about to engage in an exercise program should undergo a medical evaluation by a qualified physician. A medical history, with particular reference to cardiovascular status, is essential. Symptoms of angina, dyspnea, palpitations, and syncope should be sought. The patient should be questioned regarding the previous occurrence of a myocardial infarction, coronary angioplasty, or bypass surgery. Ideally, measurements of left ventricular systolic function and/or coronary anatomy in these patients is available and should be noted. A complete list of medications and dosing intervals must be reviewed, as these may affect the responses to exercise. Associated illnesses, including pulmonary, endocrine, neurological, and musculoskeletal conditions also should be considered in the evaluation. Social and detailed occupational history will yield valuable information such that program training and goals are tailored to meet individual needs.

Physical examination should focus on heart rate, blood pressure, and pulmonary, cardiac, vascular, and musculoskeletal areas. Signs of congestive heart failure and valvular disease should be evaluated with further work-up if deemed appropriate.

A resting electrocardiogram and physician-supervised exercise test are integral to the medical evaluation and the exercise prescription itself, as will be discussed. Exercise testing can be used to detect ischemia, whether symptomatic or silent, with particular reference to the work rate and heart rate–blood pressure product at which ischemia begins. Peak exercise capacity can be determined as well as the patient's symptomatic and hemodynamic responses to the stress of exercise. Serial exercise testing is useful to monitor functional capacity, evaluate the training effect, and assess changes in the ischemic threshold. Such follow-up testing should be done initially, after 3 months, and then every 6 months to 1 year thereafter. Should medication changes occur that may affect training parameters, it is prudent to repeat the exercise test such that the exercise prescription can be adjusted accordingly. Exercise testing also is useful in the evaluation of new or changing symptoms of chest pain or dyspnea, particularly when the etiology is not clear.

Foremost in the medical evaluation is the determination of the patient's risk for cardiovascular complications during exercise. Risk stratification using the data obtained from the history, physical examination, and exercise testing will greatly assist in the determination of the adequacy of current therapy as well as the level of supervision and monitoring necessary in a given patient. Applying this information to the risk classification guidelines as set forth by the American Heart Association[6] (Table 1) will help to ensure patient safety during exercise sessions.

Many patients with documented ischemic coronary artery disease take medications that influence autonomic tone, vascular smooth muscle tone, myocardial contractility, and many other parameters involved with physiological responses to acute exercise. Although it is clearly the purpose of these medications to reduce or eliminate the occurrence of myocardial ischemia, some of these medications may effect the exercise prescription and training response.

TABLE 1   American Heart Association Risk Classification for Exercise Training

Class A	Apparently healthy
Class B	Low risk/stable cardiovascular disease
	≤NYHA Class II angina
	Functional capacity >6 METS
	No congestive heart failure
	No exercise-induced ischemia or angina
	No sequential VPBs
	Able to self-monitor
Class C	Low risk/stable cardiovascular disease
	Unable to self-monitor, otherwise same as Class B
Class D	Moderate to high risk
	≥NYHA Class III angina
	Functional capacity <6 METS
	Exercise-induced ischemia or angina
	Previous primary cardiac arrest
	Exercise-induced ventricular tachycardia
	Low ejection fraction (<30%)
	Triple-vessel coronary artery disease
Class E	Unstable disease (exercise prohibited)

NYHA, New York Heart Association; METS, metabolic equivalents (mL/kg of oxygen consumed), VPB, ventricular premature beats.

β-Adrenergic blockers have been the most widely evaluated in this regard. It appears that these agents, in reducing exercise-induced ischemia, allow the patient to work at higher levels than they would have achieved without medications. Moreover, exercise capacity has been shown to increase in individuals who have completed an exercise training program and are taking β-blocking agents. However, this improvement appears to be relatively attenuated compared with those individuals taking placebo.[7] The influence of calcium channel-blocking agents on training has been less well evaluated, although studies to date have demonstrated no negative effects on the training response when compared with placebo.[8,9]

The Exercise Prescription

The exercise prescription is formulated based on the evaluation as detailed above. Most endurance training regimens used in healthy individuals and those with cardiac disease are designed to elicit a training effect, which refers to the ability to perform higher levels of peak work with a blunted heart rate response to submaximal work rates compared with pretraining levels. Important components of the exercise prescription include the type of exercise; limbs being used; and intensity, duration, and frequency of exercise sessions. Optimal training effects will occur when exercise is performed three to five times per week for 20 to 60 minutes' duration, at a specified training intensity.[10] For the ranges given, a training effect can be achieved by exercising at lower intensities for longer periods or higher intensities for shorter durations. Several methods may be used to determine the training intensity. For patients with cardiac disease, training intensity should be derived from the results of the exercise test using any of the following formulae:

1. Exercise at a work rate or heart rate that corresponds to 40% to 85% of peak measured VO_2
2. Using heart rate data from the exercise test:
   a. 60% to 90% of maximum heart rate achieved
   b. [(peak heart rate-resting heart rate) × 50%] + resting heart rate to [(peak heart rate-resting heart rate) × 85%] + resting heart rate (Karvonen method).[10]

If angina or ischemic ST depression develop during testing, then the heart rate at which this occurs should be substituted for the peak heart rate in the formulation. It is important to note that the use of the Karvonen method generates a target heart rate range, which usually is not far from the peak heart rate. This occurs particularly among patients taking medications that blunt the peak heart rate response. If the heart rate at ischemia is used as a peak heart rate in this situation, patients may be exercising at a rate range near the ischemic threshold. The training range should then be modified such that the peak training heart rate should not exceed 10 beats below the heart rate at onset ischemia. Careful monitoring and caution should be used here, particularly among patients who demonstrate ischemia at a low heart rate and low work rate.

Using the Rating of Perceived Exertion (RPE)[11] (Table 2), the training intensity can be tailored more finely to the patient's own interpretation of his or her exercise intensity. After careful instruction on the use of the RPE, the patient will become familiar with this method within several exercise sessions. Henceforth, the RPE should be used in conjunction with heart rate methods to determine training intensity.[12]

TABLE 2.   Rating of Perceived Exertion Scales

Category RPE scale (original)		Category-ratio RPE scale (revised)	
6		0	Nothing at all
7	Very, very light	0.5	Very, very weak
8		1	Very weak
9	Very light	2	Weak
10		3	Moderate
11	Fairly light	4	Somewhat strong
12		5	Strong
13	Somewhat hard	6	
14		7	Very strong
15	Hard	8	
16		9	
17	Very hard	10	Very, very strong
18		.	Maximal
19	Very, very hard		
20			

From Reference 11.

Telemetry systems can be used to assist in the monitoring of training intensity during exercise sessions. Although such systems are not needed for most patients, they can be particularly helpful among those with atrial fibrillation, ventricular dysrhythmias, and pacemakers. Telemetered heart rates can be used selectively to monitor patients during dynamic upper extremity exercise or resistance training, when pulse measurement of heart rate is difficult and less reliable. Telemetry systems also should be used at least during the initial stages of training in the patients deemed to be at increased risk for cardiovascular event during exercise (*ie*, AHA Class D) (Table 1 and 3).

Before beginning each exercise session, the patient should be questioned regarding new or worsening systems suggesting cardiovascular instability. Patients also should be instructed, when exercising in a supervised or unsupervised setting to be aware of these issues and address them to the appropriate medical personnel. Any changes in medication should be reported as these may affect the exercise prescription. All sessions should include 5- to 10-minute warm-up and cool-down periods. The warm-up time, which precedes the cardiovascular training period, should include range of motion and stretching exercises. This leads to greater flexibility,

TABLE 3. Suggested Uses for Telemetry Monitoring

Ventricular dysrhythmias
Atrial fibrillation
Pacemaker
Inability to self-monitor
High-risk patient
Heart rate during dynamic arm exercise

serves to ready the cardiovascular system, and, when performed properly, decreases musculoskeletal injury. Cool-down activities that follow the training period include walking or pedaling against very low resistance. This prevents venous pooling, which may lead to hypotension, lightheadedness, or syncope. The cool-down period also may decrease the risk of arrhythmias after aerobic exercise, and may help prevent muscle soreness.

Training Modalities

The variety of exercise activities that can be used for the training of cardiac patients has greatly expanded during recent years. A diverse exercise regimen can successfully use arm and leg exercise in both dynamic and static effort to provide a well-rounded, highly effective program. Dynamic leg exercises include walking, jogging, stair climbing, and stationary cycling. Many activities of daily living involve more arm work than leg work, and there is only a limited transfer of training benefits from legs to arms after a prolonged period of leg training.[13] Hence, arm training for individuals with ischemic heart disease is particularly important, since the maximal blunting of heart rate and blood pressure to any amount of arm work would be especially desirable in this group of patients. Since the ischemic threshold during arm work appears higher than that of leg work,[14,15] and the peak heart rate and blood pressure are similar, if not higher during leg work, it is reasonable and safe to derive an arm exercise prescription from information obtained from either bicycle or treadmill testing. Conversely, the arm test should not be used to establish the prescription for leg exercise. Dynamic arm exercise can be performed using an arm ergometer, combined leg-arm cycle ergometer, rowing machines, cross-country ski machines, and swimming.

Resistance exercise (*ie,* weight training) is now assuming an important place in the exercise regimen of patients with cardiac disease. Resistance training has been found to be safe while yielding favorable improvements in strength and muscular endurance. Exercise equipment includes free weights and dumbbells, wall-mounted pulleys, or exercise machines equipped with weight stacks. Resistance exercise requires careful instruction to attain the greatest benefits and reduce the potential for orthopedic injury and adverse cardiac events. Weight training should be performed in a variety of body positions to isolate specific muscle groups, using slow to moderate speed movements encompassing a full range of motion. Patients should be encouraged to exhale during the contraction phase of the movement to avoid the additive cardiovascular responses of the Valsalva maneuver during the exercise. Specific exercises should be selected to train the front and back of each major body part (eg, arm—biceps/triceps; torso—chest/back; legs—quadriceps/hamstrings). The intensity of each weight-training exercise is adjusted by varying weight load, number of repetitions per set, number of sets, and rest period between sets. A suggested routine would include 6 to 10 different exercises that use upper and lower body muscles at an intensity of 40% to 50% one-repetition maximum. Two to three sets of exercise should be performed with a 30-second to 1-minute rest period between sets. Each set should include 10 repetitions with a gradual increase to 15 repetitions, at which time the weight can be increased.

Special Considerations

Patients with heart disease often will present with a diversity of medical problems, some of which require special consideration when formulating an exercise training program. To review all of the possible combinations of associated medical conditions is beyond the scope of this chapter; however, a few select conditions will be discussed.

Recent Coronary Bypass Surgery

Patients who have recently undergone coronary artery bypass surgery usually are deconditioned upon discharge from the hospital. They often are initially anemic because of blood loss during the operative procedure, and many may suffer from mild chest (sternotomy) and leg (saphenous vein harvest site) wound discomfort. Because of these influences, initial exercise capacity is limited, and patients may tolerate a training range set only at low intensity. Interval training consisting of brief exercise periods punctuated by 1- to 2-minute rest periods may be used. As the patient's hematocrit tends to rise from compensatory erythropoesis, the heart rate responses to given work rates will diminish, requiring a readjustment of the training intensity.

Particular attention should be focused on the chest wound, which should be well healed approximately 8 weeks after surgery. Initial medical examination should include an evaluation of sternal stability. Upper extremity exercises during the early postoperative 8 weeks should be limited to range of motion exercises and, at most, isolated arm and shoulder exercises using light hand-held weights. Beyond 8 weeks, arm ergometry can be introduced and by 12 weeks, rowing and chest muscle exercise (bench press, arm-cross) can be initiated. If, however, the patient complains of increased chest discomfort with exercise or there is any evidence of sternal instability beyond 8 weeks, upper body exercises should be terminated and the patient should be referred for evaluation by the cardiothoracic surgeon.

Diabetes

Patients with diabetes require special attention, particularly if they are taking exogenous insulin or oral hypoglycemic medications.[16] Because of their susceptibility to leg and foot wounds, which may interfere with or be aggravated by exercise, initial medical evaluation should include an examination of the lower extremities. Patients should be advised to wear protective thick socks and well-fitting supportive footwear during exercise. For patients taking insulin, the expected time of exogenous insulin activity in decreasing blood glucose levels should be taken into account when planning the exercise session schedule. Patients are requested to administer insulin in the abdominal area rather than on the limbs to avoid any potential increased insulin absorption from exercising limb sites. Finger-stick blood sugars should be checked before exercise for evidence of either low (<100 mg/dl) or elevated (>300 mg/dl) blood sugars, which should preclude exercise training at that time. As exercise itself may cause a fall in blood glucose levels within several hours after the training sessions, patients should be instructed on the signs, symptoms, and management of hypoglycemia. A daily log of blood sugar measurements should be maintained and forwarded to the primary care physician to assist in diabetes management. The exercise center should be stocked with fruit juices available for patient needs should hypoglycemia ensue.

Obesity

Exercise programs aimed in part at promoting weight loss should be designed such that 300–500 kcal are expended per exercise session and 1,000–2,000 kcal are expended per week.[17] Low-intensity but extended duration activities (*eg*, walking) are ideally suited for this purpose. Patients with morbid obesity may require modification of available exercise equipment to facilitate their use, such as larger seats for stationary cycles or rowers. Patients who exceed the weight limits for treadmill equipment may alternatively walk in the exercise center's perimeter or halls, or use graded stepping exercise.

Elderly

Exercise training of the elderly patient with heart disease can greatly impact on their quality of life by increasing functional capacity.[18] A training regimen for the elderly patient should include longer warm-up and cool-down periods, with training intensities initially set at low levels. Musculoskeletal injuries can be lessened by the avoidance of high-impact activities (*eg*, running, jumping). Walking activity and treadmill exercise that use grade rather than speed are best suited for this population of patients. Arm exercise and resistance training also can be incorporated safely into a training program for the elderly, with particular attention to proper exercise technique to avoid muscle or joint injury.

Conclusion

Exercise training can yield a variety of benefits for the patient with heart disease. Initial medical evaluation and exercise testing are integral to the formulation of a safe and effective exercise program. A diverse regimen incorporating dynamic arm and leg exercises supplemented by resistance training can be formulated to yield a well-rounded, enjoyable program that promotes cardiovascular fitness and muscular strength.

Acknowledgment

I am grateful to Jane Foley for her valuable secretarial assistance in preparation of this chapter.

References

1. Sullivan MA, Froelicher VF: Maximal oxygen uptake and gas exchange in coronary heart disease. *J Cardiac Rehabil* 1983;3:549–560
2. Clausen JP: Circulatory adjustments to dynamic exercise and effects of physical training in normal subjects and in patients with coronary artery disease. *Prog Cardiovascular Dis* 1976;18:459–495
3. Asmussen E: Similarities and dissimilarities between static and dynamic effort. *Circ Res* 1981;48(suppl I):I-3–I-10
4. Franklin BA, Gordon S, Timmis GC: Fundamentals of exercise physiology. Implications for exercise testing and prescription in Franklin BA, Gordon S, Timmis G (eds): *Exercise in Modern Medicine.* Baltimore, Williams and Wilkins, 1989, pp 1–21
5. American College of Sports Medicine: *Guidelines for exercise testing and prescription.* 4th ed. Philadelphia, Lea and Febiger, 1991, pp 285–300
6. Fletcher GF, Froelicher VF, Hartley LH, Haskell WL, Pollock ML: Exercise standards: a statement for health professionals from the American Heart Association. *Circulation* 1990;82:2286–2322
7. Pollock ML, Lowenthal DT, Foster C, Pels AE, Roa J, Stoiber J, Schmidt DH. Acute and chronic responses to exercise in patients treated with beta blockers. *J Cardiopulm Rehabil* 1991;11:132–144
8. Stewart K, Effron MB, Valenti SA Kelemen MH: Effects of diltiazem or propranolol during exercise training of hypertensive men. *Med Sci Sports Exerc* 1990;22:192–198

9. Duffey DJ, Howitz LD, Brammell HL: Nifedipine and the conditioning response. *Am J Cardiol* 1984;53:908–911
10. American College of Sports Medicine: Position stand—the recommended quantity and quality of exercise for the developing and maintaining cardiorespiratory and muscle fitness in healthy adults. *J Cardiopulm Rehabil* 1990;10:235–245
11. Borg GA: Psychophysical bases of perceived exertion. *Med Sci Sports Exerc* 1982;14:377–387
12. American College of Sports Medicine: *Guidelines for Exercise Testing and Prescription.* 4th ed. Philadelphia, Lea and Febiger, 1991, pp 65–71
13. Clausen JP, Klausen K, Rasmussen B, et al: Central and peripheral circulatory changes after training in the arms and legs. *Am J Physiol* 1972;225:675–683
14. Clausen J, Trap-Jensen J: Heart rate and arterial blood pressure during exercise in patients with angina pectoris. *Circulation* 1978;53:4336–4442
15. Balady GJ, Weiner DA, McCabe CH, Ryan TJ: Value of arm exercise testing in detecting coronary artery disease. *Am J Cardiol* 1985;55:37–39
16. Leon A: The role of exercise in the prevention and management of diabetes and blood lipid disorders, in Shephard RJ, Miller HS (eds): *Exercise and the Heart in Health and Disease.* New York, Marcel Dekker, 1992, pp 299–368
17. American College of Sports Medicine: *Guidelines for exercise testing and prescription.* 4th ed. Philadelphia, Lea and Febiger, 1991, pp 113–115
18. Wenger NK: Elderly coronary patients, in Wenger NK, Hellerstein HK (eds): *Rehabilitation of the Coronary Patient.* New York, Churchill-Livingstone, 1992, pp 415–420

Index